Health Care for the Elderly: Regional Responses to National Policy Issues

Health Care for the Elderly: Regional Responses to National Policy Issues

Kathleen Gainor Andreoli, DSN, FAAN
Leigh Anne Musser, MPH
Stanley Joel Reiser, MD, PhD
Editors

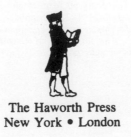

The Haworth Press
New York • London

Health Care for the Elderly: Regional Responses to National Policy Issues has also been published as *Home Health Care Services Quarterly*, Volume 7, Numbers 3/4, Fall/Winter 1986.

The Haworth Press, Inc., 12 West 32 Street, New York, NY 10001
EUROSPAN/Haworth, 3 Henrietta Street, WC2E 8LU England

Library of Congress Cataloging-in-Publication Data

Health care for the elderly.

Based on a conference held Apr. 18–19, 1985 in Houston; sponsored by the University of Texas Health Science Center at Houston and the Institute of Medicine.
Has also been published as Home health care services quarterly, volume 7, numbers 3/4, fall/winter 86—T.p. verso.
Includes bibliographies and index.
1. Aged—Medical care—Government policy—United States—Congresses.
2. Community health services for the aged—United States—Congresses. 3. Aging—Social aspects—United States—Congresses. I. Andreoli, Kathleen G. II. Musser, Leigh Anne.
III. Reiser, Stanley Joel. IV. University of Texas Health Science Center at Houston.
V. Institute of Medicine (U.S.) [DNLM: 1. Health Policy—United States—congresses.
2. Health Services for the Aged—United States—congresses. 3. Long Term Care—in old age—congresses. W1 H0502R v.7 no.3/4 / WT 30 H433407 [1985]
RA564.8.H425   1986   362.1'9897'00973   86-14869
ISBN 0-86656-607-4

Health Care for the Elderly: Regional Responses to National Policy Issues

Home Health Care Services Quarterly
Volume 7, Numbers 3/4

CONTENTS

Contributors

Henry J. Aaron, PhD, Senior Fellow, The Brookings Institute, 1775 Massachusetts Avenue, NW, Washington, D.C. 20036.

Kathleen Gainor Andreoli, DSN, FAAN, Vice President, Office of Educational Services, Interprofessional Education and International Programs, The University of Texas Health Science Center at Houston, P.O. Box 20036, Houston, Texas 77225.

Robert M. Ball, MA, Senior Consultant to Study Group on Social Security, Center for the Study of Welfare Policy, 236 Massachusetts Avenue, NE, Suite 405, Washington, D.C. 20002.

Robert Bernstein, MD, FACP, Commissioner of Health, Texas Department of Health, 1100 West 49th Street, Austin, Texas 78756.

Enriqueta Bond, PhD, Division Chief, Health Promotion, Institute of Medicine, 2101 Constitution Avenue, NW, Washington, D.C. 20418.

Elaine M. Brody, MSW, Director and Associate Research Director, Department of Human Services, Philadelphia Geriatric Center, 5301 Old York Road, Philadelphia, Pennsylvania 19141.

Leon Eisenberg, MD, Presley Professor of Social Medicine, Professor of Psychiatry, and Chair, Department of Social Medicine and Health Policy, Harvard Medical School, 25 Shattuck Street, Boston, Massachusetts 02115.

Carroll L. Estes, PhD, Professor and Chair, Department of Social and Behavioral Sciences, Director, Aging Health Policy Center, School of Nursing, N631Y, University of California, San Francisco, San Francisco, California 94143.

Jonathan E. Fielding, MD, MPH, Co-Director, Center for Health Enhancement, Education & Research, University of California, Los Angeles, School of Public Health, CHS 31236, Los Angeles, California 90024.

James F. Fries, MD, Associate Professor of Medicine, Stanford University Medical Center, HRP Building, #109, Stanford, California 94305.

Charles M. Gaitz, MD, Visiting Professor, The University of Texas Health Science Center at Houston, 7777 SW Freeway, Suite C4, Houston, Texas 77074.

Eli Ginzberg, PhD, Director, Conservation of Human Resources, Columbia University, 525 Uris Hall, New York, New York 10027.

Lawrence W. Green, DrPH, Director, Center for Health Promotion, Research and Development, The University of Texas, Health Science Center at Houston, P.O. Box 20186, Houston, Texas 77225.

James G. Haughton, MD, MPH, Director, City of Houston Health Department, 1115 N. MacGregor, Suite #178, Houston, Texas 77030-1797.

Leonard Hayflick, PhD, Professor and Director, Center for Gerontological Studies, University of Florida, 3357 GPA, Gainesville, Florida 32611.

Robert L. Kane, MD, Dean, School of Public Health, University of Minnesota, 1260 Mayo Memorial Building, 420 Delaware Street, SE, Minneapolis, Minnesota 55455.

Alexander Leaf, MD, Ridley Watts Professor of Preventive Medicine and Professor of Medicine and Chair, Department of Preventive Medicine and Clinical Epidemiology, Harvard Medical School, Massachusetts General Hospital, Fruit Street, Boston, Massachusetts 02114.

Phoebe S. Liebig, PhD, Director, Pacific Geriatric Education Center, University of Southern California Health Sciences Campus, KAM300-C, 1975 Zonal Avenue, Los Angeles, California 90033.

Mathey Mezey, RN, EdD, FAAN, Director, The Robert Wood Johnson Teaching Nursing Home Program, University of Pennsylvania, School of Nursing, 420 Service Drive, S2, Philadelphia, Pennsylvania 19104.

Leigh Anne Musser, MPH, Research Associate, Office of Educational Services, Interprofessional Education and International Programs, The University of Texas Health Science Center at Houston, P.O. Box 20036, Houston, Texas 77225.

Stanley Joel Reiser, MD, PhD, Director, Program on Humanities and Technology in Health Care, The University of Texas Health Science Center at Houston, P.O. Box 20708, Houston, Texas 77225.

Grant V. Rodkey, MD, Council on Medical Services, American Medical Association, Zero Emerson Place, Boston, Massachusetts 02114.

Steven A. Schroeder, MD, Professor of Medicine and Chief, Division of General Internal Medicine, University of California, San Francisco, 400 Parnasus Avenue, Room A-405, San Francisco, California 94143.

Ethel Shanas, PhD, Professor Emerita of Sociology, University of Illinois at Chicago, 222 Main Street, Evanston, Illinois 60202.

Karl L. Shaner, DrPH, Vice President, Research & Information Services, Texas Hospital Association, P.O. Box 15587, Austin, Texas 78761.

Charles Sprague, MD, President, The University of Texas, Health Science Center at Dallas, 5323 Harry Hines Boulevard, Dallas, Texas 75235.

Reuel A. Stallones, MD, MPH, Dean, School of Public Health, The University of Texas, Health Science Center at Houston, P.O. Box 20186, Houston, Texas 77225.

Eugene A. Stead, Jr., MD, Florence McAlister Professor Emeritus of Medicine, Duke University Medical Center, P.O. Box 3910, Durham, North Carolina 27710.

Knight Steel, MD, Professor of Medicine and Chief, Geriatric Section, Boston University Medical Center, University Hospital, 720 Harrison Avenue, Suite 1101, Boston, Massachusetts 02118.

T. Franklin Williams, MD, Director, National Institute on Aging, National Institutes of Health, 9000 Rockville Pike, Building 31, 2C-02, Bethesda, Maryland 20205.

Donald A. Young, MD, Executive Director, Prospective Payment Commission, 300 7th Street, SW, Room 702, Washington, D.C. 20024.

Preface

Probably the single most significant factor influencing the U.S. health care system for the next 50 years will be the growth in the elderly population. This demographic shift, with both numeric and proportional growth among those over age 65, has been occurring since the turn of the century and will continue well into the next century. In fact, between now and the year 2040, the proportion of those over age 65 will nearly double, expanding from approximately 11 percent to 21 percent. The most rapid growth is projected to occur between the years 2010 and 2030, when the "baby boomers" reach their sixties. Even more significant will be the increase in the "old-old," those aged 75 and over, who are expected to represent the majority of the elderly by the year 2040.[1]

The way in which health care is provided and reimbursed, who provides the bulk of care, and the philosophy of the entire system will be challenged by "The Coming Gerontocracy."[2] There will be an increased demand for health services since the elderly utilize a disproportionate amount of these services. For example, in 1981, those over age 65 accounted for 25 percent of prescription drug utilization, 40 percent of acute hospital days, 30 percent of the total personal health care expenditures, and 50 percent of the federal health care budget.[3] Other changes in the health care system will occur in response to specific characteristics of the elderly; those over 65 usually present with multiple symptomatology, are more prone to chronic disease than younger age groups, and often experience a host of social, economic and personal problems that impact greatly upon compliance with medical treatment and the ability to "get well." The philosophy of our traditional medical approach, with its emphasis on "cure" will be altered, ethical issues will become increasingly important, and the integration between health and social services will become imperative. Perhaps most importantly in this time of economic constraint, the growth in the number of elderly presents challenges to the intergenerational contract established through Medicare and Social Security, and asks us as policymakers to develop new avenues for paying for health care that do not compromise quality and do not introduce another tier, another level of inequitable access, in the health care system.

While we grapple with these momentous issues, we must remind ourselves that the elderly are not a homogeneous group, any more so than any other age group, and that broad generalizations serve to hinder the progress we seek to generate. In this context, it is important to note that the majority of elders are generally healthier, more affluent, more active, and more independent than the elderly of the recent past.[4] They report their health status as good or excellent, and over half have no activity limitations related to poor health.[5] The needs of both "well" elders and those with health problems must be addressed by health policy decisions.

In order to meet the challenges that will emanate from the geriatric imperative, we must generate a sophisticated knowledge base that is multidisciplinary in focus and establish health policy based upon it. With this directive in mind, it is fitting that two organizations whose missions reflect the stated mandate should join forces to collaborate on a conference to address the issue of health care policy for the elderly, entitled "Health Care for the Elderly: Regional Responses to National Policy Issues." The mission of The University of Texas Health Science Center at Houston is to provide a program of exemplary education, research, and service through the development of human resources, new knowledge, and the provision of health care. The Institute of Medicine, a branch of the National Academy of Sciences, has a mandate to advance and protect the health of the public by analyzing and studying critical health issues that face the nation.

The conference was conducted on April 18–19, 1985 at The University of Texas Health Science Center at Houston. Thirty-one distinguished experts in health policy, gerontology, economics, health promotion, and ethics were invited to participate in a round-table forum featuring discussion and debate on the potential impact of the growing number of elderly on the American health care system. Clearly, in a two-day period, the health, social, economic, and personal implications of the expanding elderly population and the related impact on health policy could not be adequately discussed. Thus, we selected seven timely issues for development and analysis. The topics were: issues in health and social policy for an aging society, the biological constraints on human aging, institutional versus home health care of the elderly, the impact of prospective payment on de-institutionalizing health care for the elderly, educating practitioners for the care of the elderly—the teaching nursing home, health promotion and the elderly, and lessons the U.S. can learn from other nations about health care delivery for the elderly.

Seven participants were asked to present position papers on one of the topics listed above, and three participants were asked to respond to each paper from the general, national, or regional perspective. The inclusion of regional requirements, goals, and issues was an important one. It was hoped that this focus would generate new information to be considered in the debate on national health care policy for the elderly versus a more decentralized approach that reflects different state and community needs. Following the formal presentations, all conference participants were invited to comment on the topic. Subsequently, the author of each position paper was allowed time for rebuttal. The sessions were spirited, informative, and enjoyable. At the end of the conference, the proceedings were summarized in a philosophical review of the priority issues that arose during each session.

Acknowledgement is paid to Roger J. Bulger, MD, President of The University of Texas Health Science Center at Houston, and Frederick C. Robbins, MD, President of the Institute of Medicine (1981–85) for their vision of this conference and their support in its production. The Institute of Medicine recognized the advantage of broadening their perspective on health policy issues from Washington to state and local issues, and this conference, held in the Southwestern region of the U.S., served as the first model of this approach.

The generous support of the Holmes Family Fund, Isla Carroll Turner Friendship Trust, The Moody Foundation of Galveston, and the Hogg Foundation allowed us to open the conference to the public at no cost.

The production of the conference and proceedings was made possible through the cooperative efforts of professionals dedicated to bringing to the public relevant knowledge about the elderly population that should be used to determine future health care policy. In particular, we are grateful for the cooperation, guidance, and enthusiastic support of Enriqueta Bond, PhD, Division Chief, Health Promotion, Institute of Medicine.

We hope the model presented in this conference, with its regional component, will be replicated in other parts of the nation in order to stimulate action at all levels of health policy decision-making. In turn, this will lead to a comprehensive and cohesive national health policy for the elderly that meets the needs of the increasing number of elderly, those who provide care for them, and those at the community, state, and national levels who are responsible for implementing and integrating this policy.

Kathleen Gainor Andreoli
Leigh Anne Musser

REFERENCES

1. U.S. Department of Commerce, Bureau of the Census. *Projection of the Population of the U.S.: 1982 to 2050* (Advanced Report). P-25, NO. 922, Washington, D.C.: Bureau of the Census, 1982.

2. Term coined by Ken Dychtwald, National Director of Institute of Aging, Health and Work. As reported in *Gerontology Newsletter*, 10(2):17, 1985.

3. Institute of Medicine. *Health and Behavior: A Research Agenda—Interim Report No. 5: Health, Behavior, and Aging.* Washington, D.C.: National Academy Press, 1981.

4. Kirchner, N. The elderly: Sifting fact from myth. *Medical Economics*, April 29, 1985, p. 34.

5. National Center for Health Statistics. *Vital and Health Statistics*, Series 10, No. 141, DHHS Publication No. (PHS)82-1564; Series 13, No. 72, DHHS Publication No. (PHS)83-1733; and *Advance Data* No. 92, DHHS Publication No. (PHS)83-1250. Washington, D.C.: U.S. Government Printing Office, 1982 and 1983.

CHAPTER 1

Issues in Health and Social Policy for an Aging Society Position Paper

Robert M. Ball, MA

We cannot deal adequately with the issue of health care for the elderly without considering their overall position in our society, now and in the future. The goal of a national health policy for the elderly should be additional days of life, as free as possible of physical or mental disability. Many things besides health care contribute to this goal.

For good health, both mental and physical, the retired elderly need an adequate and dependable income. They need access to activities that give them a sense of worth. They need the opportunity to make friends and the opportunity for recreation. If they are to feel secure, they also need protection against the high and unpredictable costs of illness, costs that cannot ordinarily be met from regular retirement income. And, of course, they need appropriate and good health care, which is not necessarily the same thing as insurance against the costs of care. What is the situation of the elderly in America, and what does the future hold as the proportion of older people in the population increases?

THE GOAL OF AN ADEQUATE INCOME IN OLD AGE

Since most of the topics of this conference will be focused on the issues more conventionally considered under the subject of "health care," I would like to begin with a discussion of that most important of all medicines, a reliable and adequate income. Money may not buy either health or happiness, but its absence certainly makes everything else worse. The elderly, particularly those of very advanced age, are faced with many inevitable losses: the loss of familiar roles, the loss of friends, the loss of a spouse, the loss of physical strength, a lessening of the ability to see and hear, the loss, for many of a sense of worth and function. It is intolerable and destructive to both mental and physical health if we add to these inevitable and accumulating losses, the loss of an adequate and dependable income. The foundation of success in retirement is an assured and adequate income, as an earned right, and which does not damage the self respect of people accustomed to providing for themselves.

The United States has made great progress toward this goal. This year, as we celebrate the fiftieth anniversary of the passage of Social Security and the twentieth anniversary of the passage of Medicare, it is fitting to pause and note that progress. We are celebrating one of the major achievements of this century. When the Social Security program was enacted, only about six million persons, 15 percent of those employed, held jobs covered by any sort of retirement system; only a tiny handful—perhaps 100,000 or 200,000—actually were receiving a pension. The poorhouse toward the end of life, with all its horrors, was a very real part of America.

Social Security changed all that. It created a peaceful revolution in the way older people, totally disabled people, widows and orphans live. It has been largely responsible for the fact that the proportion of those over 65 who are desperately poor is now about the same as for the rest of the population, instead of more than twice as high, as it was as recently as 1959. Without Social Security, more than half of the elderly would have incomes below the Federal government's rock-bottom definition of poverty. Instead, about 14 percent are in that category today.

But Old-Age, Survivors and Disability Insurance (OASDI), what most people mean by Social Security, is much more than an anti-poverty program. Currently, 122 million individuals contribute to the program; it is the base on which practically every family builds protection against the loss of earned income. One of the most important characteristics of the system—the absence of a means test—enables people to add private pension income and personal savings to Social Security benefits. Every private pension is planned on the assumption that the pensioner will also receive Social Security, and individuals who save on their own rely on Social

Security as a base for their efforts. Today 37 million people—elderly retired people, totally disabled people, widows, motherless and fatherless children—get Social Security benefits every month.

The Four-Tier System of Income Security for the Elderly

It has taken a long time and improvements are still needed, but our four-tier system of income security—Social Security, private pensions and career government plans, individual voluntary savings, and a national means-tested system of last resort, Supplemental Security Income (SSI)—is beginning to work well. Just about all earners are covered under tier 1, our contributory, compulsory, wage-related system of Social Security, and 90 percent of those 65 and over are getting Social Security benefits. Prior to the time benefits are payable, they are automatically kept up-to-date with wages, and thus with any increases in the general level of living. Since the benefit formula in present law gives earners credit for all the productivity gains during their working lives, real benefits per person are estimated to triple over the next 75 years for which Social Security estimates are made. Thus the ratio of benefits to recent earnings (the replacement rate) will be the same for workers retiring in the future as for those retiring today. Once benefits are payable, they are inflation-proof.

Social Security recognizes that income security in old age is not only a matter of retirement pay, but equally a matter of survivors' benefits for widows. This protection for widows is a matter of great importance. As of July 1985, it is estimated that of the 29.3 million persons over age 65 who were living in the geographical area covered by Social Security, 11.7 were male and 17.6 female. Nine million of the males and 6.9 million of the females were married. Only 2.7 million males were single, widowed or divorced compared to 10.8 million females. Nine million out of the 10.8 million were widows.[1]

Social Security payments are modest. For March 1985, the average monthly payment for a retired worker was $462, for a spouse $237 and for a widow $417. The maximum amount payable to a couple when the worker retired at 65 was about $1100.

As a result of the 1983 Amendments, OASDI is adequately financed both for the short- and long-term. It is expected to take in more than it pays out for decades. During the next five fiscal years, the trust funds are expected to grow by approximately $150 billion. If the hospital insurance fund is included, the total increase in the trust funds for five years will be nearly $200 billion, and through 1994 approximately $500 billion. The annual increases are expected to be much larger in the later part of the 1990s and well into the next century.

Although two-thirds of the over-65 Social Security beneficiaries today get more than half their total income from Social Security and over one-fourth get over 90 percent, private pensions are now an important supplement to Social Security for many, usually workers who have earned above-average wages, and more will have this additional protection in the future.

The situation of new Social Security beneficiaries gives us some idea of the future importance of these supplemental pensions. Of the new beneficiaries who retired in the two years prior to 1982, about 56 percent of the married couples and 42 percent of the unmarried couples had either a private pension or a career government pension, such as a state or local pension, a Federal civil service pension or a military pension. (Thirty eight percent of the couples and 27 percent of the unmarrieds had private pensions, while 21 percent of the couples and 17 percent of the unmarrieds had government career pensions.) For the 56 percent of the couples who had supplementary pensions, the median monthly amount was $490. The overall median pension income for the unmarrieds was $291; $400 for the men, $253 for the women.[2]

The proportion of new beneficiaries with occupational pensions is somewhat higher than for all current beneficiaries, although not dramatically so; 56 percent compared to 49 percent.[3] This is encouraging. Yet, in considering the role of supplementary pensions in meeting future income and health care needs, it is important to remember that, because of inflation, for the very old whose health needs are the greatest, these pensions will not be as useful as they may seem at first. Only the federal systems have full protection against inflation: some of the state and local plans have limited protection. Most private plans make adjustments for inflation only on an *ad hoc* basis, if at all, and the supplementary pension can lose much of its value by the time the retired person reaches advanced old age. Even with a continuation of the present "low" level of 4% inflation, an unindexed pension loses about half its value between ages 65 and 83. Moreover, private plans have focused almost entirely on retirement benefits for workers and have not been very helpful to widows. Protection for them should improve, however, since the plans under ERISA are now required to provide a survivor benefit unless both husband and wife reject the option.

The third tier of the four-tier system is individual voluntary saving. Home ownership encouraged by tax deductions for mortage interest is by far the major form of accumulated savings for the elderly. Seventy-five percent of the homes maintained by the elderly are owner occupied, and about half are owned free and clear. Income from other savings is not large for most elderly people. Looking again at the new beneficiary group, only 51 percent of the couples and 35 percent of the unmarrieds had over $100 a month in such income.

The distribution of asset income was very uneven. Couples in the top 5 percent of the asset income distribution averaged more than $2,000 a month, the unmarrieds over $1,000 a month. Couples in the lowest 25 percent of the asset income distribution averaged less than $35 a month, unmarrieds less than $18 a month.[4] The recent changes in the tax code, which allow any earner to shelter up to $2,000 a year in Individual Retirement Accounts (IRAs), are unlikely to affect this distribution very much. Average and lower-paid earners do not have the extra income to take full advantage of IRAs, and, moreover, the incentive is much greater for the higher-paid. A $2,000 IRA deduction is worth $1,000 for a person in the 50 percent bracket but only $300 to a person in the 15 percent bracket. Treasury data show that while over a fourth of those with $20,000 to $50,000 incomes, and considerably over half of those with $50,000 or more have opened IRA accounts, only 5 percent with incomes below $20,000 have done so. Asset income is not likely to be of great importance to most elderly people in the future, although home ownership will be.

Underlying these three tiers is our nationwide, means-tested system of SSI, the last resort program under which all elderly with very low assets[5] can have their incomes brought up to a federally-established minimum, which rises automatically with increases in prices. This minimum is now 89 percent of the poverty level for couples (an estimated $6,550 in 1985), 75 percent for unmarrieds (an estimated poverty level of $5,194), but for Social Security recipients with supplemental SSI, the comparable figures are 93 percent and 80 percent because part of the Social Security benefit is not counted in determining the amount of the SSI payment. If also eligible for food stamps, couples with Social Security benefits get a minimum of 101 percent of the poverty standard, unmarrieds, 86 percent.[6]

Only about 2 million people over 65, less than 7 percent of the total, are now receiving SSI payments. The fact that the percentage is so low is largely due to the success of the Social Security program. In 1950 when only 17 percent of the elderly received Social Security, Old-Age Assistance, the predecessor program to SSI, went to 23 percent of those over 65.[7]

The four tiers of our retirement income system fit well together. Social Security has a weighted benefit formula replacing a higher proportion of earnings for those with low wages, and these are the workers least likely to have private or career government pensions or asset income. For workers with low-average earnings, Social Security is just about all there is. For the worker who earns the minimum wage all of his or her life, Social Security replaces about 56 percent of recent earnings for the single worker, and 84 percent for the couples. For a worker earning average wages throughout his or her life, the replacement rate drops to about 41 percent for the single worker and 62 percent for the couple. For those who earn at the maximum all their lives, the Social Security replacement rate drops to 27 percent for the single worker, and 41 percent for the couple. Increasingly, for this group, private pension supplementation and some asset income bring total retirement income up to reasonably adequate replacement levels. For higher-paid earners, the retirement system is a combination of the first three tiers.[8]

Remaining Income-Security Problems

Although the income maintenance system for older people is increasingly successful, there are still problems. The per capita poverty rate for those over 65 is still considerably higher than for adults aged 25 through 64, 14.1 percent compared to 11.2 percent (those under 25 have a poverty rate of 20.6 percent).[9] But equally important is the fact that, considering all those over 65 as a single group is misleading. Many of the 65 to 70-year olds work at least part time, and a high proportion of women at this age still have the advantage of sharing a husband's income. Poverty among the elderly is now heavily concentrated among three groups: the unmarrieds (widowed, divorced and never married), the very old, and minorities. Among family units with one person over 65, couples have a poverty rate of 9 percent, but unmarried men have a

19 percent rate and unmarried women a 25 percent rate. And, of course, the proportion of the elderly made up of unmarried women is very large and increases dramatically at older ages. Of all family units over 65 (defining units as either a couple or a single person), 47 percent are unmarried women. By age 85, out of a total of 1.8 million units, two-thirds, or 1.2 million persons, are unmarried women, with a poverty rate of 25 percent, even when total family income is taken into account for those who live with friends or relatives. At this age, even the couples (400,000 units) have a 15 percent poverty rate, while the 300,000 unmarried male survivors have a 17 percent rate.[10]

For elderly blacks, the poverty rate is very high. For all units over 65, the rate is 40 percent, for couples 26 percent, unmarried males 38 percent and unmarried females 48 percent.[11] Poverty rates for the elderly of Hispanic origin are also very high, 23 percent overall.[12]

So in spite of progress toward an adequate system of income maintenance for the elderly, we are a long way from being able to claim complete success. The high rate of poverty among unmarried women, the very old and minorities and the fact that two-thirds of the very old are unmarried women need to be kept very much in mind as we plan for improvements in our four-tier system of income maintenance and in improvements in health care for the elderly.

Can We Pay for What We Have Promised?

But before we get to improvements, what about the argument that we can't afford what we have already promised, that when the "baby-boomers" reach retirement age in the next century Social Security, Medicare and other promises to today's workers will need to be cut back?

This notion, which I believe is wrong, is based primarily on the expected increase in the ratio of persons over 65 to those 20 to 64, as the "baby boom" generation retires and the "baby bust" generation that follows makes up the largest part of the work force. Here are the figures. Today there are about 20 people over 65 for every 100 persons age 20 through 64. The ratio will rise slightly to 21 per 100 by 1990 and stay approximately level until after the year 2005. But it will then rise rapidly and by 2035, peak at 41, flattening out after that. In the 30-year period from 2005 to 2035, the over-65 population is estimated to rise from 38 million to 71 million (an 87 percent increase), while the 20–64 age group stays just about the same, rising slightly from 173 million in 2005 to 179 million in 2015, but dropping back to 173 million in 2035.[13]

Now, of course, these ratios are not a direct measure of retirees to workers. Not all people over 65 will be retired, and not all 20 through 65 working. Labor-force participation rates of older people, the level of unemployment in the future, the extent to which people are disabled for work or elect early retirement (before age 65), and the extent to which women will prefer work in the paid labor force to work at home are all important factors affecting the ratio of retirees to workers. The demographic shift is so large and so rapid, however, that it, more than anything else, will govern the worker/ retiree ratio.

In all probability, the ratio of the retired aged to those at work will be much larger in 2035 than it is today. However, this is not the whole story. At the same time, the number of children to be supported by the working age group will be declining. While the ratio of non-working elderly to those at work will rise, the ratio of all non-workers to workers is not expected to rise above rates of the recent past. The various assumptions which produce an increasing ratio of older people to those 20 through 64 also result in a declining ratio of those under 20 to the 20–64 group. Thus, if instead of the ratio of those over 65 to those 20–64, we take what has been called a *total* dependency ratio—the ratio of those over 65 plus those under 20 to the group 20–64—we get a much different picture than if we look only at the elderly. It just isn't true that reasonable demographic assumptions show a large increase in the number of dependents per worker after the early part of the next century. Instead what they show is a shift in the composition of the dependency group; fewer children, more elderly.

Today we have about 70 persons either over 65 or under 20 for every 100 in the age group 20 through 64. Over the next 25 to 30 years, this ratio drops steadily until it reaches a low point of 65 per 100 around 2010. Up to that year there are actually fewer dependents per person age 20–64 than we have now. Then the ratio rises, reaching where we are today in about the year 2017, but even at the high point beginning about 2035, we get a ratio of only 85 per 100 as compared to 90 in 1970, and 95 in 1965.[14] Moreover, productivity increases—even modest ones—will make it easier for workers to support non-workers. Modest increases of one and three-quarters percent a year, on the average, translate into a doubling of real wages by about 2025. In the future, people may need to shift some of the resources that would once have been spent to raise children to building the kind of world they want for themselves and others in retirement, but they will have the means to do so.

Let us look narrowly at OASDI for a moment. Not only is it adequately financed over the next 75 years in technical actuarial terms by the financing in present law, but as a percent of Gross National Product. OASDI fluctuates within a relatively small range over the entire 75 years. In 1985, 4.9 percent of GNP is going to this program. Under the trustees' immediate estimates, the percentage will drop steadily until it reaches 4.3 percent in 2005, and then rise gradually, until by the year 2015, it will be about where it is today. It will go up somewhat after that, the maximum being a little under 6.3 percent in the year 2030, and then drop back to 5.7 percent in 2060.[15] The financing in present law, which provides for a maximum OASDI contribution rate of 6.2 percent of earnings beginning in 1990 (compared to 5.7 percent today), fully takes into account the demographic changes described.

RECOMMENDATIONS

Over time, assuming even modest productivity gains, present workers can afford to improve the four-tier system of income security for themselves and the present elderly if they want to. As first priorities, I would suggest raising the pay standard in SSI to the poverty level, particularly for single persons[16] and liberalizing the asset test. This would help the very poorest of the poor among the elderly.

In OASDI, I would recommend improved benefits for single workers, divorced women and widows, while leaving benefits for couples at the levels provided by present law. This can be accomplished by a 7 percent increase in the retirement and widow's benefit concomitant with a reduction in the spouse's benefit from 50 to 40 percent. (Other changes would be needed to improve benefits for divorced homemakers.) This change could be financed by an increase in income equivalent to a contribution rate increase of about one-third of 1 percent each on employees and employers (0.66 percent of payroll). Such a change would increase benefits where increases are needed most.

In the private pension area, I would stress the need for at least limited protection against inflation.

THE POLITICAL DIMENSION

This is a difficult time to improve government programs, however, whether cash benefit programs or medical programs. This administration has been the most successful since the New Deal days in changing the direction of government and the terms of political debate. The administration of Franklin Delano Roosevelt moved the federal government toward taking a degree of responsibility for the well-being of all citizens. The Reagan administration has been moving the federal role back to the narrow one that prevailed before the Great Depression. The strategy has been to promote large tax cuts and accompanying cuts in domestic spending. But increases in military spending have more than offset the cuts in domestic programs, so that the reduced tax income nowhere near meets total spending; the resulting large deficits create still further pressure for cutbacks in domestic programs. If Social Security and the hospital part of Medicare (Part A) are eliminated from both expenditures and receipts (a reasonable adjustment since they are self-financed programs), receipts as a percent of GNP will average 12.9 percent in the period 1986–90, according to Congressional Budget Office projections, and outlays 18.4 percent, as compared with 15.8 percent and 16.9 percent respectively in 1961–70. Under present law, the deficit in the 1986–90 period will average 5.8 percent of GNP as compared to 1.1 percent in 1961–70, and 2.6 percent in 1971–80.

These large deficits have changed the political question from "To what extent do we want to improve programs to meet the needs of the American people?" to "How can we get the deficit down?" The argument now is largely over how much more to cut in domestic programs and how *fast* the military should be increased.

In discussions of the entire domestic budget, there is much talk of adjusting to a period of "scarce resources." Yet the facts are that as compared with, say, 1965 when the two big health service programs, Medicare and Medicaid, were passed, we as a people have much more, on average, than we did then. To take one measure: real per capita disposable income has risen by over 50 percent. This administration has been remarkably successful in turning back the clock. It has created a situation in which the first priority will be to reduce the deficit, and those who want to improve programs have to first bear the onus of advocating tax increases just to stay even. This is a reality we need to face. There is no more important public policy issue before the country than how to gradually restore the tax base. Tax reform with accompanying tax increases in tax revenues has to be the major goal of those who believe in using government for the common good.

MEDICAL CARE INSURANCE

Let me turn now to the specific question of medical care insurance for older people: what we have and what we should have. Medicare has recently come under attack from both conservatives and those who are not so conservative. It has been seen as financially out of control and headed for "bankruptcy," and it is criticized for putting too much emphasis on acute care and not enough on the long-term care needs of the elderly and practically none on prevention and health promotion.

Medicare is up for serious review. The continuing large federal deficit and the size of the program (a projected $72 billion for fiscal year 1985) would, in any event, result in scrutiny. The fact that the part of the program intended to be fully self-supporting, hospital insurance, is predicted to be short of funds before the turn of the century, and the fact that general revenue financing of the coverage of physicians' fees is projected to increase from $17.5 billion in fiscal year 1985 to $25.6 billion in fiscal year 1988 will help to assure a comprehensive review some time in the next few years.[18]

During such a review, it will be important to keep certain considerations in mind.

Medicare is an Immensely Successful Program

The most common concerns of elderly retired people are their health and their income. Medicare contributes importantly to maintaining both. It has greatly increased the ability of older people to secure quality health care, and it has gone a considerable way toward protecting their incomes (and, equally important politically, the incomes of their sons and daughters) against the high and unpredictable costs of illness.

With the passage of Medicare, for many of the elderly, medical care that improves functioning and contributes to the quality of life—such as cataract removal, hernia repair and hip replacement—became affordable for the first time. And although the dramatic improvement in life expectancy for those over 65 (two and one-half years since 1960) has many causes, it is likely that Medicare is at least partly responsible.

Medicare Shares a Crisis of Rising Costs With All Health Insurers

The financial problems of Medicare are more visible than those of private programs because Medicare is part of the federal budget in a time of unprecedented deficits. Also, the long-range costs of Part A are more visible than those of other programs since they are made for 25 years ahead, whereas private insurance, like Part B of Medicare, looks ahead only a year or two. Yet all payers have been affected by the extraordinarily steep increases in health care costs, and consequently current workers under private plans, not just Medicare beneficiaries, are threatened with benefit cuts.

Medicare has had some success in reducing its own costs. The date for Medicare bankruptcy keeps being postponed. The trustees now say 1998 as compared to 1989 or 1990 a short time ago, and if reasonable cost control measures are applied, the date could well move to sometime in the next century. Yet, the go-it-alone approach of Medicare may shift costs to other payers, and in the long run, as providers react to lower payment for Medicare beneficiaries, may reduce the quality of care. The universal nature of the cost problem argues for measures that apply across-the-board to all payers.

Many of the elements of a successful cost-control plan applied to all have been spelled out in the Kennedy-Gephardt bill, although there are additional ideas that also deserve consideration, including strengthening control of technology diffusion, curtailing the use of tax-free bonds for hospital capital, controls over the number of training slots for physicians in some specialties, making it easier for beneficiaries to make out living wills, and providing a different way of compensating for loss in cases of medical malpractice.

Medicare Has Special Problems of Financing and Benefit Design Because of the Aging of the Population

Medicare costs, particularly over the long run, will rise some-what more than the cost of programs covering workers and their families. The need for medical care increases with age and is higher for the disabled under age 65 than for those who are not disabled.

The aging of the population will be an important factor in health care costs for the elderly as the numbers of the very old continue to increase disproportionately to the total number over 65.

In the next 15 years, the total number of persons over 65 is expected to increase by about 23 percent, from 29.3 million to 36.2 million, but the number over 75 is expected to increase by about 46 percent and the number over 85 by 81 percent—from an estimated 2.9 million in July, 1985, to 5.2 million in 2000. If we take the estimates out to the year 2020, we have an increase of about 82 percent for all those past 65 as compared to today, but a 150 percent increase for those past 85, for a total of 7.1 million. Of this number, 5.1 million, or 72 percent, will be female, including 3.8 million widows.[19]

The elderly tend to take longer than younger people to recover from episodes of acute illness, but more importantly, they are subject typically to chronic illness from which there is no recovery. And the chronic conditions typical of the elderly require continuing medication, a variety of health care and social services at home, and, more often than for younger people, long-term institutional care.

Today Most People Die in Old Age and Care of the Terminally Ill Is a High Proportion of Medicare Costs

Some 30 percent of Medicare costs go for medical expenses in the last year of life, and half of these expenditures occur in the last 60 days. The issues that surround medical treatment for terminal illness, therefore, are much more important to Medicare than to programs covering current workers and their families.

Medicare Today Is Inadequate

Medicare pays for only about 45 percent of the total cost of health care services for older people. In 1984, cost-sharing and beneficiary premiums came to a little over $500 a year per enrollee, and it is estimated that the average beneficiary had additional costs of about $550 for non institutional services, mostly prescription drugs and dental care. If the costs of nursing home care were averaged over all beneficiaries, it would add another $650 per person for a total of over $1700 of uncovered care.[20] (Although only about 5 percent of the elderly are in nursing homes at any one time, about 20 percent will be in a nursing home sometime before they die.)

Benefit cuts are not a reasonable option. The cost of health care for the elderly and the disabled will need to be met in one way or another. If the present inadequate level of protection under Medicare is further reduced, major consequences will include increased costs for the federal and state governments under the Medicaid program, increased costs for the high proportion of beneficiaries who buy medigap policies and greater exposure to risk for those who cannot afford to purchase medigap coverage. The states are already spending 40 percent of Medicaid for the care of 3.5 million elderly and, partly as a consequence, their efforts to meet the needs of the younger low income population are totally inadequate. And shifting more cost to the medigap policies hurts beneficiaries and is socially inefficient because of the high selling and administrative costs. Medicare expenditures can be cut back through cost control, but there is nothing in the benefit package that should be reduced. In considering new kinds of protection under Medicare, they should be thought about as additions not substitutes.

RECOMMENDATIONS

Beyond cost control and the defense of what exists, what should we be doing about medical care insurance for the elderly? I believe, first, we have to recognize the political reality I have described. Improvements in government programs have to pay their own way. In fact, the best strategy would be to combine advances in health care coverage for the elderly with plans to reduce the deficit.

Unlike cash benefits under OASDI, Part B of Medicare is a large and growing burden on the general revenues of the federal government and is a legitimate part of the debate on how to reduce the budget deficit. Unlike OASDI, this puts Part B of Medicare in competition with all other programs supported by general revenue and makes the defense against raising the premium paid by beneficiaries or cutting Medicare benefits more difficult than would otherwise be the case. It also makes attempts to improve Medicare almost out of the question. Moreover, with three-fourths of the support of Part B of Medicare coming from general taxes, the defense of the program against means-testing is more difficult than if the program were more nearly self-sustaining. Financing from earmarked taxes would help remove Medicare from the budget deficit argument, just as self-financing of OASDI has made it possible to consider changes in that program largely in terms of the internal needs of OASDI rather than the general budget.

At the same time, substituting new earmarked taxes for general revenues now going to Part B would reduce the overall deficit and relieve pressure on programs supported by general revenues. This might be a relatively popular way to increase income to the government. Reluctant as people are to pay increased taxes, they are more willing to do so if the taxes are earmarked for a purpose that is widely approved and that has tangible benefits for them or their families. All through the recent past, when taxpayers were supporting cuts in general purpose taxes, there was strong support for Social Security tax increases. The polls showed consistently that people of all ages were willing to pay in earmarked taxes what was necessary for an adequate Social Security program. Medicare is just as popular. Not only elderly people but their sons and daughters oppose cutting benefits. Cost control is the first priority, but there is good reason to think that people would also be willing to pay higher taxes for an improved program.

Some new income sources to consider are:

1. Applying the Medicare tax to the 30 percent of state and local employees (4 million persons) not covered under Social Security. Since many of these employees now become eligible for Medicare without paying the Medicare tax while in state or local employment, extending the tax improves Medicare financing.
2. Covering new state and local employees under Old-Age, Survivors, and Disability Insurance in those jurisdictions that have not elected coverage and, since such an extension of coverage saves OASDI money, reallocating part of the 1990 presently scheduled OASDI tax increase to Medicare.
3. Including employer contributions to group health and life insurance in the Social Security tax and benefit base and reallocating the increased income to Medicare. Although this change increases OASDI benefits in the long run, because of the weighted benefit formula there is a net gain to the system.
4. Raising alcohol and tobacco taxes and dedicating the proceeds to Medicare as an advance payment for the higher Medicare cost for those who drink or smoke.

5. Including the general revenue subsidy for Part B of Medicare (currently three-fourths of the total cost) in the personal income tax of higher-income persons and dedicating the proceeds to Medicare.
6. If employer contributions for group health insurance are included in the income tax for workers, including one-half the value of Part A of Medicare protection in the income tax of higher-income persons and dedicating the proceeds to Medicare.
7. Following a reform of the income tax, dedicating a surtax on the income tax to Medicare.

There is an additional possibility for partial financing of health insurance that should be kept in mind. If, instead of the present plan of financing the long-range costs of OASDI by building huge trust funds over the next 25 years, the program were to continue on a more or less pay-as-you-go basis (although with a sizeable contingency reserve, say 150 percent of the next year's outgo) it would be possible to reallocate to Medicare much of the tax increases now scheduled for OASDI in 1988 and 1990. Retaining a pay-as-you-go approach for OASDI would require additional income equivalent to about a 1 percentage point increase in the contribution rate from about 2020 on.

With additional funding, Part B could be made self-financing, improved in many ways and extended to additional groups. Parts A and B should be combined into a single program with one annual deductible and administered by a single contracting agent. The entire program should be mandatory, as Part A is today. People have as much neeed for physician coverage as for hospital coverage, and both should be mandatory. Currently 99 percent of the elderly and 92 percent of the disabled eligible for Part A also elect Part B.

The present Medicare program provides reasonable good insurance against the cost of hospital stays, paying overall about three-fourths of the hospital cost of beneficiaries. The program, however, provides no protection against the cost of very long hospital stays or the other costs associated with very expensive illness. Catastrophic insurance should be added so that no beneficiary would have to pay more than a specified amount, say $2,000 a year, for all medical expenses covered by the new combined Part A and Part B plan.

Over time, benefits should be expanded to include prescription drugs, long-term care benefits and health promotion and disease prevention.

Medicare has not been designed to pay for either the cost of long-term care in a nursing home or to provide many of the services that would allow more elderly and disabled people to remain in their own homes instead of going to the nursing home. This needs to be changed. Long-term care insurance under Medicare should cover home health services, including an assessment service and case-management, as well as nursing home benefits. The assessment service should be open to all Medicare beneficiaries, as the need arises, to determine medical and other needs and to help develop disease prevention and health promotion activities. It should be required when major changes in health status call for a choice between additional community services and institutional care.

Some of the home services that might be included are those already available as home health care visits to Medicare beneficiaries, but the services would be provided as well to those who are not homebound. In addition, social services necessary to keep an individual from having to enter a nursing home could be provided, particularly homemaker services, chore services, help with the activities of daily living, such as bathing, eating, helping with food preparation, and others. The cost of a plan for home health services should not exceed the average cost of care in the nursing home in the area.

Nursing home care is an essential part of a long-term care program. Present arrangements are very unsatisfactory. Half the care is paid for by the means-tested federal-state Medicaid system, and frequently Medicaid is unable or unwilling to pay for quality care. The cost of the other half of nursing home care falls mostly on the individual and on relatives. Few people can pay for extended stays in a nursing home, and a high proportion of those who start out as private payers end up on the Medicaid rolls with their funds exhausted and, in many instances, after considerable expense to friends and relatives. Private insurance and Medicare play almost no part in protecting people against long-term nursing home costs. Medicare pays less than 3 percent of nursing home costs; private insurance less than 1 percent. Yet, as we look ahead to a much older population, provision of nursing home care and other long-term care services will become increasingly important. The fear of exhausting resources and ending up in a Medicaid nursing home is a major concern of elderly people.

A way of greatly reducing the cost of extending Medicare to nursing homes would be to separate out the basic room and board component of nursing home costs and include as part of a health insurance payment only the nursing home costs in excess of room and board. Room and board would be paid for by the recurring retirement income of the patient, supplemented, if necessary, by SSI. The purpose of Social Security, private pensions and government career retirement plans is to meet the ordinary living expenses of the recipients. After retention of a small allowance for personal expenses, it would seem reasonable to devote these payments to meeting the room and board part of nursing home charges. The goal of Medicare should be to insure only for average expenses above average room and board costs. Exactly how to do this—perhaps just through a large deductible or coinsurance instead of the actual determination of room and board costs—needs further study, but it seems to be the best approach to providing nursing home care on a non-means-tested basis.

The present prohibition against paying for prevention should be removed from the Medicare law and a well-planned effort made to encourage disease prevention and health promotion. A professional advisory board should be established to recommend, on the basis of health effectiveness and cost effectiveness, which preventive services should be paid for, how often they should be provided and under what conditions.

In time, the improved Medicare protection described should be extended to all Social Security beneficiaries: all those receiving disability benefits, not just those who have been receiving benefits for two years; all persons age 62 or over eligible for Social Security, rather than those 65 or over; and younger beneficiaries, principally widows and motherless and fatherless children.

Cost controls applied to all payers should bring Part A of Medicare into long-run actuarial balance over the 25 years for which estimates have been made traditionally. Additional sources of income earmarked for Medicare should be used to reduce or eliminate Part B's dependence on general revenue, thus reducing the deficit. At the same time, the additional earmarked revenue should be sufficient to improve and extend a new combined Part A and Part B Medicare Program.

OTHER HEALTH AND SOCIAL POLICY ISSUES

It has not been possible in one short paper to discuss many of the important health and social policy questions raised by the aging of our society. Let me just mention some of them. The health needs of the elderly would be best served if they were part of a health plan covering all ages. Health promotion and disease prevention obviously help the elderly and everyone else most if they start early, and appropriate therapy should be available at any age. It is of high-ranking importance to provide protection for the approximately 35 million persons who are not now covered by any health insurance program. And how are we to deal with the cost of the major technological advances to be expected unless we develop an overall health plan?

What proportion of the elderly in the future will be able to afford retirement communities that provide a guarantee of life-time care? Are social HMOs practical on a large scale? Would it be desirable for large numbers of the elderly to increase their current incomes by home equity conversion arrangements that allow them to remain in their own homes? What about the issues that surround the cost of dying?

With less pressure on the labor market from new entrants because of lower birth rates, will more older people find attractive job opportunities? With compulsory retirement prohibited before age 70 and with recent Social Security changes that will gradually remove penalties for working,[21] more older people may want to work longer and employers may want them.

Will the much talked of generational conflict actually develop, with younger workers wanting to spend more currently and less on supporting a system of income and health care guarantees for their parents and, in turn, for themselves as they grow older? Can this threatened conflict be lessened by avoiding special privileges for the well-off elderly, such as the double exemption under the income?

And there are more issues that need attention. The demographic changes described will have profound effect on many aspects of American life.

CONCLUSION

The United States will enter a period of great social change some 25 years from now when the long-range trend of an increasing number and proportion of the elderly in the population takes a dramatic leap upward. We have developed good income support systems for older people which should serve the country well, not only now, but when that period arrives. Some changes are desirable, but progress in the last 50 years has been phenomenal and we have good arrangements in place.

Provision for health care for the elderly is also much advanced from 20 years ago when Medicare was established. But in this area, the list of unfinished business is much longer. And because of increases in the length of life and the fantastic technological developments that have occurred and are to be expected, health care for the elderly will present ever-changing issues of cost, appropriateness and ethics.

REFERENCE NOTES

1. Social Security Administration. *Social Security Area Population Projections, 1984: Actuarial Study No. 92*. Social Security Administration Publication No. 11-11639, Table 20a.

2. Maxfield, Linda Drazza, and Virginia P. Reno. *Social Security Bulletin*, January 1985.

3. Munnell, Alicia H., Retirement Income Security in the United States, Testimony before Subcommittee on Social Security and Subcommittee on Oversight of the Committee on Ways and Means, U.S. House of Representatives, July 18, 1985, Table 2.

4. "Distribution of Income Sources of Recent Retirees: Finding from the New Beneficiary Survey," Op. Cit.

5. With the exception of a home, life insurance policies of less than $1,500 face value, household goods and personal effects of less than $2,000 and the first $4,500 of the market value of an automobile, all other assets must total less than $1,600 for an unmarried person, less than $2,400 for a couple in 1985, increasing gradually to $2,000 and $3,000 by 1989. Partly because of this stringent asset test and partly because of the low-income threshold, of all the households headed by elderly persons that are below the poverty level only half are receiving SSI.

6. Committee on Ways and Means, Background Material and Data on Programs within the Jurisdiction of the Committee on Ways and Means, U.S. House of Representatives, Washington, D.C. 1985. Tables 6 and 7, pp. 444–445.

7. Annual Report of Federal Security Agency, 1950. Tables 5 and 6, pp. 91–92 and author's calculation.

8. It should be noted that these replacement rates do not represent the true situation of most workers. For example, workers who end up with a career average that equals the average wage at the time of retirement have typically had wages that were below the average when young and well above the average in the years shortly before retirement. Thus these "average" workers get benefits that do not replace nearly as much of their recent earnings as the illustrations imply. The same over-statement of the ratio of benefits to earning just before retirement occurs at all wage levels (except for the consistently maximum earner), with the result that there is more need to supplement Social Security than would appear from looking at these commonly used illustrations.

9. Bureau of the Census, Characteristics of the Population below the Poverty Line, 1983, *Current Population Reports* P60-147, Table 11, p. 40. Washington, D.C. 1985.

10. Bureau of the Census, *Current Population Survey*, March 1983, unpublished data.

11. U.S. Department of Health and Human Services, *Income of the Population 55 and Older, 1982*. Table 48, p. 82, Washington, D.C. 1984.

12. *Characteristics of the Population Below the Poverty Line*, 1983.

13. 1985 Annual Report of the Board of Trustees of the Federal Old-Age and Survivors

Insurance and Disability Insurance Trust Funds. Washington, D.C. 1985. Assumptions 11-A and 11-B, Table A1, p. 77.

14. Ibid.

15. Ibid. Table 31, p. 69.

16. Both SSI and Social Security seem to have overstated the needs of couples compared to those living alone. Although the poverty measure for singles is 80 percent of the measure for couples, these programs pay the single person only two-thirds of the amount paid the couple.

17. Some of the material that follows was first published in: Ball, Robert M., Medicare: A strategy for protecting and improving it. *Generations*, Summer, 1985, p. 9.

18. Derived from Budget of the United States, Fiscal Year 1986. Washington, D.C. 5-111.

19. Social Security Area Population Projections, 1984. Tables 20a, 20d, 20e. The assumptions underlying the projections differ somewhat from Census Bureau assumptions.

20. Congressional Budget Office, Changing the Structure of Medicare Benefits: Issues and Options, 1983, Washington, D.C.: U.S. Congress.

21. The 3 percent per year increment for working past 65 that now applies to Social Security benefits is to gradually increase beginning in 1990 to the actuarial equivalent amount so that those who retire will, on average, receive the same lifetime benefits as those who retire early.

Issues in Health and Social Policy for an Aging Society
A General Policy Perspective

Leon Eisenberg, MD

In this era of open disclosure and informed consent, I find myself obliged to acknowledge that I owe Bob Ball three debts: as an aging citizen, for his singular contribution to the nation as Commissioner of Social Security; as an erstwhile cynical citizen, for his having restored my faith that dedicated public servants do exist; as a sometimes confused citizen seeking to understand the complexities of government policy, for his lucid analyses of where we are, how far we have come, and where we need to go with respect to health and social policy for older Americans. I shall endeavor to repay those debts in the only currency he accepts: by joining his campaign for social justice.

Bob has made clear that government programs *can* work and, in the case of Social Security and Medicare, *do* work. That is important news in an era when the perceived wisdom has many believing that "you can't solve social problems by throwing money at them." The facts are otherwise. Targeting government expenditures in an appropriate fashion diminishes the misery resulting from poverty and sickness.

What kneejerk conservatives really object to is diverting funds from the "haves" to the "have-nots"; they are remarkably indifferent to the money thrown, for example, at military contractors charging $748 for a pair of pliers.[1] With one in seven of the elderly below the poverty line, shall we agree to cut supports still further at a time when, as the Assistant Secretary for Manpower in the Defense Department acknowledges, military "pork barrel" costs "the taxpayer at least $10 billion a year."[2]

Bob has documented for us that Social Security and Medicare underpin minimal decency in the lives of the elderly. Yet, today's political rhetoric treats these programs as unacceptable drains on the

23

treasury. Thus we see proposals to omit the Social Security cost of living adjustment and to control Medicare costs by methods which are not applied to other health care sectors.

Medicare is said to be "in crisis." But "crises" are not matters of "fact," they are social constructions. As Carroll Estes has pointed out in the case of the so-called Social Security crisis,[3] the perception of a crisis legitimates the rejection of previously shared assumptions; it affords public officials authority to act in ways that would ordinarily be strongly resisted. Thus, the social legislation of the New Deal and the Great Society, surely among the proudest accomplishments of this nation, is under attack, despite the long-term solvency of Social Security and the postponement of Medicare's ostensible "bankruptcy" until the end of this century.[4]

Those who seek to reduce social welfare benefits assert that this country cannot afford them. The fact is that total government expenditures constitute a smaller proportion of the Gross National Product in the U.S. than in many other industrialized nations.[5] The real issue is how much we are willing to spend, and for what. Agreed, resources are not infinite. Trade-offs are inevitable—trade-offs between stockpiling weapons in an arsenal of nuclear destruction and preserving the democratic policy which that armory purports to "defend." Recall what Representative Wright of Texas said in the MX debate: "We are spending more . . . on military might this year than we spent in any year during the Viet Nam war, in any year during the Korean war, and, yes, in any year during World War II."[6]

Recall that President Regan: "who promised to balance the Federal budget, has added more to the national debt in four years than all the other Presidents combined in the 192 years of the Republic."[6] The terms of the political debate must be recognized for what they are. Unless we challenge the rhetoric that resource constraints arise from fiscal "necessity," we become accessories to a crime against older Americans.

Capping Medicare will hold down costs, no question about it. But caps do not discriminate between needed and effective care and unnecessary or even harmful medical practices. If we keep the focus on the *health* in health policy, there is a very considerable potential for human benefits as well as savings. Consider only the following anachronisms in our present health care system: the three- to seven-fold variation in population rates for medical and surgical procedures among comparable geographic areas;[7] the perversity of a physician fee reimbursement schedule which rewards doctors disproportionately for technical procedures as against clinical care;[8] the lack of an adequate mechanism for technology assessment so that costly new devices are introduced before their efficacy has been demonstrated;[9] and purchases of hospitals which increase per diem rates by inflated depreciation and pass-through of interest on borrowed funds.[10] Effective interventions to reverse these irrationalities in the health care delivery system would benefit patients *and* tax payers.[11,12]

Contrast that approach with the single-minded focus in Washington on containing Medicare costs and the willingness to tolerate a two-tier system of care, which has led to measures targeted solely at Medicare beneficiaries. Out-of-pocket costs per hospital admission doubled between 1981 and 1984 and are slated to rise another 60% by 1990.[13] DRGs imposed on Medicare patients invite hospitals to shift costs and to dump the "losers" onto the public system.[14] It does not require a very sophisticated computer program to identify the demographic characteristics of potential admissions who will be costly outliers—in order to turn them away at the door. Caps on Medicare physician fees will have one predictable outcome: they will impair access to services for the elderly. Physician participation rates in Medicaid programs have been shown to be highly sensitive to fee levels. Freezes on payment rates, in contrast, have proved ineffective in controlling program expenditures because physicians respond by increasing the quantity and complexity of services billed for.[15]

The latest panaceas, attractive to both political parties, are Medicare voucher plans to prod beneficiaries into the prepaid HMO market despite the fact that HMOs do not currently offer extensive long-term care benefits.[16] Elders are ill-equipped to choose between health insurance policies and providers; this is evident in the extent to which they have purchased worthless medigap policies from unscrupulous insurers.[17] Unless legislation mandates comprehensive coverage for chronic illness as a condition for eligibility for Medicare vouchers and regulatory agencies monitor compliance, elders will once again be naked in the marketplace.

And what shall we say of the "Alice-in-Wonderland" logic employed by the Inspector General of DHHS? Richard Kusserow has justified an increase in the deductibles for Part B Medicare beneficiaries on the grounds that: " . . . an increase in the deductible would impact only on the consumers of health care, not the nonusers."[18] *Mirabil dictu!* The Red Queen would have understood: off with insurance altogether! After all, why should the healthy pay for the sick?

Once costs take precedence and the nation accepts a lifeboat mentality, cost-benefit analysis, which reduces all question of interest to dollars, is at hand to demonstrate that providing medical care to elderly patients is a losing proposition because they, along with housewives and minorities, are not economically "productive."[19] Bias against the elderly has become so pervasive in the health field that even so excellent an institution as the Centers for Disease Control employs age 65 rather than average life expectancy as the cut-off point for computing years of life lost by cause of death.[20] This system of computation sharply reduces the apparent impact of diseases which strike at older ages, implying that years lost after 65 are irrelevant in public health calculations.

Bob Ball has shown us how Social Security and Medicare, appropriately expanded and financed, can enhance lives and dignity and quality for older Americans. I have tried to spell out how current proposals for retrenchment in these programs threaten the foundations of equity in our society. Which is it to be? The answer will depend on the strength of our commitment, as health professionals, to the proposition that neither age nor poverty forfeits the right to care.[21]

REFERENCE NOTES

1. Boeing cuts price of $748 pliers, but contract total remains same. *New York Times*, March 23, 1985.
2. Military "pork barrel" wastes billions a year, official says. *New York Times*, April 1, 1985.
3. Estes, C. L., Social Security: The social construction of a crisis. *Milbank Memorial Fund Quarterly*, 61:445-61, 1983.
4. Pear, R., Medicare trust fund is seen as healthy until '98. *New York Times*, March 29, 1985.
5. Kravis, I. B., Heton, A. and Summers, R. *World Products and Income: International Comparisons of Real Gross Product*. Baltimore: John Hopkins University Press, 1982.
6. Reston, J., What's "security" anyway? *New York Times*, March 31, 1985.
7. Wennberg, J. E. and Gittelson, A., Variations in medical care among small areas. *Scientific American*, 126:120-34, 1982.
8. Almy, T. P., The role of the primary physician and the health care "industry." *New England Journal of Medicine*, 304:225-228, 1981.
9. Institute of Medicine Conference Report, *Evaluating Medical Technologies in Clinical Use*. Washington, D.C.: Institute of Medicine, 1981.

10. Comptroller General, *Hospital Merger Increased Medicare and Medicaid Payments for Capital Costs*. Washington, D.C.: Government Accounting Office, 1983.

11. Wennberg, J. E., Bunker, J. P. and Barnes, B. A. The need for assessing outcomes of common medical practices. *Annual Review of Public Health*, 1:227–95, 1980.

12. Institute of Medicine Study, *A Manpower Policy for Primary Care*. Washington, D.C.: Institute of Medicine, 1978.

13. Sullivan, R., Medicare hospital bills for elderly soar. *New York Times*, March 8, 1985.

14. Stern, R. S. and Epstein, A. M., Institutional responses to prospective payment based on diagnosis-related groups. *New England Journal of Medicine*, 312:621–27, 1985.

15. Gabel, J. R. and Rice, T. H., Reducing public expenditures for physician services: The price of paying less. *Journal of Health Politics, Policy and Law*, 9:595–609, 1985.

16. Winn, S. and McCafree, K., Issues involved in the development of a prepaid capitation plan for long term care services. *The Gerontologist*, 19:184–90, 1979.

17. Pegels, C., *Health Care and the Elderly*, Rockville, Maryland: Aspen Systems Corporation, 1980.

18. Inspector General backs increase in Medicare deductible. *Washington Health Costs Letter*, January 18, 1985.

19. Avorn, J., Benefit and cost analysis in geriatric care: Turning age discrimination into health policy. *New England Journal of Medicine*, 31:1294–1301, 1984.

20. Centers for Disease Control, Table V: Years of life lost, death and death rates, by cause of death, and estimated number of physician contacts, by principal diagnosis, United States. *Morbidity and Mortality Weekly Report*, 34:139, 1985.

21. Eisenberg, L., Rudolf Ludwig Karl Virchow, where are you, now that we need you? *American Journal of Medicine*, 77:524–32, 1984.

Issues in Health and Social Policy for an Aging Society
A National Policy Perspective

Henry J. Aaron, PhD

Reading Bob Ball's paper reminded me of my youth and a story I read in a collection of Jewish humor. A class on English language was being held for immigrants. As part of their lessons, they were asked to write a short essay on "The Elephant." A Frenchman wrote on "The Love Life of the Elephant," a German on "Military Uses of the Elephant," an Indian on "Hunting Elephants in the Punjab," and a Jew from the Polish *shtetl* wrote an essay entitled "The Elephant and the Jewish Problem." Reading Bob Ball's paper made me realize that if in that class, his essay would be "The Elephant and Social Security."

His paper is divided into two main parts. The first concerns income of the aged and the role that Social Security plays in maintaining it. The second deals with health care for the aged and the role Medicare plays in paying for it. I will divide my comments along those lines and conclude with some thoughts on other issues that Mr. Ball treats lightly if at all.

INCOME

The paper recounts the achievements of Social Security and it does so very well. No other law in American history has played so important a part in transforming and improving the lot of Americans. The Social Security Act is the most important legacy of the New Deal. A comprehensive program of social assistance to begin with—including from the start old age insurance, unemployment insurance, and public assistance—it has been broadened to encompass survivors benefits, disability insurance, social service grants, Medicare, Medicaid, and other provisions as well.

29

Bob Ball points out the dramatic improvement in the living standards of the aged and correctly in my view, attributes much of that gain to Social Security. He notes that the aged have achieved economic parity with the non-aged. Mr. Ball points out that the incidence of poverty among the aged is no greater than among the non-aged. In fact, one can make a strong case that the average income of the aged has surpassed that of the non-aged. Data indicate that if one adjusts income data for family size, possession of household durables, and several other factors, the aged had reached income parity with the non-aged by the early 1970s. Since then, the relative status of the aged has improved, largely because Social Security benefits have been fully protected against inflation, while earnings have not. Mr. Ball points out that some groups among the aged have higher poverty rates than others and suggests that this fact establishes the desirability of higher benefits. But the same would be true for the non-aged. Only the opposite finding—would be surprising, indeed incredible. Despite what Garrison Keilor says, not all children can be above average.

Bob Ball goes on to argue that the burden of maintaining benefits is clearly sustainable. He employs the concept of the "total dependency" ratio, the ratio of the sum of children and aged persons to the working age population, and shows that this ratio rises far less than the ratio of the aged to prime age population. While the total dependency ratio is a useful concept, we should not forget that the per capita cost of the aged is much greater than that of children.

But there is a genuine issue of intergenerational equity, which Mr. Ball addresses only by inference and, in my opinion, incorrectly. Social Security has been managed on the "pay-as-you-go" principle. According to that principle, Social Security taxes are paid out immediately as benefits; a negligible reserve is maintained that would be sufficient to preclude the need to raise taxes if there was a revenue shortfall, for example due to recession. If the ratio of the retired to the active population is roughly constant, all generations pay taxes that bear the same relation to the benefits they later receive. If there is a big bulge in the number of retirees, pay-as-you-go financing forces one generation—the one that is active and paying taxes when the large cohorts are claiming benefits—to pay much higher taxes in relation to the benefits they will receive than other generations.

It is precisely to reduce this inequity that current law calls for taxes over the next twenty-five years well in excess of those needed for current benefits. In effect, the baby-boom generation is being asked to pay some extra taxes now to minimize the extra burden that strict pay-as-you-go financing would place on their children later. Mr. Ball would use those extra taxes not to build up a reserve to support future retirement and disability benefits, but to make up the projected deficit in Medicare. Such a step would recreate the very inequity eliminated by the financing reforms successfully urged upon Congress by the National Commission on Social Security Reform, on which Mr. Ball served with extreme distinction.

I confess that the line of argument I have just presented seems to be torpedoed below the waterline by the massive deficits that have resulted from the tax cuts enacted in 1981. From one standpoint, it seems pointless for the federal government to go through the charade of saving for a rainy day by building up reserves in its Social Security pocket while at the same time it empties several other pockets, the closet, and the cupboard to pay for current spending through fiscally irresponsible deficits. It is doubly pointless when federal prodigality causes the United States to surrender its role as the leading creditor nation and to slide into being the leading debtor nation in the world, as current policies are now doing. The burdens of these debts will have to be shouldered by, among others, the children of the baby-boomers, the very generation that Social Security reserves are meant to spare.

In fact, however, preserving the Social Security surpluses that have been forecast to start in 1988, helps combat the deficit. Spending them to patch up Medicare, rather than raising additional taxes or even curtailing Medicare benefits, a course I do not recommend, will make the fiscal situation worse. I believe that the accumulation of Social Security trust funds should be protected. Financing health care is a distinct problem which should not be avoided because of the historical happenstance that both cash benefits and Medicare are financed with payroll taxes.

HEALTH

I have little to add or to criticize in Mr. Ball's examination of Medicare. I would only call attention to the subtext. Mr. Ball's Medicare story is played out in a world where national health policy toward the non-aged is largely confined to cost-containment. To be sure such programs as the Indian Health Service and CHAMPUS continue; but the only health programs for the non-aged that Mr.

Ball mentions are the Kennedy-Gephardt bill and other programs which aim to slow the growth of spending. Any realistic prospect of a national health plan is conspiciously absent from Mr. Ball's vision. I think that this perspective is the politically right one, subject to a speculation I will come to in a moment.

Bob Ball notes correctly that the day of insolvency for Medicare has been receding. The same trustees of the Medicare trust funds who in 1982 foresaw reserves vanishing by 1987 now predict sufficient revenues *with no changes in current law* until 1998. This respite means that Congress will not have to amend the Medicare system any time soon unless it wishes to use cuts in Medicare benefits or increases in payroll taxes to cut the deficit. And that means program cuts will be the only items on the agenda until either the budget deficit is safely behind us or the financial condition of Medicare worsens.

Despite this forecast of continued and extreme tight-fistedness toward federal spending, Mr. Ball reminds us of a number of serious social problems still unsolved or now emerging that will afflict the aged. The most notable is the cost of long-term care. In principle, with careful financial planning, people could save for the costs of long-term care, but they don't; in principle, they could act as informed buyers of the extraordinary range of services called long-term care, but they don't; and in principle, the market could respond to such informed demand, but it doesn't. Like Bob Ball, I see an important federal role, but unlike him, I am unpersuaded that Medicare is the optimum or even a desirable vehicle to deal with these problems. In particular, closed-end grants to states or other providers, rather than entitlements merit close scrutiny. But I think he is dead on target to place long-term care first on the agenda for federal action.

OTHER ISSUES

The title of Bob Ball's paper is "Health and Social Policy for an Aging Society." But to keep things manageable he has written a paper that would be more accurately entitled "Federal Income and Health Expenditures on the Aged." Fair enough, especially because the paper does what it does so well.

What is largely missing, however, is explicit emphasis on what the United States can do to deal with the burden of a rising dependent population. In macroeconomic terms, the most important thing we can do is save, thereby building up productive capacity and assets that can be used to meet rising costs of income support and health. That is precisely the argument that the Japanese, facing demographic shifts even more dramatic than our own, use to justify their high saving and capital export. They are acting with foresight. We are consuming our inheritance.

Secondly, the conservative shift in political opinion makes likely a continuing debate on the relative roles of social security, private pensions, and voluntary saving. With the rejection of President Reagan's 1981 proposal to cut the Social Security program more than 20 percent, frontal efforts by the President to shift the balance ended. But the 1983 Social Security amendments promise large benefit reductions. And a move away from complete indexation of benefits for retirees threaten more.

These latest proposals represent a truly absurd retirement policy—why one would want to assure people a steady drop in living standards from retirement until they die is hard to fathom. If this is the quality of proposals to change the relative importance of Social Security on the agenda today, then action should be put off until the agenda improves.

I would like to close with a speculation that a national health plan may not be as removed as some believe, but that it may come about in a completely unforeseen way. Medicare has recently begun to pay hospitals prospectively. The best informed supporters of the DRG system recognize, however, that this system must evolve. The game of shifting costs to other payers will increase pressures to cover all payers. The game of shifting services pre-admission or post-discharge will create pressures to extend budget control outside the hospital. All of these steps will keep narrowing the opportunities to provide uncompensated care, raising pressures to provide direct support for services to the 20 percent of the population lacking adequate third-party coverage. If we respond to these pressures, we will wake up one day and find that budgetary control of health care resides in state or federal regulatory bodies. In short, we will have all of the administrative elements of a national health plan.

Issues in Health and Social Policy for an Aging Society
A Regional Policy Perspective

James G. Haughton, MD, MPH

Early in the decade of the 1960s Walter Reuther, then President of the United Auto Workers and a devout advocate of the principle of social insurance, invited 100 Americans to serve on what he termed "The Committee of 100 for National Health Insurance." It was a "many splendored" group which included such luminaries as E. G. Marshall, a leading television star of the time, Isidore Falk, a grand old man of health care issues, and Jim Brindle, the President of the Health Insurance Plan of Greater New York; but it also included a few unknown neophytes like me who was just beginning a medical administrative career in New York City.

Walter Reuther knew the history of our national approach to the financing of health care and had come to the conclusion that only by addressing the problems of all the people could we effectively address the problems of any segment of the people.

Almost 20 years ago I came to the conclusion that programs designed specifically for the poor are inevitably destined to become poor programs because they have no powerful constituency to protect them nor to be their advocates. Furthermore, because of their specificity and high profile, they easily become political targets when budgetary constraints dictate financial retrenchment. At the time I reached those conclusions, I was referring specifically to Medicaid and to the health programs created by the "War Against Poverty."

My observations were soon proven correct when in 1969 President Nixon created the Medicaid Task Force to study the "problems" of the three-year old Medicaid program, the problem being the nation was spending too much on health care for the poor. Just three years after its implementation Medicaid had become the political target some of us had predicted, and has remained so ever since.

Two years ago the Governor of Texas appointed a Task Force on Indigent Health Care to study the problems of health care for the poor—almost 20 years after passage of national legislation which was supposed to catapult the poor into the "mainstream" of health care. The Task Force has produced a report highlighting the problems of health care for the poor and has proposed a number of initiatives to address them. The legislature has taken its lead from this report and is now discussing legislation tailored to the health care needs of poor women and children.

This proposed legislation, while unquestionably well-intentioned, completely ignores the national history of defection from continued, committed support for programs designed expressly for the poor.

In the national debate over Medicare and its financing we are repeating history. We are focusing on the problems and costs of health care for the elderly. I fully agree with Bob Ball that "the health needs of the elderly would be best served if they were part of a health plan covering all ages." This was what Walter Reuther perceived more than 20 years ago when he proposed a national health insurance plan with universal coverage. It was also what was perceived by President Truman and the sponsors of the Murray-Wagner-Dingle bill in 1948.

Because we have not learned that lesson, we now find Medicare the target of administration and hear it being discussed in the context of solving the problem of the national deficit. Medicare was an incomplete program at its conception, as Bob Ball points out, and has, therefore, always been subsidized by the individual as well as by the Medicaid program. The result is that all actions at both national and state levels that affect the Medicaid program have a halo effect on the Medicare program.

It appears from the current local and national dialogue that we are not yet ready to address the health care needs of all the people. As long as that is true the elderly will be underserved.

With a rapidly growing elderly population, the problem is not merely one of providing and financing acute health care for this cohort of our citizens. We have relied very heavily on institutional interventions in addressing the needs of this group. Nursing homes have become accepted as a part of our national response, but even this limited response has not achieved its fullest and best potential because nursing homes have often become warehouses where we abandon our elderly. Not only have we not provided the funds to support this response, but we have ignored the development of non-institutional responses which would reduce the need for institutionalization of our older citizens.

National policy does not seem to encourage expenditures for non-institutional alternatives such as home health services, homemaker services, or Meals on Wheels as investments in the reduction of the high cost of institutional care. In Houston and Harris County, for example, the Area Agency on Aging delivers meals to 2,100 home bound elderly citizens five days per week. It is estimated that another 900 could legitimately be served if funds were available, and more than 1200 actually need two meals a day instead of one, but available funds do not permit this.[1]

Foster homes for adults are another approach to non-institutional care of elderly citizens which has been proven effective, but this, too, has had limited financial support.

While medical care is important, we may never adequately come to a resolution of the problems of cost until we find ways of reducing our reliance on institutional responses. It is conceivable that the only ultimate solution will be the reallocation of existing resources to invest more in community networks of social support and less in high cost institutional medical care.

Clearly, such social responses will not empty our nursing homes given the increasing longevity of our population, just as DRGs are not going to empty our hospitals. But surely the existence of socially acceptable alternatives can delay the need for institutionalization which very often occurs only because there are not alternatives. Many older citizens enter nursing homes not because they are ill and need nursing care, but because they do not have the stamina to perform the household chores which living alone requires. This is the group for whom institutional responses can be delayed or even completely prevented.

It is time that we do more than discuss these policy issues. Furthermore, it is time that we stop proposing pilot projects and instead review past documented successful experiences and begin to pursue ways of making them a permanent part of our response to the care of the elderly.

REFERENCES

1. Area Agency on Aging of Houston and Harris County, April, 1985.

Issues in Health and Social Policy
for an Aging Society
Panel Discussion

Dr. Stanley Reiser: There is an interesting link between Dr. Aaron's remarks and those of Dr. Haughton. They both cite the threat to securing health benefits for the elderly as if this group is left conspicuously standing as one of the major recipients of federal dollars and they thereby connect Medicare to the issue of national health insurance. If I remember correctly, Wilbur Cohen, discussing the passage of the Medicare Act, said he and others around him had never envisioned Medicare to stand alone. They hoped that it would be the first policy of a long-range strategy which would ultimately lead to national health insurance.

I would like to believe that Dr. Aaron is right, that a successful cost containment policy would in fact evolve into a national health plan. However, a fundamental reason that we stopped thinking about a national health insurance plan in the late 60s and early 70s, in addition to the higher cost of Medicare and Medicaid than we anticipated, was a decline in the capabilities of European medical systems, based on total national health insurance, to deal adequately with the problems of illness. These suspicions of failure have grown in the 70s and early 80s as some Europeans themselves consider ways of getting out of the national health insurance business. I wonder, therefore, if the people around the table and the speakers would like to comment on how the European experience affects our vision of whether we can take the elderly out of this conspicuous "standing alone" and convert our system into a more national one.

Dr. Henry Aaron: I interpret the history of the 1960s and 1970s somewhat differently. The principal reason why the national health insurance effort stalled in this country was that national health insurance existed for most people. It didn't exist as part of a nationally-legislated plan; rather, it existed in the form of a

crazy-quilt of employer-based insurance and national health programs such as Medicare. As a result, too few people lacked
coverage to have much direct clout, and not enough people were
upset about the inadequacies of health insurance to mobilize the
majority for action.

The high water mark of the national health insurance effort was the
1965 legislation which created Medicare and Medicaid. What was
left after that legislation was a politically vestigial, uncovered
population. The effort for a nationally-legislated health insurance
plan died and remains dead. It could be rekindled if we start
squeezing out uncompensated care sufficiently ruthlessly, but it
seems possible that if we move in the direction of national controls,
it may come in a completely different fashion. We have a system of
third-party coverage with tremendous technological change, which
is increasing costs very rapidly. Concern about costs might push us
in a direction, incrementally, that would lead to having all of the
control mechanisms needed for a national health plan.

Dr. James Haughton: I have a totally different perspective than Dr.
Aaron about what happened in the late 1960s and 1970s because I
happened at that time in my life to be running large public hospital
institutions. There was a great need never met by Medicare or
Medicaid. Every state in this Union had established eligibility
standards for Medicaid that left a large proportion of the population
totally uncovered. Those people fell to the services of the public
system that was locally funded, highly exposed, and politically
threatened. The people who were just above those defined as
"medically needy" were not frequently covered by their employers
because they worked in marginal industries. They were not eligible
for Medicaid and were out there struggling to get their care from
underfinanced public systems. So, it was not for lack of need that
the steam fell out of the national health insurance push.

Dr. Aaron: We don't disagree. Tens of millions of people had
inadequate protection. The remark I was making referred to political
salience. It is simply that the groups both of us would have liked to
have seen receive more adequate health protection were without the
political clout to make their will felt.

Dr. Eli Ginzberg: There are three statements that have been put on
the table: that the U.S. never adequately covered anyone with health
insurance, that the U.S. got nervous about the European experience

in their attempts to give everybody coverage and backed away from national health insurance, and that we really have most people covered. I would like to point out that we don't have a kind of structure in this country through which the federal government can deliver a single standard of any kind of service throughout the entire United States, acting alone. It cannot do it in education, it cannot do it in health, it cannot do it in environmental protection. That's not the kind of structure we have. So there are inherent problems to any kind of singular national response to local service delivery. That's the first point and I think it is very important to keep it in mind as we have this discussion.

Secondly, in a country in which there are gross differentials in income and a strong resistance to programs that transfer income from those who have it to those who don't, it is impossible to get a decent health care system for everybody—I don't care who they are, either a part of the population or the total population—because there is no value consensus to do that. So we are just talking in the wind. I am amazed how well we did with both Medicare and Medicaid, not how poorly we did. Some of the states have done much better than others. The state I come from does a lot better than Texas has done with its poor.

Ms. Elaine Brody: Since it is early on in the conference, I wonder if it wouldn't be useful to draw a distinction between medical care, which is really what Medicare addresses, and the kind of social health services that we have come to call long-term support services, which Medicare does not address. I would be very much interested in Mr. Ball's and some of the other people's notions about how long-term health care services, not medical *per se*, can be financed.

But before I hand over the microphone I would like to respond to one thing that Dr. Haughton said, with respect to the kind of services that would keep people out of institutions. I think it is a really bad idea to try to sell community care services and long-term social health services using this argument. Certainly there is a minority of older people in institutions, nursing homes, who could be kept out if we had a complete network of services. But community care and nursing homes should not be viewed as opposing propositions. Certainly "Meals on Wheels" should stand on its own, as should all other health services, because they are useful to people and help them maintain themselves at better levels of health and well-being. But "Meal on Wheels" or five "Meals on Wheels" never really kept anybody out of a nursing home.

Dr. Grant Rodkey: In one part of Mr. Ball's paper, he talks about the limitations of Medicare coverage of catastrophic and long-term care, to which Ms. Brody just referred. In his proposal, there might be a maximum cap put on the expenditures per individual or per family in an annual term before this kicked in. I wonder if we should give Mr. Ball an opportunity to discuss his views about this and comment on his idea about dedicated taxes that might be used to bolster the Medicare program.

Dr. Eugene Stead: One of the problems that we have here is that there is no insurance for long-term care. One of the suggestions that has been made is to create a market which would bring in the insurance industry if only there were a way in which part of IRAs could be used to purchase long-term care during the period of time in which the IRA was being accumulated. Is there any virtue in that notion?

Dr. Mathy Mezey: We have heard discussions in terms of national health insurance and I think it quite interesting that one group of people well able to pay for services are in fact interested in a pooled-risk arrangement, i.e., the life care community. A lot of interest has been generated among homogeneous groups of upper middle income older people in this type of pooled-risk insurance commitment which allows them to have control over the environment in which they are going to live. I would like to have Mr. Ball comment on whether he believes this is a potential model for long-term care services.

Dr. Robert Kane: Dr. Eisenberg has presented some very important challenges early on with regard to the value structure of the society. If we are going to look at questions on how to fund care for the elderly, we have to look at what are the implications behind the strategies that we use to do that. For example, if we begin to approach a question of the potential for some kind of universal delivery system that may or may not have multiple streams of funding coming from different sources, we move in a very specific direction for society. If we begin to pursue the question of privatization of fund-raising in areas of long-term care, that has implications with regard to things like dual stream and dual levels of quality, dual levels of systems provision, questions about how you set thresholds of eligibility when one system kicks in and another one stops.

It seems to me that we ought to pause for a moment before we get caught up in arguing some of the technical minutiae of whether or not we ought to have life care communities or "Meals on Wheels" and look at what we are saying about how the way we approach the care of a sub-population reflects on the values of the country. Are we willing to accept one set of standards for performance for defense contractors and another set of standards for performance for social services providers? I think that this is probably the one chance we are going to have in this session to look at some of those issues, and I hope we take it.

Rebuttal

Robert M. Ball, MA

Before getting to the specific questions that have been raised, it might be useful for me to give my perspective on how Medicare came about. It seems to me that history may shed light on what's possible now. Medicare is typically American. It follows a famous dictum of Lincoln's, that the government should do only what the private sector cannot do, or cannot do as well. Before Medicare was adopted, there was a very convincing demonstration that, although private insurance was able to sell both group insurance and individual insurance to people at work, it really was not very successful in protecting retired people against the cost of health care. The reasons were that older people used hospitals about two and one-half times as often, but had only about half as much income as the average worker. Thus, if you tried to charge the elderly a current premium covering their cost, most were priced out of the market. So in spite of a tremendous effort made by the insurance companies made to off Medicare by selling private policies, more than half the elderly population never bought private insurance, and what they did buy frequently wasn't very good.

Thus, the government came in, in the absence of other solutions. Most of us who had anything to do with the creation of Medicare, including myself, hoped very much that it was a first step, that we would gradually enlarge it in various ways. But, unlike Social Security, in general, Medicare has not been improved. As a matter of fact, in recent years it has been cut back.

I dismiss the notion that benefit cuts are a solution to the cost problem. If you include nursing home care as a part of health care, then Medicare today is covering a little less than 45 percent of the total health costs of the elderly. So the administration says that if you have a problem in financing, cut benefits. That doesn't make sense. Sixty-six percent of people over 65 are buying so-called "medi-gap" policies in an attempt to fill in the inadequacies of the Medicare program. Often, they are not very good policies, and typically, they don't cover the things important to the elderly that Medicare is not covering. They don't touch long-term care. They fill in co-payments and deductibles and some extra days of care, frequently using the same definitions as Medicare does. Because of the inadequacy of Medicare, the elderly have been led into buying policies that do not provide good coverage and are inefficient.

I would prefer to extend Medicare to cover the things that these medi-gap policies are trying to cover plus additional long-term care benefits, or, second best, have the government offer a medi-gap policy on a voluntary basis. Such a policy could be sold at a lower price than through private insurance because of savings in selling costs and administration. Cutting benefits would just increase medi-gap purchases by those who can barely affort it, and shift more costs onto Medicaid for those who can't possibly buy a private policy.

The first job that needs to be undertaken is to control costs in the medical system overall, and thus avoid the cost-shifting problem that arises when we focus on Medicare alone. One of the biggest barriers to expansion of Medicare coverage has certainly been the rapidly rising cost for the whole system, not just Medicare. That's perhaps the first priority before we get down to talking about improvements and more money to pay for them. I think people might be willing to put more money into Medicare extensions if they were convinced it would be well spent.

The cost control proposals in the Kennedy-Gephardt bill are a nice finesse of a lot of the policy debate that has been going on about how to control cost, and meets Dr. Ginzberg's point that you can't do it all from Washington. The country has not come to an agreement on how to control health care costs. As a country, we haven't decided how far to push regulation or whether we should encourage and rely on competition. So, the bill proposes to let each state decide. It encourages each state to take its own approach to cost control, as long as the national goals are met. If a state doesn't meet the national standard, the federal government's own plan will come into effect for that state. The bill won't pass the way it is, but it is a fairly good idea at this stage of disagreement on how to go about cost control. I argue in the paper that this is a high priority item.

An idea that has not caught on, but one which I like and will keep talking about until it does, is that it's possible to raise money to do some good beyond cost control, if you do it in a way that reduces the deficit at the same time. Now that's a neat trick. Sooner or later, we will decide that more income for the federal government is a large part of the answer to reducing the deficit. More, it is easier to get increases in taxes if they are earmarked for a purpose that people feel good about. For example, all the time that people were resisting general taxes, polls showed that they supported Social Security taxes, earmarked taxes for a special purpose that they believed in. Part A of Medicare is supported in the same way, but I am afraid that Part B, with three-fourths of the cost paid for from general revenues, is inherently vulnerable. It is legitimately part of the general budget discussion.

Let's assume we are going to raise taxes anyhow. Let's raise them in a way that dedicates part to Medicare Part B. This will reduce Medicare's dependence on general revenue and reduce the deficit. I make a series of tax suggestions in my paper that reduce the deficit. Overall, I think the plan to reduce the deficit through tax increases is more salable if combined with benefit improvements. I would combine Parts A and B of Medicare and earmark some funds derived, for example, from increasing the cigarette and liquor tax and extending medicare taxation to the four million state and local employees who are not under Social Security, but many of whom nevertheless, will derive benefits from Medicare. There are many other possibilities. Some of the increased income would go for deficit reduction by substituting new earmarked taxes for general revenues now going to Part B and some would go for benefit improvements.

Perhaps the most important way to improve Medicare is to include long-term protection. This will not be easy; the definition of at-home benefits is difficult. You also need an assessment plan to learn whether people belong in a nursing home or what at-home benefits they need. I have come to the conclusion that the private approaches to this problem are not likely to work in the long run. There are some inherent difficulties in selling long-term care insurance on an individual voluntary basis and group insurance is not being widely explored.

Extending the coverage of Medicare can occur in two ways. You can hold out the goal of a National Health Plan for everyone and work directly for that or you can take one step at a time in that objective. One step in an incremental approach would be to extend Medicare to cover Social Security beneficiaries. The disabled are now covered after two years. There is no reason why they should not be covered after six months, as soon as they come on the Social Security program. The same general reasons for Medicare coverage apply to the motherless and fatherless children who are on Social Security as to the elderly and disabled. They tend to be greatly underinsured compared to the population as a whole. The same can be said about young widows who are on Social Security. This starts to move the coverage into groups that go beyond just the elderly and the disabled. I would use this approach for the unemployed, as well. Block grants to the state level do not seem to me the best way to take care of the unemployed.

I am still very much interested in a national health plan, whether we get there through cost control, or incremental increases in expansion of Medicare, or all at once.

Now to specifically address some of the questions that have been raised, let me take first the fundamental one of whether we should be trying to save, during the next 15 or 20 years, for the inevitable greater cost for the elderly. I don't really know the right answer, but we don't have to decide right away. Even if we remain on a "pay as you go" plan, you need a major contingency reserve and you need to keep the scheduled 1988 rate increase to build a sufficient contingency reserve by about 1995. The issue then becomes whether you build a big earnings reserve beyond that, as would happen under present law. If you stay with the "pay as you go" system, it would mean you would have to begin in about the year 2025 to increase the income to Social Security the equivalent of about 1.5 percentage points in the contribution rate, each, on employers and employees. That would make up for the interest you lose from an earnings reserve. It has the advantage of being enough indefinitely into the future. Under the present arrangement, you start to use up the fund, say, about 2045, and run out around 2060.

However, I would not mind saving large amounts for the future in one way or another. I think running surpluses in the federal budget is a good way, but to make the Social Security surpluses produce real savings, you have to balance the rest of the budget. Otherwise, you are, in effect, using the Social Security tax to finance defense and other general revenue expenditures. If we had confidence that Social Security savings would not be offset in other parts of the budget, a good case could be made for building the surplus. We have until 1995 to decide.

On the question of whether the rest of the world is beginning to back away from a commitment to providing equitable access to health care, I'm not expert enough to answer for many nations. I would like to hear what other people have to say about that. I am somewhat familiar with the Canadian situation and find absolutely no retreat there. When some of the provinces started to retreat, the central government pushed them back to the original idea. I think it is absolutely disgraceful the way we treat poor people in this country when it comes to health care. They either don't get the care or are made to beg for it. I don't understand how a country as rich as this could leave thirty million people with no kind of health coverage they can count on. It is a national disgrace! Medicaid covers less than half of the people below the poverty level. We are going to have a return of conscience on this, and we will fix it. I hope we don't fix it just on a means-tested basis, but through some universal plan.

I want to respond to the question about the life care community idea, which I think has a good possibility of being extended to more people. This is the place where you make a major down payment, $50,000 for example, and pay a monthly fee, to move into a retirement community in which you live in your own apartment as long as you are able, with a commitment on the part of the organization who runs the community to take care of you no matter what happens. If you need nursing home care, that is available, usually on the campus, but if not on the campus, somewhere nearby. It is long-term care insurance combined with current living arrangements. I think it will grow in popularity because we now have a large number of older people who could afford the down payment by selling their home. Seventy-five percent of the elderly own their homes. This approach is obviously not for the poor, but I wouldn't be surprised if 20–25 percent of the elderly population could afford it. Still, many people don't like to live in a community arrangement like that. It is not for everyone. The average age is 80 or more in those communities.

To respond to Dr. Stead's question about IRAs, their existence was a terrible idea, I think. Keogh plans for the self-employed who didn't have pensions on their own and IRAs for people who didn't have pensions were okay, but when they were extended to everybody, IRAs ending up costing the federal government a great deal of money. It is very clear that only people who have relatively substantial means go into them and, of course, they're worth more the higher the income bracket you are in. And there is no evidence that it has increased the savings rate significantly. People probably just use them to shelter savings they would have made anyway.

Returning once again to Medicare, we must make it clear that Medicare is not just hospital insurance for old people and the long-term disabled. It is protection for the middle-aged and young as well—a way of pooling the costs that the elderly and everyone else would otherwise have to take care of. I am concerned about the reliance of Medicare Part B on general revenue. I think it is vulnerable in the same way that a program just for the poor is vulnerable, as Dr. Haughton pointed out. We all have charitable instincts, but they are not very consistent and not something you can count on year by year and across political elections. That's why dedicated taxes are a great idea.

CHAPTER 2

The Biological Constraints
on Human Aging:
Implications for Health Policy
Position Paper

James F. Fries, MD

The ultimate constraint within which we must develop health policy for the future is, of course, the limit of life itself. Human beings are mortal, and the limits to what presently may be accomplished in decreasing mortality are set by the life span of our species. In the following discussion, we will examine natural limits to the life span, develop an incremental model of chronic disease and of aging which focuses upon the postponement both of disease and of senescent change, and examine the implications of improvement of vitality in a finite world.

The compression of morbidity represents a new theoretical structure for describing disease, infirmity, and death, and carries with it substantial implications for health policy, planning and decisions. Since the onset of significant morbidity may be postponed while termination of the genetic life-span may not, the period of infirmity may be compressed into a shorter period toward the end of life.[1] A more comprehensive definition[2] states that the average age of onset of a significant permanent infirmity may increase more rapidly than does life expectancy, thus shortening both the proportion of life spent infirm and the absolute length of the infirm period. The strategy for postponing infirmity involves social, individual, and medical changes; the most important elements are preventive

---

This paper was adopted with permission, from Fries, J. F. The compression of morbidity, *Milbank Memorial Fund Quarterly*, 61:397–419.

approaches to premature chronic diseases, and changes in prevalent social expectations for the elderly which include "detraining" and social withdrawal.[3]

This model has attracted considerable attention, as it suggests a positive program for reducing the burdens of illness and contrasts with negative predictions of a coming geriatric catastrophe. Neither of the two underlying principles (the fixed human life span and the ability to postpone chronic illness) is individually very controversial, yet their conjunction has been disturbing to some.

It is important first to define some terms. The "maximum life potential" is approximated by the oldest age achieved by any human being. In the United States this age is 113 years, 214 days.[4] This figure represents a point far out on the "tail" of a distribution of genetically different individuals. "Life expectancy" is the average length of life which we may expect, given current age-specific death rates, for an infant born today. This figure is 74 at present, approximately 70 for men and 78 for women. The "lifespan," on the other hand, represents the average longevity in a society without disease or accident. The life expectancy can rise toward, but cannot exceed, the life span. The human life span appears to be approximately 85 years, with a broad distribution in which natural longevity for individuals falls nearly entirely within the range of from 70 to 100 years. Much misunderstanding in discussion of this topic comes from confusion of the mean of a distribution with its extremes.

THE FINITE LIFE SPAN

National mortality figures demonstrate a smooth decline in number of deaths and a smooth increase in mortality rates as we move toward higher ages.[3] The 41,000 deaths per year in the United States in the eighty-fifth year of age decreases to 24 deaths per year by age 110, in a smooth progression which shows no exceptions. The absence of exceptions carries important implications since it demonstrates that particular lifestyles or particular food or vitamin intakes which have been promoted as aids to longevity and which have been used extensively througout the culture do not, in fact, prolong the genetically-determined life span. If vitamin C or lifelong aerobic exercise extended the life span, we should expect to have seen exceptionally long lives (beyond 115 years) in at least a few practitioners of such habits. The ultimate limits appear to apply to the aerobically fit and to the megavitamin faddist, to the farm or city dweller, and to all societies.

Examination of mortality rates in different societies confirms the actuarial "law" first proposed by Benjamin Gompertz.[5] Gompertz noted a linear increase in mortality rates with age when rates were plotted on a logarithmic scale. That is, the mortality rate increases exponentially with age, doubling approximately every eight years of age. Gompertz's law is an empirical observation which fits closely with the observation of smoothly and rapidly declining numbers of individuals alive at successive ages.

At least 10 general lines of evidence confirm the existence of a finite human life span:

1. There are no exceptions to the declining numbers of individuals present at successive ages.
2. Gompertz's law appears to hold in all human populations and assures an exponentially increasing mortality rate and, therefore, death for the entire population within a decade or two past the age of 100.
3. There has been no historical change over several centuries of observation with regard to maximum life potential as underscored by studies of centenarians; this observation has been repeatedly made in the United States with good data since 1939 or earlier.[6,7] Life expectancy at age 100 has changed at most 0.7 years over 80 years,[6] and much of this improvement must have been due to reduction of premature death, not change in life span.
4. There is no biological reason to assume that any change in genetic longevity characteristics should have occurred merely because we have improved infant mortality, cleaned up water supplies, or invented penicillin.
5. The difference in species life span among animals is a commonplace daily observation.
6. Anthropological analyses[8] suggest a formula by which mammalian life spans may be predicted by the brain size/body weight ratio; such models suggest an approximately constant life span for the human species for the past 100,000 years.
7. The linear decline in organ reserve, repeatedly the subject of physiologic observation, mandates a point at which function must be inadequate to support life, that point apparently

being when organ reserve is reduced to approximately 20 percent over that function required for the maintenance of basic life processes; reserve of this magnitude is required for daily functions outside of bed.

8. The increasingly rectangular life expectancy curve demonstrates the barrier to immortality.

9. We have the important phenomenon of *a priori* aging, the daily evidence of our senses. People do grow older, with changes that are apparent to all of us, as we age. And these changes—from hair color to hearing—are not the result of disease as we usually define it. A new group of Americans has become a subject of increasing concern, the "frail elderly." This term is a new one; it refers to individuals, often without demonstrable disease, who have manifestly limited organ reserve and increased frailty to external perturbation.

10. The Hayflick Phenomenon[9] may represent these limiting events at the cellular level.

There are several methods of estimating the human life span. One may use the anthropological formulas, reconstruct an ideal survival curve from the tail of the present curve using the assumption that these individuals have been essentially free of disease, make extrapolations from the rectangularizing survival curve, or use estimates based on observed decline in organ reserve. All suggest an average life span of approximately 85 years, with a distribution which includes 99 percent of individuals between the ages of 70 and 100 (Figure 2-1). It is not clear whether this distribution is "normal," based on the Gompertz function (which gives a slightly sharper drop-off) or some other distribution. For policy purposes, these distinctions are minor.

Different species, however, have very different life spans; the obvious fact that we tend to outlive our pets is not due to increased disease or accident among the animals, but rather to the difference in species life span.[10] Rodents live, at best, a few years, while some of the Galapagos tortoises, which formed a part of Charles Darwin's observations about the origin of the species, were still alive on the 100th anniversary of Darwin's death.

While the process of senescence certainly has biochemical and cellular underpinnings, it is presently best understood by decline of maximal function of the vital organs.[11,12,13] The organ reserve

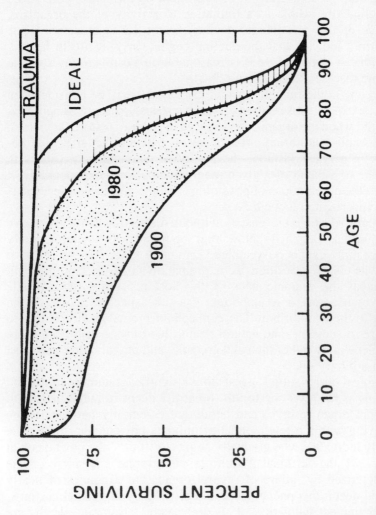

Figure 2-1. Ideal survivorship curve. Trauma plays a large and potentially reversible role. Chronic disease accounts for almost all of the approximately ten-year-wide area of premature death remaining over ages 60-90. Reprinted with permission from J. F. Fries and L. M. Crapo, *Vitality and Aging* (San Francisco: W. H. Freeman, 1981).

potential, greatest in early life, shows a functional decline which is essentially linear and roughly parallel for all major organs. The decline is in the "reserve power" of the particular organ, and thus, is apparent on measurement of maximum performance well before it is clinically visible as a limitation to activity of the organism. Studies of this physiologic decline, about 1.5 percent per year, uniformly indicate that the decline begins early in life in healthy individuals—well before it is reasonable to postulate any specific chronic disease effects (Figure 2-2).

Decline in the function of multiple organs may be considered in the context of preservation of homeostasis. Reserve function is required when the organism is stressed in order to restore the normal homeostatic equilibrium. As the reserve of individual organs declines in a linear fashion, the ability to maintain homeostasis in the face of a threat of a given magnitude declines exponentially,[13] hence, the observations of physiology and the actuarial observations of Gompertz are reconciled.

Natural death must ensue, without disease, when the reserve function has declined below that point at which routine daily perturbations cannot be weathered, probably about 20 percent above basal levels. A transition from premature death to natural death occurs as the characteristics of the host resistance (homeostatic reserve) become more important than the specific nature of the insult to the equilibrium. The concepts of premature death (due to disease or accident) and natural death (due to senescent frailty) are complementary rather than antagonistic, and any dividing line must be an arbitrary one.

Clinical observation suggests that a significant number of deaths, perhaps as many as one-fourth, presently occur in individuals with minimal organ reserve, and hence are essentially natural deaths, occurring within a few months of ultimate physiologic limits. The elderly individual who gradually begins to "fail," the quiet death at home, or the terminal "multiple catastrophe" hospital course characterized by failure of several organs are examples of nearly natural death; this phenomenon is obscured by our social customs, which prevent tabulation of natural death. "Natural" deaths are hidden in the statistics for bronchopneumonia, heart failure, generalized atherosclerosis, and other categories, since there is no death certificate category for natural death, and everyone must be assigned. When the number of natural deaths is relatively low, projections ignoring these classification errors are reasonably accu-

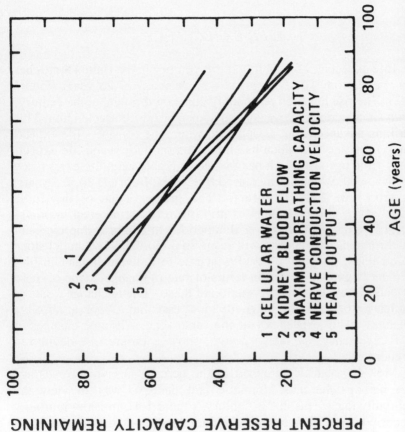

Figure 2-2. Linear decline in organ function with age. Based on Shock 1960 and Strehler and Mildvan 1960. Reprinted with permission from J. F. Fries and L. M. Crapo, *Vitality and Aging* (San Francisco: W. H. Freeman, 1981).

rate, but as their frequency increases, such models increasingly underestimate future mortality at advanced ages. If there is a major force for mortality, natural death, with a hazard function increasing rapidly from essentially zero at age 70 to nearly 99 percent at age 100, and the demographic model does not include this term,[7] then the projections will be wrong.

LIFE EXPECTANCY

Life expectancy from birth in this century in the United States has increased from 47 to 74 years[1]—an increase of 26 years (Figure 2-3). The rise has been reasonably constant throughout the century, with some periods of plateau and some periods of acceleration. This striking advance is not as apparent when one considers life expectancy from age 20, which has increased only 13 years; life expectancy from age 40, which has increased eight years; life expectancy from age 60, which has increased five years; from age 80, 2.5 years; or from age 100, 0.7 years.[7] The greater slope of the curve representing life expectancy from birth reflects the great improvement in infant mortality over this period. In contrast, improvement in chronic disease control will result in a more nearly parallel slope to all lines, since these benefits accrue to individuals later in life. We are beginning to see, in terms of rate of change, some of these effects. To avoid misinterpretation of these "rate of change" data as indicative of galloping longevity, it is essential to look at absolute changes in life expectancy at the same time. Absolute changes in life expectancy, as shown above, show a progressive decline at higher ages.

Mortality statistics graphed as the percent surviving versus age are perhaps the most dramatic and decisive way to view the mortality rate events in this century (Figure 2-4). In 1900, mortality occurred at a relatively steady rate throughout the life span. In successive decades, the curves have begun to bend upwards and to the right, each considerably different from the last. The form of the curve is increasingly rectangular, having an increasingly flat top and an increasingly sharp downslope. This observation is frequently referred to as "rectangularization of the survival curve." The point on the age axis at which the curves intersect has remained approximately the same, the differences lying within the width of the lines used to plot such curves. The progressive shape of these

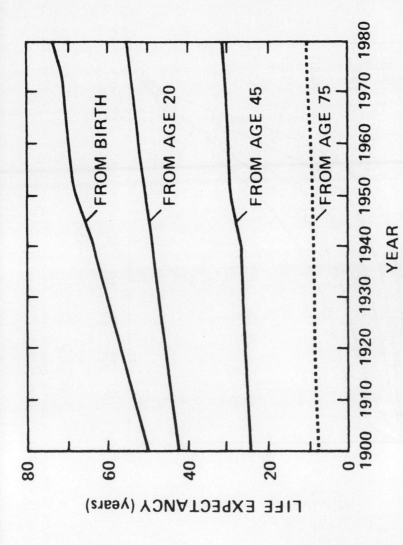

Figure 2-3. Changes in life expectancy from different ages in the twentieth century. Reprinted with permission from J. F. Fries and L. M. Crapo, *Vitality and Aging* (San Francisco: W. H. Freeman, 1981).

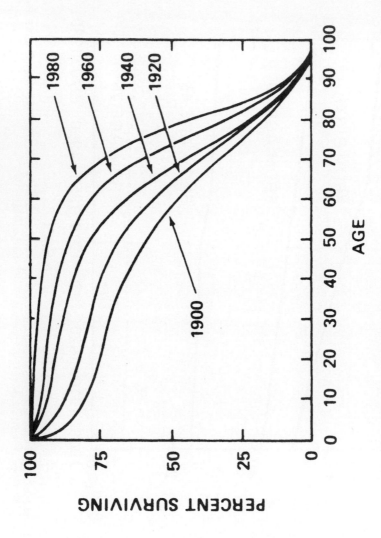

Figure 2-4. Changes in survivorship curves in United States in the twentieth century. Reprinted with permission from J. F. Fries and L. M. Crapo, *Vitality and Aging* (San Francisco: W. H. Freeman, 1981).

curves allows visual prediction of future trends. The ideal curve must lie in its initial 60 years within a very narrow flat zone, and then must plunge quite precipitously if it is to meet the historical lines at the bottom of the graph (Figure 2-1). The increasingly rectangular survival curve, with the clear convergence of curves from different decades, demonstrates visually the limits of the human life span.

Even the most optimistic calculations[7] project that life expectancy at age 100 is projected to increase from 2.45 years in 1980 to only 3.01 years in 2000, and 3.35 years in 2020. Reduction of premature death, as opposed to change in life span, must account for at least part of such projected change. But such an increase of eleven months over the next forty years, even if due entirely to a change in the genetic life span, does not distort the policy implications of the "compression of morbidity."[1]

THE COMPRESSION OF MORBIDITY

The compression of morbidity occurs if the age at first appearance of aging manifestations and chronic disease symptoms can increase more rapidly than life expectancy. This statement of the thesis recognizes that increases in life expectancy, whether or not associated with minor changes in the life span, are likely over the next 25 years. The question of whether the period of morbidity may be shortened depends upon whether the average onset age of a marker of morbidity (first heart attack, first dyspnea from emphysema, first disability from osteoarthritis, first memory loss of a certain magnitude) can increase more rapidly than does life expectancy from the same age. If it does, then the period between that marker and the end of life is shortened. Absolute compression of morbidity occurs if age-specific morbidity rates decrease more rapidly than age-specific mortality rates. Relative compression of morbidity occurs if the amount of life after first chronic morbidity decreases as a percentage of life expectancy.

The Characteristics of Chronic Disease

The acute infectious diseases have ceased to be statistically major causes of mortality in the United States. Tuberculosis, small pox, diptheria, tetanus, polio, typhoid fever, and others have declined by

99 percent to 100 percent in this century.[14] The major medical problems today are chronic illnesses: atherosclerosis in all of its guises, cancer in its many forms, emphysema, diabetes, cirrhosis, osteoarthritis. These illnesses are not well conceptualized under the medical model of diseases with single causes and specific cures. These present health problems are characterized by "risk factors" which accelerate their course or which increase the probability of their occurrence. Their "cause" is thus multifactorial, and no single cause is essential. Even more importantly, these illnesses have other characteristics which are not those of the acute diseases. They are, to one degree or another, universal. Every individual has, to a greater or lesser degree, the potential for increasing atherosclerosis, an increasing statistical possibility of malignant change, and slow degeneration of the articular cartilage. Moreover, the chronic illnesses have their onset early in life; signs of such problems may be found in autopsy studies of individuals in their twenties. The severity of the conditions increases progressively with age (Figure 2-5).

Thus, the current most important illnesses are universal, have early onset, are progressive, are generally characterized by a symptom threshold at which time they become clinically obvious, and are multifactorial in cause.[3] The differences between individuals are manifested not so much by the presence or absence of the condition as by the rate at which the condition progresses. This rate may be low, as in atherosclerosis in native Japanese on native diets, or higher, as in Japanese on American diets.

As a caveat, there are a number of major chronic diseases, less important statistically, which do not have these characteristics, and which are not the subject of this discussion. Such illnesses include rheumatoid arthritis, Hodgkin's disease, systemic lupus, ulcerative colitis, and multiple sclerosis. They are not universal, not age-related, "risk factors" are few or none, and they have a definite onset point. These illnesses may ultimately fit the traditional medical model quite closely. Alzheimer's disease, a major problem currently increasing in prevalence, is difficult to classify, and clearly deserves both preventive and curative study. This condition is heavily age dependent, and may have a specific pathology.[15,16]

The multiple risk factor universal susceptibility model fits our prevalent health problems, with important implications. In this model, as risk factors are modified, the slope of the progression is decreased. As the slope decreases, the date of crossing the symptomatic threshold (Figure 2-5) can be postponed; death due to the

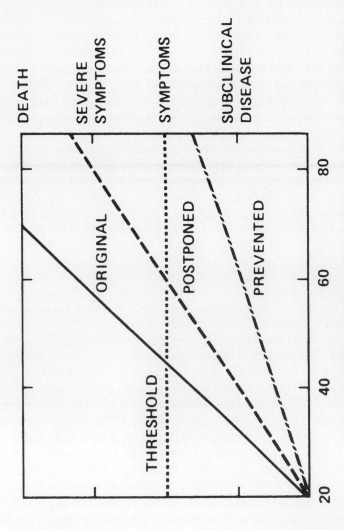

Figure 2-5. An incremental model of chronic disease. The model is characterized by early age of onset, progression at various rates, and passage of a symptomatic threshold at which time a clinical diagnosis may be made. Reprinted with permission from J. F. Fries and L. M. Crapo, *Vitality and Aging* (San Francisco: W. H. Freeman, 1981).

disease can be postponed or even prevented; and the severity of symptoms experienced can be decreased. If the slope is sufficiently reduced, the disease may be said to be "prevented," since the symptom threshold may not be passed during life.

A model of universal progressive disease with a symptom threshold allows one to divide life into a "firm" portion, occurring before the threshold is passed, and an "infirm" portion following passage of that threshold. As the slope is decreased, the "firm" period of adult vigor is prolonged and the "infirm" period of disease or senescence is compressed against the natural barrier at the end of life. Both the absolute amount and the percentage of life spent in less than good health may, thus, be decreased.

Another significant attribute of this model is that any reduction in the average slope of lines, representing individuals in a population will result in a decreasee in age-specific mortality rates. And, it will also result in an increase in the average age at which the first symptom is experienced. Thus, as improvement in the rate of accretion of chronic disease occurs, an effect on morbidity is linked to the effect on mortality. Importantly, this model may be used to describe the senescent changes of aging in multiple organ systems as well as the accelerated decrepitude in a particular organ associated with a chronic disease.

Consider two brothers (Figure 2-6), one of whom smokes three packages of cigarettes daily while the other smokes one-half package of cigarettes a day. The top line represents the life of the heavy-smoking brother. Moving life expectancy toward the right along such a life history provides insights into many of the phenomena of contemporary medicine and its interactions with society. In 1900 perhaps this individual would have encountered pneumonia at age 30 and have died, after a life of 30 years and an illness of three days—premature death, to be sure, but inexpensive (at least in terms of direct medical costs), with relatively little illness burden upon the society, and with a high proportion of vigorous life to sickness. Now, with penicillin, the man survives to begin to develop a cough, wheezing, and shortness of breath at age 40. If he continues to smoke, he will be increasingly short of breath for the remainder of his life. In his fifties he has a heart attack; perhaps, prior to modern management, he might have died at this point. Now his arrhythmia is controlled and he goes on to encounter a stroke a few years later, requiring intensive rehabilitation efforts. Throughout, he remains short of breath. Finally, a lung cancer

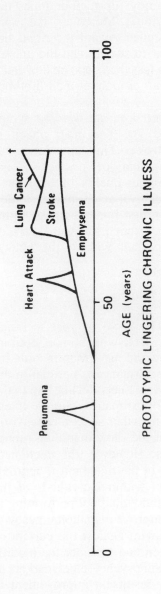

PROTOTYPIC LINGERING CHRONIC ILLNESS

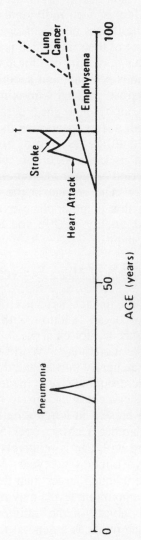

EFFECTS OF THE POSTPONEMENT OF CHRONIC DISEASE

Figure 2-6. The compression of morbidity. Two health-lives are diagrammed, the upper with poor health habits and the lower with better health habits. The period of adult vigor prior to infirmity is reduced in the lower example. Reprinted with permission from J. F. Fries and L. M. Crapo, *Vitality and Aging* (San Francisco: W. H. Freeman, 1981).

develops and he dies, in a crescendo for chronic disease. Such patients appear to require, not surprisingly, up to four times the medical resources of the average individual. Moreover, the more that the life of such individuals is extended toward the right, the greater the illness burden they represent to society and the greater the amount of their life which is spent in less than good health. Such individuals may "linger" for actually half or more of their lifetime, at enormous personal and social cost.

In contrast, the light-smoking brother does not develop symptomatic emphysema until perhaps age 70. The heart attack is postponed a few years, as is the stroke. The lung cancer is postponed all the way out of his lifetime and does not occur. This individual is more vigorous, with a higher quality of life, for a longer period of time, and represents socially a much smaller burden on society. The change in the point of first breathlessness represents, in this commonplace example, as much as thirty years of improved quality of life for the individual without the heavy-smoking habit.

The Plasticity of Many Senescent Phenomena

The same linear senescence observed by Shock in cross-sectional studies of organ function with age is seen with human optimal performance as, for example, with the world age-group records for men in the marathon.[1,3] World-class performance is optimal in the twenties and early thirties and then shows a linear decline[1] up to the point where sample size is inadequate for estimation. Similar linear decline is evident in age-group records for other athletic endeavors. It is also present in longitudinal data of the same marathon runner (e.g., Clarence DeMar) over 50 years. However, the decrement associated with age is relatively small; in the marathon it approximates two minutes per year. Variation within individuals of the same age is much larger than this; the individual not performing at personal maximum levels may readily improve marathon times with age. This ability of the individual to swim against the current of senescence holds as a general truth when one consider the modifiability (or lack thereof) of the physical and psychological markers of aging. Training in a particular faculty results in improvement in performance in that faculty, at any age.

Human potential may be conceptualized within the following paradigm. There is a level of optimal human performance in each faculty, approximated by world-class performance at each age. Athletic performance is only the most measurable faculty; optimal performance is possible for almost any endeavor, from shopping to playing chess. The decline in optimal performance is linear. The mean performance of a population, on the other hand, has also been measured to show a linear decline, at a level of performance markedly below that of the best human performance (Figure 2-7).

By inference, each individual must have his or her own particular curve of optimum performance. That is, with maximum training and effort, there is a theoretically optimum performance for each individual, and this curve should be expected to have the same characteristics as do the measurable curves. The same individual, untrained and expending less than maximal effort, will show a similar curve but at a lower level of performance. For each individual, the area between the line of present performance and that of potential performance enables the plasticity of aging. With time and age, one may improve, regress, or stay the same within surprisingly broad limits of performance; the limits are evidenced by the wide variation in interindividual performances, and by the increase in such variation with age.[17] If one is not performing near an individually optimal level with regard to a particular faculty, then improvement, despite increasing age, remains possible.

Some aspects of the aging process appear to be nonmodifiable. For the most part, these have in common the slow accumulation of fibrous tissue, replacing tissue which previously functioned. Thus developing rigidity of the arterial wall, cataract formation, the graying of hair, the gradual loss of glomeruli in the kidney, the thinning of hair, and the loss of elasticity of skin. These capacities appear to be insidiously and irreversibly lost with age, according to present data.[3] Given present knowledge, there is little reason to expect that lifestyle or theraputic interventions will reduce decrements in these areas.

When questioned about fears of growing old, individuals over the age of 50 usually do not cite fear of death.[18,19] As more significant concerns, they first describe a dread of approaching chronic illness, pain, and inability to physically get around. Second, they report fears of approaching senility and loss of memory. And third, they describe a fear of total dependence upon others.

In these areas, there is good reason to expect improvement from preventive and lifestyle approaches. There are convincing studies which indicate that cardiac reserve, dental decay, glucose tolerance,

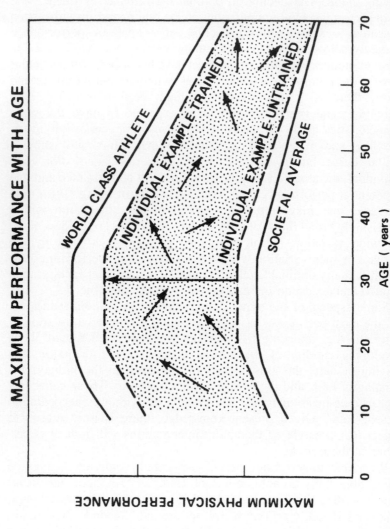

Figure 2-7. The plasticity of aging. Within the biological potential of the organism are multiple possible pathways to improvement of performance with age bounded by present performance and maximum potential performance. Reprinted with permission from J. F. Fries and L. M. Crapo, *Vitality and Aging* (San Francisco: W. H. Freeman, 1981).

intelligence test performance and memory, osteoporosis, physical endurance, physical strength, pulmonary reserve, reaction time, social ability, and blood pressure, among other variables, are modifiable by the individual at any age. This modifiability is sometimes termed the "plasticity of aging."[19] Modification consists in most instances of training and practice in the specific faculty.[3,20-26] In many instances, there is relatively little cross-over from training in one attribute to success at another.

The ability both to postpone chronic disease,[27] and to utilize the plasticity of aging affords an approach to the major fears of chronic disease, loss of intellect and memory, and total dependence upon others. The compression of morbidity and the plasticity of aging are related concepts, and are applicable both to the problems of chronic disease and the problems of senescence.

Some emerging data suggest that the compression of morbidity may be a present, as well as a future, phenomenon. Conclusive data are difficult to come by because data on the incidence of markers of morbidity have not been systematically collected, nor do we have, even in cross-sectional studies, prevalence figures for the "quality of life." Indeed, it is not even clear what measures of morbidity should be used. If we accept as such measures the age at first heart attack or the age at development of identifiable lung cancer or the average age at admission to nursing homes, available data suggest that the onset age of these markers may be increasing more rapidly than is life expectancy from age 40 in the United States. For example, the average age at first heart attack for men appears to have increased approximately four years in the past sixteen, while life expectancy from age 40 increased only two years over the past 20. Despite the decreasing prevalence of heart attack over the period of 1968 to 1978, the percentage of hospital discharges for this condition over the age of 65 has risen from 47 to 52 percent of the total.[7,28,29,30] The ratio of fatal and nonfatal heart attacks appears to have remained constant during this period, suggesting that morbidity and mortality from this cause have both been reduced.[31] The stroke data are more equivocal, but appear to show the same thing.[32,33] Lung cancer age-specific incidence rates appear to have similarly changed and the risk-factor model based heavily on cigarette smoking (pack/years) suggests that as smoking decreases the effect will first be postponement of onset; that is, the requisite number of pack/years will be reached later in life. Life-time medical costs of heavy smokers and/or heavy drinkers, inferred from studies of high-cost hospital users,[34] appear to be as much as four times those of individuals with moderate habits, even though the duration of life is shorter. The rate of admission to nursing homes has remained essentially constant for those over 65 or over 85,[18] despite empty beds and an increasing age as the population gradually drifts older.

Policy Implications

Human variability, the compression of morbidity, and the recognition of untapped human potential at advanced age contain implications for research and public policies. They suggest need for development of some new research directions. First, a broad biopsychosocial model of health must be utilized, since many of the interventions important in affecting senescent phenomena are certain to be outside of a traditional biological model. Second, there is a lack of good data on the "quality of life," and efforts at systematic accumulation of such data must be accelerated. Initially, there needs to be decisions on those specific measures of "quality of life" to be collected and cross-sectional data on these measures needs to be gathered. Third, longitudinal studies need to be initiated at the same time, and these need to include biologic, psychological, and social variables in the same studies. Fourth, the means for affecting positive change in an aging population are to be found in the variability of the population, as well as in the average values. Studies need to identify and quantitate interindividual variation for specific marker variables at particular ages, identify the factors which predict the variability, and design rigorous prospective intervention trials based upon identification of associated risk factors.

On the public policy side, there are several implications. First, there should be no mandatory retirement age. Studies of plasticity suggest strongly the health and vitality benefits of continuing challenge, problem solving, perception of productivity, continued activity, and more money; for some these features will be best obtained by continued employment. Second, creative vocational opportunities should be available, with multiple and flexible pathways toward optimal use of the later years. Third, health enhancement programs must begin early in adult life and be continued throughout. Aging programs directed only at the aged will have less impact than those addressing the same problems earlier. Fourth, to the extent possible, we should seek deinstitutionalization of long-term care programs, which in their most severe forms prevent individual initiative. Usually this will consist of seeking the most independent living alternative possible for the individual. It will require better development of home health care services, a redevelopment of the role of the family, and a more peripheral distribution of needed care away from large impersonal institutions. Fifth, programs should stimulate the independence of individuals. A false dichotomy is sometimes raised between "caring" and "curing," and there is some risk that our elderly may be smothered by good intentions. The elderly have a right to an independent life and to the execution of personal choices within the broadest possible framework. Finally, solutions are hampered by the existence of certain adverse incentives within our society. We subsidize bad health habits and we encourage disuse of the mental and physical faculties of older individuals. Our health insurance programs take money from those with good health habits and give it to those with poor health habits. We need to look closely at how our laws and our customs may affect the independent expression of vitality in the older individual.

The rectangular morbidity curve represents, in many ways, a social ideal—a long, vigorous life culminating, as in Oliver Wendell Holmes' "one-hoss shay,"[35] with a sudden terminal collapse; vitality until at the end, and death coming without fear or fury at the natural end of the individual life span. It will not happen this way, of course. Utopias may be envisioned, but not totally achieved. Increasing birth cohorts will continue to discharge even larger numbers of individuals into the older age groups until equilibrium is reached after some 50 years, and the problems we have been experiencing will grow worse before they grow better. Clinical observation of our most vital older citizens suggests a usual terminal decline of months to even a few years, not an abrupt collapse as that of the one-hoss shay. But the compression of morbidity is an achievable phenomenon; it is already occurring in some areas, and it can be made to grow importantly. Projection of health needs under the scenario presented are more favorable than sometimes supposed. But the many problems of our increasingly elderly population continue to exist and require vigorous attack from many directions. The paradigm of increasing vitality and finite life, with the consequent compression of morbidity into a shorter period prior to the end of life, offers a framework within which to view these problems, and within which we may begin to develop some constructive solutions.

REFERENCES

1. Fries, J. F. Aging natural death, and the compression of morbidity. *New England Journal of Medicine*, 303:130–35, 1980.

2. Fries, J. F. The compression of morbidity, *Milbank Memorial Fund Quarterly*, 61:397–418, 1983.

3. Fries, J. F., and Crapo, L. M. *Vitality and Aging: Implications of the Rectangular Curve*. San Francisco: W. H. Freeman, 1981.

4. McWhirter, N. *Guiness Book of World Records*. New York: Bantam Books, 1980.

5. Gompertz, B. On the nature of the function expressive of the law of human mortality. *Philosophical Transactions of the Royal Society of London*, 1:513–85, 1825.

6. Bowerman, W. G. Centenarians. *Transactions of the Actuarial Society of America*, 40:360–78, 1939.

7. Faber, J. F. *Life Tables for the United States, 1900–2050*. Actuarial Study No. 87, Office of the Actuary. SSA Pub. No. 11-11534, Washington, D.C., 1982.

8. Cutler, R. G. Evolution of human longevity: A critical overview. *Mechanisms of Aging and Development*, 9:337–54, 1979.

9. Hayflick, L. The cell biology of human aging. *Scientific American*, 242:58–65, 1980.

10. Rockstein, M. Heredity and longevity in the animal kingdom. *Journal of Gerontology*, 13:7–12, 1958.

11. Finch, C. E. The regulation of physiological changes during mammalian aging. *Quarterly Review of Biology* 51:49–83, 1976.

12. Shock, N. W. Discussion on mortality and measurement. In: Strehler, B. L., et al. (editors), *The Biology of Aging, A Symposium*. Washington, D.C.: American Institute of Biological Sciences, 1960.

13. Strehler, B. L. and Mildvan, A. S. General theory of mortality and aging. *Science* 132:14–21, 1960.

14. Fries, J. F. and Ehrlich, G. E. *Prognosis: Contemporary Outcomes of Disease*. Bowie, Maryland: Charles Press, 1980.

15. Beck, J. C., Benson, D. F., Scheibel, A. B., Spar, J. E., and Rubinstein, L. Z. Dementia in the elderly: The silent epidemic. *Annals of Internal Medicine*, 97:231–41, 1982.

16. Blass, J. P. and Weksler, M. E. Toward an effective treatment of Alzheimer's Disease. *Annals of Internal Medicine*, 98:251–52, 1983.

17. Dittman-Kohli, F. and Baltes, P. B. Toward a neofunctionalist conception of adult intellectual development: Wisdom as a prototypical case of intellectual growth. In: Alexander, C. and Langer, E. J. (editors) *Beyond Formal Operations: Alternative Endpoints to Human Development*, Oxford: Oxford University Press, 1983.

18. Neugarten, B. L., and Havighurst, R. J. *Extending the human life span: Social Policy and Social Ethics*. Washington, D.C.: National Science Foundation, 1977.

19. Baltes, M. M. Environmental factors in dependency among nursing home residents: A social ecology analysis. In: Willis, T. A. (editor), *Basic Processes in Helping Relationships*, New York: Academic Press, 1982.

20. Bortz, W. M. Disuse and aging. *Journal of the American Medical Association* 248:1203–8, 1982.

21. Dehn, M. M., Bruce, R. A. Longitudinal variations in maximal oxygen uptake with age and activity. *Journal of Applied Physiology*, 33:805–7, 1972.

22. Farquhar, J. W. *The American Way of Life Need Not Be Hazardous to Your Health*. New York: Norton, 1978.

23. Labouvie-Vief, G., and Blanchard-Field, F. Cognitive aging and psychological growth. *Aging and Society*, 2 (Spring), 1982.

24. Langer, E. G., and Rodin, J. The effects of choice and enhanced personal responsibility for the aged: A field experiment in an institutional setting. *Journal of Personality and Social Psychology*, 34:191–98, 1976.

25. Paffenbarger, R. S., et al. Energy expenditure, cigarette smoking, and blood pressure level as related to death from specific disease. *American Journal of Epidemiology,* 108:12–18, 1979.

26. Baltes, P. B. and Baltes, M. M. Plasticity and variability in psychological aging: Methodological and theoretical issues. *Determining the Effects of Aging on the Central Nervous System.* Berlin: Schering, 1980.

27. Walker, W. J. Changing United States life-style and declining vascular mortality: Cause or coincidence. *New England Journal of Medicine,* 297:163–65, 1977.

28. National Center for Health Statistics. *Inpatient Utilization of Short-stay Hospitals by Diagnosis: United States.* Series 13, Numbers 6, 12, 26, 46. Washington, D.C.: NCHS, 1965, 1968, 1974, 1978.

29. Elvebach, L. R., Connolly, D. C., & Kurland, L. T. Coronary heart disease in residents of Rochester, Minnesota, 1950 to 1975. II. Mortality, incidence, and survivorship. *Mayo Clinic Proceedings,* 56:665–71, 1981.

30. Connolly, D. C., Oxman, H. A., Nobrega, F. T., Kurland, L. T., Kennedy, M. A., and Elvebach, L. R. Coronary heart disease in residents of Rochester, Minnesota: 1950 to 1975. I. Background and study design. *Mayo Clinic Proceedings,* 56:661–64, 1981.

31. Paffenbarger, R. S. *Proceedings of the Conference on the Decline in Coronary Heart Disease Mortality,* p. 298–311. NIH Publication No. 79-1610, Washington, D.C., 1979.

32. Kramer, S., Diamond, E. L., and Lilienfeld, A. M. Patterns of incidence and trends in diagnostic classification of cerebrovascular disease in Washington County, Maryland, 1969–1971 to 1974–1976. *American Journal of Epidemiology,* 115:398–410, 1982.

33. Robins, M., and Baum, H. M. Incidence of stroke. *Stroke,* 12:145–57, 1981.

34. Schroeder, S. A., Showstack, J. A., and Roberts, H. E. Frequency and clinical description of high cost patients in 17 acute care hospitals. *New England Journal of Medicine,* 300:1306–11, 1979.

35. Holmes, O. W. The Deacon's masterpiece; or, The wonderful "one-hoss shay." From: *The Autocrat of the Breakfast Table,* 1857–1858. In: *The Complete Poetical Works of Oliver Wendell Holmes.* Boston: Houghton Mifflin, 1908.

The Biological Constraints
on Human Aging:
Implications for Health Policy
The Human Lifespan

Leonard Hayflick, PhD

More than sixty years ago, the pioneer gerontologist Raymond Pearl recognized that with the elimination of deaths in the early years of life, survival curves constructed at intervals were becoming more rectangular.[1] This phenomenon subsequently was discussed extensively by Comfort,[2] Strehler,[3] Kohn[4] and Hayflick.[5,6,7] More recent reviews on the accuracy of rectangular survival curves and their interpretation for future geriatric planning[8,9,10,11] have met with considerable controversy.[12,13,14,15]

Fries has argued that the continuing rectangularization of human survival curves for developed countries is compressing the period of time in which most mortality occurs in later life. He has now broadened this interpretation to include the compression of morbidity as well as mortality.[16] As the increase in life expectation and delayed clinical manifestations of chronic diseases approach what for Fries is a fixed lifespan, then compression occurs. He interprets this[8] to mean that:

1. the number of very old people will not increase,
2. the average period of diminished vigor will decrease,
3. chronic diseases will occur in a smaller proportion of the total lifespan, and
4. this will result in a reduction in the need for medical care in the elderly.

If the human lifespan is fixed and the diseases causing death occur at increasingly older ages, then morbidity and mortality will occupy an increasingly smaller proportion of the human lifespan.

This scenario, if true, has important implications for planning present and future allocations of health care resources. But the probability that it is true is questionable.

IS THE HUMAN LIFESPAN FIXED?

The first premise on which this scenario rests is the belief that the human lifespan is fixed. Although what little data that exists has been interpreted by Fries[16] to argue for a fixed human lifespan, there are important qualifications.

Most gerontologists will not accept a maximum human lifespan that exceeds about 115 years of age. The reason for skepticism is simple. First, unlike tree rings and fish scales, there are no reliable biomarkers for accurately determining the chronological age or biological age of humans. Lacking this, it is necessary to assess written, or worse, oral records. If the scientific method is applied, few, if any, birth records of very old people alive today can be authenticated. Most records that are accepted simply prove that cherished beliefs, or faith, are greater persuasive forces than are scientific data.[17,18]

Since there are so few authentic centenarians, a correct determination of the maximum human lifespan is not possible. The reliability of non-contemporaneous records is even more questionable. Thus the uncertainty of birth dates and the small number of very old people conspire against accuracy.

This uncertainty not only compromises a determination of the maximum human lifespan itself, but also prevents knowing whether it is changing. For example, if the human lifespan increased by as much as five or even ten years during this century, the likelihood is remote that it could be detected. Consequently, as good an argument could be made for a fixed human lifespan as could be made for one that has increased or even decreased.

Evolution of Lifespan

Nevertheless, on an evolutionary scale, there is good evidence that the human lifespan increased rapidly until about 100,000 years ago, when it slowed down considerably. The evidence for this is the remarkable concordance found to occur when the ratio of the weight of the adult mammalian brain to the weight of the adult body is expressed as a function of lifespan.[19,20,21,22] By this criterion it is possible to say with confidence that early hominids had a lifespan far less than modern humans because their brains were considerably smaller than ours in relation to body weight.

The brain weight/body weight ratio of humans slowed considerably about 100,000 years ago when the human lifespan became what it is today. However, on an evolutionary scale, the human lifespan still may be increasing because the sensitivity of brain weight/body weight measurements are insufficient to detect small differences that may have occurred over the last 100, 1000 or even 10,000 years. However, on an evolutionary scale, the human lifespan *has* increased. This fact is important because it implies that the human lifespan, even if it has been fixed for millenia, has the potential to increase in the future. Studies with animals also show that lifespan can be manipulated by reducing caloric intake.[23,24,25]

Demography of Lifespan

Tantalizing evidence that the human lifespan may be increasing comes from the recent work of several demographers. Myers and Manton have argued that the population dynamics of the elderly have *not* been subject to the effects of the rectangularization of the survival curve.[14] Survival curves for the United States show a large gain in life expectancy from 1900 to today. The greatest increases have occurred in the younger age groups until about 1960. Since 1960 there has been a substantial increase in life expectancy in the older age groups.

Fries[16] states, in respect to the rectangularization of survival curves, "The point on the age axis at which the curves intersect has remained approximately the same, the differences lying within the width of the lines used to plot such curves. The progressive shape of these curves allows visual prediction of future trends."

Rectangularization of the survival curve is apparent if one includes data from the birth of all members in a cohort to the last survivor. Meyers and Manton[14] point out that "this, however, combines two different types of mortality reduction, i.e. those due to declines in infant and child mortality and those from chronic disease mortality at later ages." These phenomena are not only different in their biological origins, but they have occurred at different times in this century as indicated above. Meyers and

Manton[14] argue that the vertical slope of the rectangular curves derived from the aforementioned data do not all intersect the abscissa at the same fixed point. They are rather more asymptotic and curves for succeeding years intersect at later points.

Meyers and Manton, however, do not comment on the possibility that what they believe to be an advancing lifespan may, in fact, be the creep of advancing life expectation. It may also reflect the advance of that elusive concept of "specific age" mentioned by Comfort[2] or what Fries[16] defines as lifespan "or the average longevity in a society without disease or accident." For Fries this is "approximately 85 years, with a broad distribution in which natural longevity for individuals falls nearly entirely within the range of from 70 to 100 years." One value of this concept is to eliminate those rare persons who outlive the vast majority of the cohort and, by so doing, reveal more about the maximum human lifespan than about life-expectation.

If one constructs survival curves by eliminating the influence of mortality at earlier ages as Meyers and Manton have done for 60 years-old females in 1900, 1960 and 1980, there is little tendency for the curves to rectangularize.[14] Crimmins[12] examined female survival curves for ages 65 to 85 for the years 1967 and 1978. She found no rectangularization, but rather parallelism, and no steeper slope in this age range in 1978 after survival rates increased. She concluded that there was "no empirical evidence for recent rectangularization of the survival curve up to age 85."

However, what might be expressed in these two studies is the well-recognized increasing life expectation and not increasing maximum lifespan. The failure of many authors to define their use of the terms life expectation and the life-span or to understand the difference has led to much unnecessary controversy and many erroneous conclusions.[26]

Meyers and Manton[14] also provide data that show "a slow progression toward later average ages of death for *all* five diseases (that are the leading causes of death), an increasing gap between males and females, and *greater variation* in age of death about the mean levels." These findings argue against the compression of mortality, hence morbidity.

Fries[11] has presented arguments against most of the conclusions reached by Meyers and Manton,[14] but the latter, in turn, have rebutted Fries.

Conflicting Views

Schneider and Brody's[15] interpretation of the rectangularization of survival curves is diametrically opposite to that of Fries. They argue that: (1) the number of very old people is increasing rapidly, (2) the average period of decreasing vigor will increase, (3) chronic diseases will occupy a larger portion of the lifespan, and (4) requirements for medical care will increase in later life. Schneider and Brody say, "One important cornerstone to Fries' predictions is that there is a genetically defined human lifespan that we are rapidly approaching." They cite the work of Hayflick and Moorhead[27] and Hayflick[28] in which we reported that the ability of normal human cells to proliferate and function in vitro is finite as the evidence used by Fries to support his belief that there is a genetically defined program.

Schneider and Brody[15] state that " . . . it has been amply demonstrated that some replicating cell populations have lifespans that far exceed the replicative lifespan of the parent organism, often by severalfold." They cite the work of Harrison[29] and Daniel and Young[30] in support of their contention.

The fact that grafted normal tissue may survive longer than cultured normal cells from the same species, or longer than the lifespan of the species itself, is a spurious argument against the genetically-determined program. Transplanted tissue simply has a much smaller pool of replicating cells and those cells that do replicate do not do so at in vitro rates. Even cultured cells can be made to replicate slower by decreasing the incubation temperature. This results in a longer calendar time before the cells age and die, but it does not change the number of population doublings. The logical conclusion to be drawn from Schneider and Brody's statement is that because normal human cells can be held at cryogenic temperatures, apparently indefinitely, then humans must be immortal. This has been discussed more fully elsewhere.[31] The essential point is that when normal cells are cultured or transplanted, they have a finite ability to replicate and function. A genetically-determined program, as championed by Fries, is, on this basis, tenable.

Even if compelling in vitro evidence for a genetically-determined finite lifespan did not exist, the in vitro evidence for a genetically-determined lifespan is significant. The wide range of lifespans for each animal species provides strong evidence for this. A fruit fly is old in 30 days, a mouse in 30 months, and a human in 75 years. When deaths in young members of these species are eliminated, survival curves reveal a remarkable constancy in time of death that is characteristic for each species. If this constancy were not at least partly attributable to a chronometer, one would expect random appearances of old animals in each species over a much broader span of time.

The Gompertz Equation

In support of the compression of morbidity and mortality hypothesis, Fries invokes the Gompertz equation stating that it "fits closely with the observation of smoothly and rapidly declining numbers of individuals alive at successive ages."[16] However, Bayo,[32] using the must reliable mortality data for single years of age above 85, has shown that the Gompertz equation does not hold above the age of 85 and that, after 90, mortality increases at a progressively smaller rate. Manton concurs[13] and Bourgeois-Pichat[33] reach similar conclusions. If these studies are to be believed, then decompression of mortality is occurring, not compression.

In defense of fixed lifespans, Fries draws attention to the consistent differences in the fixed lifespans of several different animal species.[16] Yet there are animals in which aging is rare or has never been demonstrated. Some fish and amphibians that have an indeterminate size may also have an indeterminate lifespan.[2] Thus a fixed lifespan, and even the universality of aging in vertebrates, remains unproven. Animals of indeterminant lifespan are not immortal. They will die eventually of diseases, predation or accidents at an actuarily determined annual rate which is not true aging.

In fact, the occurrence of aging arguably is restricted to humans and the domestic and zoo animals that we choose to protect. The extreme manifestations of old age that are found to occur in humans simply do not occur in feral animals. If aging occurs at all in wild animals its expression is brief because the physiological decrements of aging quickly make feral animals vulnerable to disease and predation. They simply do not live long enough to get really old.

In developed countries, humans have been so successful in resolving the causes of death that their aging is expressed to an extreme unattainable by wild animals. Civilization has produced life expectations that were unknown in prehistoric times, revealing a plethora of physiological decrements that perhaps teleologically, were never intended to be revealed. Aging may be an artifact of civilization or domestication because these "unnatural conditions" have permitted the expression of aging that otherwise would not have occurred.

COMPRESSION OF MORBIDITY

The second condition that must be satisfied if compression of morbidity is to occur is that diseases leading to death become clinically manifest in succeedingly later years. Although Fries[16] believes that this is not controversial, some believe that it is. What may not be controversial is that *deaths* attributable to chronic diseases are being postponed by medical intervention so that they are occurring at succeedingly advanced ages. This might produce a compression in mortality but not in morbidity. If the start of morbidity and death itself are both postponed equally, then there is no absolute gain in healthy years.

Although Fries[16] maintains that "Some emerging data suggest that the compression of morbidity may be a present as well as a future phenomenon," others dispute this claim. For example, Colvez and Blanchet[34] have analyzed data from the National Health Interview Survey conducted annually since 1957 by the National Center for Health Statistics. They report a disturbing general increase in recent years in morbidity and disability in all age groups. The increase was found to be greatest in mid-life. Thus while life expectation increases, morbidity may also increase.[34]

Aging and Disease

The phenomena of aging must be distinguished from the phenomena of disease. Biological changes attributable to aging are frequently referred to as "normal age changes," (as if there was a category of "abnormal age changes"). Age changes are not diseases, they are natural losses of function. Loss and greying of the hair, reduced exercise capacity and stamina, wrinkled skin, menopause, presbyopia, loss of short-term memory and hundreds of other similar decrements of aging are not regarded as diseases. They do not increase our vulnerability to die. Analagous "normal" decrements in vital organs *do* produce increased vulnerability to pathological change. For example, normal age-related decrements in immune system functions increase vulnerability to diseases that in youth would be easily resolved. Or, antigen recognized as "self" in youth might be recognized by an aging immune system as "nonself," thus producing the chronic autoimmune diseases of old age.

Schneider and Brody,[15] argue that there is no evidence that "natural death" can occur without disease because no functional decline associated with aging " . . . is compromised sufficiently, even at extreme ages, for death to result in the absence of disease. Therefore, the compromised physiology of the elderly still requires a specific pathologic insult . . . for death to occur."

Whatever Happened to Natural Causes?

There is much confusion on this important point. The confusion results from the blurred distinction between death attributable to natural causes and death attributable to pathological processes. It is further compounded by the fact that deaths attributable to natural causes were once frequently written on death certificates. That has not been true for many years. Physicians, apparently have felt that to write "natural causes" on a death certificate, even when the cause of death is truly unknown, is an admission of ignorance and hence undesirable, in an era of scientific enlightenment. Thus cardiac arrest, stroke, pulmonary infarct or some other guessed-at cause is thought to be more professionally acceptable than to admit that the cause of death is natural or unknown. The impact that this non-medically based, sociologically determined phenomenon has had on the statistics of true causes of death in the past fifty years can only be speculated upon.

It follows from this that one of the really significant triumphs of biomedical research in the twentieth century has been the resolution of deaths attributable to "natural causes." Despite the magnitude of this achievement, the scientific literature describing the resolution of "natural causes" of death is nowhere to be found. The extraordinary modesty of the discoverers of the cure, if not the etiology, of "natural causes" is awesome. The mystery is further compounded when one considers that this monumental accomplishment occurred, apparently, without grant support. Certainly if it had, the sponsors themselves hardly would have been expected to keep it a secret.

Causes of Death in the Very Old

The term "natural causes" represents the very category that should be defined to mean "death in the absence of disease."

Functional decline does occur during aging, as Schneider and Brody[15] admit, but they conclude that a specific pathologic insult is required to administer the coup de gras. The fact that functional decline is recognized to occur, as are pathological insults, implies that a distinction can be made between the two concepts. I believe that this distinction is crucial. The distinction may be subtle but it is important. Functional decline is believed to be a normal process. Pathology is not a normal process. The subtlety is that functional decline—a normal process—increases the vulnerability to pathology—an abnormal process. As a consequence of this it is just as likely that causes of death written on the death certificate of the elderly are *all* in error—including those attributable to accidents.

The true cause of deaths in the aged are normal functional decrements that increase vulnerability to a pathological process. Thus whatever is written on the death certificates of the aged should be preceded with the disclaimer that whatever the ultimate cause of death might be, the penultimate cause is normal loss of function.

Schneider and Brody[15] argue that " . . . the compromised physiology of the elderly still requires a specific pathologic insult, such as pulmonary edema or pulmonary infarction, for death to occur." They provide no evidence for this statement. Their belief that it is true probably rests on the questionable assumption that, since virtually all death certificates of the aged contain a cause of death attributable to a pathology, natural causes or loss of function alone cannot be the ultimate cause. Their reasoning thus is circuitous because the fact that deaths attributable to natural causes do not appear on death certificates does not mean that they do not occur.

Schneider and Brody, ignore the important work of Kohn[4] who autopsied 200 people 85 years of age and older. He found no acceptable cause of death other than "complications of the aging syndrome in at least 30% of the cases." He comments further that:

> vital statistics for the aged are misleading because diagnoses are not definitive. Physicians accept causes of death in the aged that would not be acceptable in younger persons, and the role of aging processes themselves as cause of death are not appreciated. Aging is characterized by a universal progressive decline in physiological function to the point where life cannot be maintained in the face of otherwise trivial tissue injury.

Kohn's autopsy data are in strong disagreement with the causes of death listed in the "Vital Statistics" where it is found that the major causes of death in those over 85 are ischemic heart disease and cerebrovascular disease. In only 20 percent of the autopsied cases were these causes justified. No cause of death could be found in 26 percent of the autopsies and this category does not even exist in the "Vital Statistics." If the 3.5 percent of cases in which uncomplicated trauma was followed by death are included then 30 percent of the autopsied cases were found to have no acceptable cause of death. Kohn concludes, as I have,[5,6,7] that the normal physiological decrements of aging are the ultimate cause of death in this large fraction of individuals. Despite this, the normal consequences of aging are, today, not an "acceptable" cause of death.

If our understanding of the important factors that cause death in old people is to be based on the truth and not on bias and faulty data then we must mount a major program with the goal of collecting reliable autopsy data at the deaths of old people. Until that is done on a national scale, we cannot formulate reliable health programs and policies for the elderly. Today, two-thirds of all deaths occur in persons over the age of 65 and almost one third occur in persons over the age of 80,[35] yet only 15 and 5 percent, respectively, are ever autopsied.

How much longer will we continue to base important research decisions, program development and health policies on misleading and outright erroneous information on the fastest growing segment of our population? The irony is that for the price of a tiny fraction of the cost of existing programs, it *is* possible to obtain the reliable data on which plans for sound future research and health policies could be based.

Kohn also observes that a cause of death chosen from a standard list must go on a death certificate and, for persons over 80, deaths are attributed in descending order of frequency to cardiovascular disease, cancer, infections, and accidents (33). These data then comprise the "Vital Statistics" used to formulate our concepts about disease in the very old and to plan programs and formulate health policy. Deaths without a significant cause, or deaths due to the normal decrements of old age, do not appear in the "Vital Statistics." If we are to obtain reliable data on the causes of death in older people many more autopsies must be done on this growing segment of our population. Kohn (1982) has demonstrated that the percentage of autopsies done on individuals in this country drops almost linearly from about 65% done at age 30 to 5% done at age 85.

Kohn concludes from his studies on 200 autopsies done on individuals over the age of 80 that one or a small number of fundamental age-related biological processes occur and that the causes of death found on the death certificates of these individuals are merely "complications of the basic process." He observes that although it cannot be predicted what disease an old person may die of, it is not important because they will die at about the same time of one of the usual pathologies currently put on death certificates.

It is very likely that a significant number of deaths in older people should be attributed to loss of function in some vital organ and not to some unproven pathology. Even those causes of death in the elderly that are reported to be accidental bear some scrutiny in this context. If the ultimate cause of death was a fall or a failure to avoid an approaching vehicle, the penultimate cause was normal loss of function in which such normal decrements as reduced reaction time, presbyopia or presbycusis actually led to the accident. A younger person probably would have escaped death under similar conditions because those normal decrements would not have been manifest.

The Morbid Years

It does not necessarily follow that if the average age of *onset* of chronic diseases is delayed the remaining morbid years will be reduced. In fact, if this does occur, it is just as likely that medical science will be able to offset that gain by maintaining these chronically ill patients for an equivalent period on life support systems. People with chronic diseases simply might be incapacitated for the same absolute period of time thus making greater demands on our health care system rather than less as Fries suggests. The decision to place dying people on life support systems and for how long is precisely one of the most complex moral dilemmas that presently confronts us.

Furthermore, even if we grant that compression of morbidity might occur, the suggestion that this would lead to less demand on biomedical resources does not necessarily follow. Since there is no dispute that the number of people over the age of 65 will increase dramatically in the future, this will quite obviously lead to much greater absolute numbers of aged individuals with chronic diseases. Thus even though the years in which morbidity may occur might be compressed, the absolute number of individuals resident in that compressed compartment will increase dramatically. This enormous number of older people will require far more medical and other services than reasonably could be gained by delaying the clinical expression of chronic disease for several years. It also must be appreciated that the burden for health care is far less in the early years of chronic diseases than in the years preceding death. Fuchs estimates that about ten percent of all medical costs are incurred during the last year of life.[36]

A good example of the certainty that morbidity will not be compressed in at least one major area is the absolute increase in numbers of old people who will require health services for cognitive impairment. Recent data from the Bureau of the Census show that by the year 2050, persons 85 years of age and older will have increased from the present 2.3 million to about 16 million.[15] Today about 20 percent of persons over 85 have severe cognitive impairment and require long-term care.[37] Even if that value were to be halved by 2050, the number of these individuals requiring long term care would increase from about 500,000 today to about 1.6 million in 65 years.

Increase in Absolute Numbers

There is at least one other phenomenon overlooked by Fries that will work against any putative reduction in years spent with chronic disease. Medical science has been enormously successful in postponing the deaths of many individuals who would have otherwise died in youth of one of a growing number of genetically-based chronic diseases including such common pathologies as diabetes. The results of our success in postponing deaths in these individuals with inborn errors of metabolism is to permit them to live long enough to pass on those undesirable traits to their offspring. The consequences of this have been variously referred to as an increasing rise in the contamination of the human gene pool or gene pollution.

Few people would advocate that individuals possessing these undesirable traits should not be helped medically but others would argue that they should not be permitted to transmit those undesirable genes. The fact that they are means that the chronic diseases that these genes express have been, and will continue to be, transmitted to greater numbers of humans as the generations pass. Even if a compression of morbidity could be made to occur in non-genetically based diseases, the growing number of individuals, with inborn errors of metabolism will probably offset whatever gain might occur in reduced health services to others. Indeed the leading causes of death in most developed countries are cardiovascular diseases, stroke and cancer and they are believed to have a genetic component. About thirty human cancers are now known to be associated with cytogenetically demonstrable chromosome anomalies.[38] It might very well be that the genetic predisposition of these pathologies already is so widely distributed in the human gene pool that there is little possibility for eliminating them.

CONCLUSION

Our present concern with the growing number of elderly in this country and the impact that this will have on many of our health, economic and other institutions is in danger of obscuring at least one major concept. The reason that so many people in this and other developed countries are reaching old age is absolute proof that the medical, public health, economic, social and educational advances that have been made in the last hundred years have been successful. Every old person alive today is testimony to that fact.

Instead of bemoaning the likelihood that more of us are destined to reach old age, it seems to me that every old person should be a cause for the celebration of our success and not for lamentation. Why have we striven to improve biomedical research, health and social services over the last decades if it was not to reach the goal of allowing more people to become old? Every success in biomedical research has the potential net effect of increasing human life expectation. If that goal is undesirable, then why do biomedical research at all?

REFERENCES

1. Pearl, R. and Pearl, R. D. *The Ancestry of the Long-lived*. Baltimore: The Johns Hopkins Press, 1934.

2. Comfort, A. *The Biology of Senescence*. New York: Elsevier North Holland, Inc., 1964.

3. Strehler, B. *Time, Cells, and Aging*. New York: Academy Press, 1977.

4. Kohn, R. R. *Principles of Mammalian Aging*. Englewood Cliffs, New Jersey: Prentice-Hall, Inc., 1971.

5. Hayflick, L. The biology of human aging. *American Journal of Medical Science*, 265:433–45, 1973.

6. Hayflick, L. The strategy of senescence. *The Gerontologist*, 14:37–45, 1974.

7. Hayflick, L. The cell biology of human aging. *New England Journal of Medicine*, 295:1302–08. 1976.

8. Fries, J. F. Aging, natural death, and the compression of morbidity. *New England Journal of Medicine*, 303:130–35, 1980.

9. Fries, J. F. and Crapo, L. M. *Vitality and Aging: Implications of the Rectangular Curve.* San Francisco: W. H. Freeman, 1981.

10. Fries, J. F. The compression of morbidity. *Milbank Memorial Fund Quarterly/ Health and Society*, 61:397–418, 1983.

11. Fries, J. F. The compression of morbidity: Miscellaneous comments about a theme. *The Gerontologist*, 24:354–59, 1984.

12. Crimmins, E. M. Life expectancy and the older population. *Research on Aging*, 6(4):490–514, 1984.

13. Manton, K. G. Changing concepts of morbidity and mortality in the elderly population. *Milbank Memorial Fund Quarterly/Health and Society*, 60:183–244, 1982.

14. Myers, G. C. and Manton, K. G. Compression of mortality: Myth or reality? *The Gerontologist*, 24(4):346–53, 1984.

15. Schneider, E. L. and Brody, J. A. Aging, natural death, and the compression of morbidity: Another view. *New England Journal of Medicine*, 309:854–56, 1983.

16. Fries, J. F. The biological constraints on human aging: Implications for health policy. In Andreoli, K.G., Musser, L.A., and Reiser, S.J., editors: Health Policy for the Elderly: Regional Response to National Policy Issues, New York: The Haworth Press, 1986.

17. Mazess, R. B. Health and longevity in Vilcabamba, Ecuador. *Journal of the American Medical Association*, 1781, 1978.

18. Medvedev, Z. A. Caucasus and Altay longevity: A biologic or social problem? *The Gerontologist*, 14:381, 1974.

19. Friedenthal, H. Ueber die Giltigkeit des Massenwirkung fur den Energieumsatz der lebendigen Substanz. *Zentralbl. Physiologie*, 24:321–27, 1910.

20. Hofman, M. A. Energy metabolism, brain size and longevity in mammals. *Quarterly Review of Biology*, 58(4):495–512, 1983.

21. Sacher, G. A. Relation of lifespan to brain weight and body weight. In: Wolstenholme, G. E. W. and O'Conner, M. (editors). *The Lifespan of Animals*, Boston: Little, Brown, and Company, 1959, pp. 115–141.

22. Sacher, G. A. Maturation and longevity in relation to cranial capacity in hominid evolution. In: Tuttle, R. H. (editor). *Interdisciplinary Topics in Gerontology*, 9:69–83, 1975.

23. Masoro, E. J. Extending the mammalian life span. In: Gaitz, C. and Samorajski, T. (editors). *Aging 2000: Our Health Care Destiny.* New York: Springer Publishing Co., 1985.

24. McKay, C. M., Crowell, M. F., and Maynard, L. A. The effect of retarded growth upon the length of life span and upon the ultimate body size. *Journal of Nutrition*, 10:63–79, 1935.

25. Weindruch, R. and Walford, R. L. Life span and spontaneous cancer incidence in mice dietarily restricted beginning at one year of age. *Science*, 215:1415–18, 1982.

26. Yin, P. and Shine, M. Misinterpretations of increases in life expectancy in gerontology textbooks. *The Gerontologist*, 25(1):78–81, 1985.

27. Hayflick, L. and Moorhead, P. S. The serial cultivation of human diploid cell strains. *Experimental Cell Research*, 25:585–621, 1961.

28. Hayflick, L. The limited in vitro lifetime of human diploid cell strains. *Experimental Cell Research*, 37:614–36, 1965.

29. Harrison, D. E. Normal production of erythrocytes by mouse marrow continuous for 73 months. *Proceedings of the National Academy of Sciences*, 70:3184–88, 1973.

30. Daniel, C. W. and Young, L. J. T. Influence of cell division on an aging process: Life span of mouse mammary epithelium during serial propagation in vivo. *Experimental Cell Research*, 6527–32, 1971.

31. Hayflick, L. Biological determinants of the human lifespan. In: Bergener, M. (editor), *Innovations in Psychogeriatrics*, New York Springer Publishing Co., 1986. (In Press.)

32. Bayo, F. Mortality of the aged. *Transactions of the Society of Actuaries*, 24:1–24, 1975.

33. Bourgeois-Pichat, J. Future outlook for mortality decline in the world. *Population Bulletin of the United Nations*, 11:12–41, 1978.

34. Colvez, A. and Blanchet, M. Disability trends in the United States population 1966–76: Analysis of reported causes. *American Journal of Public Health*, 71:461–63, 1981.

35. Brody, J. A. Facts, projections, and gaps concerning data on aging. *Public Health Reports*, 99(5):468–475, 1984.

36. Fuchs, V. R. Though much is taken—reflections on aging, health and medical care. *Milbank Memorial Fund Quarterly/Health and Society*, 62:143, 1984.

37. Hagnell, O., Lanke, J., Rorsman, B., and Ojesjo, L. Does the incidence of age psychosis decrease: A prospective longitudinal study of a complete population investigated during the 25-year period 1947–1972; The Lundby Study. *Neuropsychobiology*, 7:201–11, 1981.

38. Rowley, J. D. Human oncogene locations and chromosome aberrations. *Nature*, 301:290–91, 1983.

The Biological Constraints
on Human Aging:
Implications for Health Policy
A National Policy Perspective

Alexander Leaf, MD

I have been following Dr. Fries' views with great interest. It seems that his thesis is logically unassailable. If preventive interventions can increase the age of clinically manifest disease more rapidly than the biological limit of life is extended, then morbidity will be compressed. One has to assume, of course, that nature will not invent new chronic diseases—such as AIDS—for the elderly to confound the situation. One also must be exceedingly optimistic (excessively optimistic, I would say), in expecting preventive measures to eradicate the chronic ills of the elderly. It seems to me that today we lack adequate knowledge of the pathogenesis of many of these diseases to know what interventions will prove preventive, and we certainly don't know, for diseases that are preventable with today's understanding, how to motivate people to adhere to healthful lifestyles that potentially will reduce risk for future disease.

I am also aware of the writing of Schneider and Brody[1] who see no evidence that morbidity in the elderly is being compressed. On the contrary, they document their increasing need for medical care. Thus, the Fries thesis, appealing as it seems, still has empirical hurdles to overcome. Perhaps when preventive interventions become more ideally effective than they currently are, we will see the logic of the Fries thesis become reality.

What are the consequences for national health policy if Dr. Fries' thesis is correct? Is medical care today, as practiced by its high priests, the medical profession, pursuing such a route or is it moving in the opposite direction? I would like to examine the path our profession is taking with regard to the chief cause of death and a major cause of morbidity in the United States, to see if this direction is in our best interest, and to propose an alternative consistent with the thesis proposed by Dr. Fries.

In the United States and other affluent industrialized countries, coronary artery disease (CAD) is the leading cause of death and a major cause of morbidity. CAD alone accounted for 29 percent of U.S. deaths in 1982, despite a gratifying reduction in mortality rates since 1967. According to the most recent figures,[2] there are some 4.7 million Americans who have CAD, either a past myocardial infarction or angina pectoris. Some 1.5 million Americans will suffer a heart attack this year, of which about 550,000 will die. Furthermore, nearly 350,000 will die before being able to reach a hospital. Thus, despite a very gratifying 25 percent reduction in mortality rate from CAD in the United States since 1967, CAD remains the leading cause of death and a major cause of morbidity in the United States. The costs of CAD in medical care—hospitalization, physicians' charges, medications, and lost output due to disability—will be some $72.1 billion this year. But the situation with respect to CAD is not unique to us. Other industrialized developed countries suffer a similar burden of illness, some even greater than ours. Furthermore, the reduction in mortality rate that has occurred in the United States in the past 20 years has not occurred in all afflicted countries. Some have continued to experience increasing CAD mortality rates.

With this brief description of the burden of illness caused by CAD, let us examine the response of the medical profession. For the most part we wait in our offices until patients come to us complaining of chest pain or other symptoms of ischemic heart disease. Occasionally we meet the ambulance at 3 a.m. at the emergency room. Management consists largely of monitoring, drug treatment of arrhythmias, vasodilator drugs, beta-blockers, now slow calcium channel blockers, thrombolytic therapy, percutaneous transluminal coronary angioplasty. If these measures fail to relieve signs or symptoms of CAD, patients are sent for cardiac angiography and frequently to the operating room for coronary artery bypass surgery.

In 1982, the last year for which figures are available,[2] there were 170,000 coronary bypass operations done at $25,000 a piece or some $4 billion. Since the CASS study[3] has shown that benefits from this surgery are limited to a few special conditions, there probably has been a decline in the rate of increase in coronary bypass surgery, but it remains a large and active enterprise. The technological imperative has produced even more costly interventions in the "curative" approach to CAD. Heart transplants and artificial hearts are the fad despite the obvious fact that the former can benefit at best only a very few persons at very high cost and the latter despite expenditures of upward of $200 million in research, has so far, and for the foreseeable future, yielded no benefits.

In listing the response of the medical profession to CAD, I don't mean to be derisive or denigrating. Undoubtedly these "curative" interventions have, in many instances, relieved pain and anxiety, and, in some, have postponed death. It seems important, however, to place our response in perspective and recognize what we are doing and where our actions are leading us. Limitations of our present medical approach may be listed as:

1. One has to survive the heart attack to be treated and the odds for this are not too encouraging.
2. The treatments barely scratch the surface of the health problem; 170,000 coronary bypass operations, were they curative, represent a small fraction of the 1.5 million heart attacks this year.
3. The treatments are expensive.
4. More importantly, the interventions are all palliative; they do nothing about the underlying disease process, atherosclerosis, which causes CAD.
5. Most importantly, even if current interventions were curative and affordable they do nothing for the next generation of 20, 30 and 40 year olds who will be destined to the same fate.

It appears, therefore, that a more rational response is required to control this major cause of death and morbidity in industrialized countries. Preventive cardiology seems to offer such a rational approach. Over the last 50 years a small number of dedicated epidemiologists have been identifying risk factors for CAD. Today these include:

Nonmodifiable	Modifiable
family history	high plasma LDL cholesterol
male sex	low plasma HDL cholesterol
age	cigarette smoking
	hypertension
	physical activity
	obesity
	diabetes (Type II)
	stress

Recognition of the modifiable risk factors for CAD comes largely from epidemiologic studies. In the case of cholesterol, it has been demonstrated in a randomized prospective trial that reduction of plasma LDL cholesterol decreases mortality from CAD.[4] Cigarette smoking, hypertension and physical inactivity are also well established risk factors, and preventing them will lower the probability of CAD. Undoubtedly there will be other interventions that will prevent CAD as we understand better the pathogenesis of atherosclerosis. Studies are already in progress to determine whether prevention of platelet aggregation by low dose salicylate or by n-3 polyunsaturated fatty acids from fish oils will prevent CAD.

The modifiable risk factors, which are so prevalent in our affluent society, are responsible for the majority of instances of CAD. Genetic factors of such penetrance as alone to doom an individual to CAD are uncommon—e.g. homozygous familial hypercholesterolemia, homocystinuria, or progeria. The modifiable risk factors, superimposed on a variable polygenic constitution, must account for the majority of CAD in our country.

There has been a popular movement in the United States toward adoption of behavior and lifestyles which reduce cardiac risk factors. These changes account for most of the reduction of CAD mortality rates that have occurred in the past two decades.[5] The medical profession has not played a major role in fostering this change. In fact, until recently many physicians have been skeptical about the value of reducing these risk factors and proponents have often been faddists. It is only in the past few months that a consensus statement has been issued by physicians advocating reduced saturated fats and cholesterol in the American diet.[6]

Actually there is a major role for careful research to establish a more solid basis of knowledge regarding the risk factors and the effects of their reduction on health. Behavioral sciences have much to do to learn about how to change life styles. Knowledge that smoking cigarettes is injurious to health is not sufficient to eradicate this major health risk. Changing behavior and sustaining adherence to healthful life styles are the limitations on preventive cardiology and preventive medicine generally. A great advance in preventive medicine would also occur if means were discovered to identify the individuals who are at risk from cigarette smoking or from ingesting high saturated fat and cholesterol diets so that preventive measures could be concentrated on such individuals rather than imposed upon the entire population.

A greater involvement in preventive measures by the health professions could do much to reduce the burden of chronic illness that plagues our aging population. Cardiovascular diseases are particularly amenable to preventive strategies. A redistribution of expenditures from very expensive technologic interventions that at best can benefit only a very few of the many individuals in need, to preventive measures, makes sense to me. I am not critical of our traditional role as physicians to relieve suffering and to cure illness, but I think the current almost total preoccupation with end-stage "curative" medicine is not a rational response to the major health problems confronting us today. Some redress and better balance is needed.

Today most health insurance plans specifically proscribe reimbursement for health promotion activities. We need a health policy that provides reimbursement incentives to engage health workers to provide more preventive medicine and health promotion services. But we shouldn't get caught in the trap of expecting preventive medicine to reduce national medical costs. It may or may not accomplish this desirable goal. The purpose of health care is not to save money but to optimize the quality of life by allowing more of it to be spent in a state of vigorous health. We should at least spend our health dollars in ways that optimize health and I believe that health promotion is likely to buy us more good health per dollar spent than will current expenditures on established, serious and often irreversible disease.

With a national health policy that incorporates an appropriate balance of preventive medicine, the question of how much of our resources should also be devoted to high technological interventions in established disease will still be with us. I have no preformed response to this question. Once we are maximizing our efforts to prevent disease, we can examine available resources and assess possible benefits and make a decision at that time.

REFERENCES

1. Schneider, E. L. and Brody, J. A. Aging, natural death, and the compression of morbidity: Another view. *New England Journal of Medicine*, 309:854–856, 1983.

2. American Heart Association. *Heart Facts*. Washington, D.C.: AHA, 1985.

3. CASS principal investigators and their associates. Coronary Artery Surgery Study (CASS): A randomized trial of coronary artery bypass surgery. Survival data. *Circulation*, 68:939–50, 1983.

4. Lipid Research Clinics Primary Prevention Trial Results II. The relationship of reduction in incidence of coronary heart disease to cholesterol lowering. *Journal of the American Medical Association*, 251:365–74, 1984.

5. Goldman, L. and Cook, E. F. The decline in ischemic heart disease mortality rates: An analysis of the comparative effects of medical intervention and changes in life style. *Annals of Internal Medicine*, 101:825–836, 1984.

6. National Institutes of Health, *Consensus Development Conference, Lower Blood Cholesterol*, December 10–12, 1984.

The Biological Constraints
on Human Aging:
Implications for Health Policy
A Regional Policy Perspective

Reuel A. Stallones, MD, MPH

Dr. Fries' 1980 paper in the *New England Journal of Medicine*[1] bore the seductive title, "Aging, natural death, and the compression of morbidity." Seductive because coupling an unfamiliar term with two very familiar ones leads one to believe that the unfamiliar one will be readily understandable. The familiar terms are kind of Judas goats, leading us to an etymological slaughter. Aging I understand all too well with the passing of the years, and can identify with the old man in John Steinbeck's "Sweet Thursday" who said, "I knew growing old was going to be bad, but I didn't know it would be this bad." Natural death is more difficult to understand; I wish my own death to be unnatural, long deferred, of course but unnatural. With these terms leading the way, we can pursue the meaning of compression of morbidity.

The greying of America has engendered much discussion and much concern; concern over the effects of a higher proportion of aged persons on our culture, our politics, our economy, and our medical care system. Medical care costs rise so rapidly with advancing age, that the prospect of a significant increase in the proportion of older persons in the population has led to speculation that the medical care burden would be insupportable. Among the alternatives that have been considered are rationing and restriction of services, uncomfortable choices for a society that professes egalitarian ideals. However, that the costs of medical care for individuals rise with increasing age does not necessarily mean that the costs of medical care for a society increase as the age structure on that society changes. An alternative, presented by Dr. Fries, is that the overall burden of morbidity may not increase, or may even decrease, the result of a phenomenon he has designated the compression of morbidity.

For those of us who choose to practice preventive medicine, a signal point is that the concept of compression of morbidity depends upon the prevention of disease, the deferral of onset of illness. Improved and extended medical care may prolong life, but, with only a few exceptions, the lives that are prolonged are damaged and the burden of morbidity in the community is increased.

Few of the matters addressed by Dr. Fries have regional peculiarities attached to them. Lifespan is defined as a species characteristic, and we have enough examples of successful cross-breeding to assure us that although Texans are different from other people they are not a separate species. One of the special demographic features of Texas is the tri-ethnic character of its population, with 12 percent black, almost 20 percent Hispanic and 65 percent other white, sometimes imprecisely designated Anglo. The age structure of different ethnic groups is sharply different; in 1980, 12 percent of the white population was over the age of 65 years, as compared with 8 percent of blacks and 5 percent Hispanics. The population subsets of Hispanics and blacks not only are younger, but have larger families, a higher rate of unemployment, and lower incomes. However, none of these ethnic and racial differences should have effect on the concept of compression of morbidity, for their consequences should be quantitative, not qualitative.

I have found so little to say about regional considerations in a geographic sense, that I am impelled to consider the matter in a regional scientific sense, exploring the implications of the compression of morbidity in the region of epidemiology. The central issues are whether the notion of compression of morbidity is correct, and whether it is useful, correct or incorrect. Evidence as to its correctness is scanty to non-existent, but the idea is so attractive that one would strongly wish for it to be true, and this should serve as an adequate stimulus to seek evidence. The evidence might be of three kinds, direct measures of the deferral of onset of illnesses of special relevance, more global assessments of the total burden of morbidity in a community, or demonstration of improved health.

DIRECT MEASURES OF ILLNESS

The diseases of special concern include ischemic heart disease, stroke, hypertension, diabetes, cancer, arthritis, and other major causes of disability in older persons. Data on the occurrence of these illnesses that are other than anecdotal and highly selected are extremely sparse. For example, in seeking explanations for the prolonged decline in mortality from ischemic heart disease in the United States, information on whether the incidence had declined in parallel with the death rates is needed. If both were declining, then medical care need not be invoked as a cause of the decrease; however, if incidence were constant while mortality decreased, then improved medical care would be a candidate for the explanation. The few data that have been brought forward are equivocal and contradictory.[2] If we are unable to determine whether the incidence of heart attacks has decreased by some 30 to 40 percent over a period of twenty years, then we surely do not have in hand information on the rather more refined question of whether the age at onset of first myocardial infarction is increasing. Obtaining more information on some of the other causes of disability will be much more difficult than is true for heart attacks.

GLOBAL ASSESSMENTS

Some indices of change in the total burden of illness and disability in a community might be derived from the records of organizations, such as the Kaiser-Permanente Health Plan, that provide fairly comprehensive medical care to a fairly unselected population group. These data are seriously deficient with respect to minor illness and the set of pleasures incorporated in the jargon term, "quality of life." Another major problem with this source of information is that changes in medical care procedures may entirely obscure trends of illness. For example, advances in the treatment of stroke patients have resulted in many cases coming to medical attention that previously would not have been seen. Thus, the records of a medical care system may reflect an apparent increase in the frequency of a disease which may in actuality be unchanged or even decreasing.

DEMONSTRATIONS OF IMPROVED HEALTH

If morbidity is deferred, and thus compressed into a fewer number of years preceding death, then the antecedent years might well be a time of enhanced health, and that should be a researchable matter. Nothing establishes more sharply the need for a clear and precise definition of a phenomenon than a proposal to make it the subject of research. Research is based on counting things, and a thing cannot be counted very well unless it is given a name and differentiated from all those other things. If someone wishes to study health, then health must be defined, and health shares with many other matters the characteristic that although everyone knows what it is, a useful definition is difficult to propound. Relatively few population-based studies of health have been conducted, and the first of these of which I am aware was the study of the epidemiology of health of ten and eleven year old school children conducted by the Kent Pediatric Society in the early 1950s.[3]

In that research, the World Health Organization's (WHO) definition of health was used as the philosophical starting point. It declares that health is a state of complete physical, mental and social well-being and not merely the absence of disease or infirmity. This may serve well enough as a statement of intent or aspiration, but it cannot be incorporated directly into a research protocol. The pediatricians of Kent evolved a multipart solution: a clinical examination, chest x-ray, tests of muscular strength and endurance, an intelligence evaluation, and a personality assessment. Taking the results of these examinations jointly, the study group was divided into three subsets, from not so healthy to super healthy, and allocation to those classes was related to information obtained by questionnaire on characteristics of family, growth, and development of the children, health and habits of parents, and the home environment, all matters hypothesized to have something to do with determining the state of health.

Whether the children at the upper ends of the distributions of the measured traits and abilities satisfy the WHO definition of health is, I suppose, arguable. I find the WHO definition uncomfortably vague; too vague to evaluate. However, it was used in another important study of human health, that was conducted in Alameda County, California, by Breslow, Belloc, and colleagues.[4]

Morbidity and disability data were obtained by questionnaire, and deaths were ascertained by searching the State files. The well-being included in the WHO statement was studied by asking people how energetic they were, how happy and pleased with themselves they felt, and the extent to which they participated in social and community affairs. However, for the most part, other reports emanating from this study have presented the relations between various personal attributes and habit and the risk of illness and death. Thus, despite espousal of the WHO verbiage, in practice, health was equated with longevity and the absence of disease.

Reed and colleagues have undertaken some analyses of the healthy members of a cohort of Japanese-Americans enrolled in a study of ischemic heart disease in Honolulu.[5] Persons with clinically manifest disease and with high values on some biochemical and physiological variables were excluded, and the remainder were declared to be healthy. This implicitly defined health as the absence of disease and absence of the best identified immediate precursors of disease.

Dubos wrote[6]: "Clearly, health and disease cannot be defined merely in terms of anatomical, physiological, or mental attributes. Their real measure is the ability of the individual to function in a manner acceptable to himself and to the group of which he is a part." This introduces some concepts different from the positive sense of wellbeing. It is very similar to the definition offered by Talcott Parsons, that health is the ability to perform socially valued categories of tasks.[7] These are, I think, very attractive as starting points for the study of health, but as with the WHO definition, they require the explication of tests, examinations, and measures before any research can be initiated. These definitions suggest two very different approaches, one based on measurement of the abilities or accomplishments of individual study subjects, and the other based on some external perception of the social value of an individual. With either approach a further option exists; whether a single scale shall be applied to all persons, or whether a person should be evaluated on a scale unique to himself/herself, or to some subset of peers. The point is that a person of limited endowment may function extremely well within those limitations, and may be as socially useful as another person in a more exalted role. Value judgments are likely to serve up a higher score for the latter person if a single scale is employed.

Whatever decisions are made on these matters, the measurements needed do not reduce to one or a few axes, but must be multifactorial.[8] Health, in these terms, cannot be considered to be unidimensional. I believe that it is, however, definable in terms that can be used in the conduct of research into the nature and the determinants of health. This may promote the exploration of the concept of the compression of morbidity and allow an evaluation of the benefits of deferring illness.

Whether the compression of morbidity hypothesis is correct or not is unknown. I suspect that the effect, if present, will not be large. However, the value of an hypotheses is a function of the extent to which it stimulates useful research. Compression of morbidity should stimulate research.

REFERENCES

1. Fries, J. F. Aging, natural death, and the compression of morbidity. *New England Journal of Medicine*, 303:130–135, 1980.
2. Havlik, R. J. and Feinleib M. (editors). *Proceedings of the Conference on the Decline in Coronary Heart Disease Mortality*. MIH Pub. No. 79-1610. Washington, D.C.: U.S. DHEW, 1979.
3. The Kent Pediatric Society. *A Study in the Epidemiology of Health*. Kent, England: Kent Health Department, 1954.
4. Berkman, L. F. and Breslow, L. *Health and Ways of Living*. New York: Oxford University Press, 1983.
5. Reed, D., personal communication.
6. Dubos, R. *Mirage of Health*. Garden City, New Jersey: Anchor, 1959.
7. Parsons, T. Definitions of health and illness in the light of American values and social structure. In: Jaco, E. G., (editor): *Patients, Physicians, and Illness*. New York: The Free Press, 1958.
8. Stallones, R. Human ecology and human health. Presentation: Life Planning Center Symposium, Tokyo, 1975.

The Biological Constraints
on Human Aging:
Implications for Health Policy
Panel Discussion

Dr. Henry Aaron: There are two questions which were confused in the preceding discussion. One is whether, biologically, we are heading toward rectangularization. The second concerns the implications such a biological development would have for health care costs. Let me state my hypothesis at the outset; one can infer nothing about health care costs from the alleged rectangularization of mortality.

I am willing to give Dr. Fries his biology. I found the discussion of Dr. Hayflick thought-provoking, but for this purpose I want to put those aside. There are a number of reasons why I think one can infer nothing about the future of health care costs from rectangularization. First, there is the fundamental question of what causes the rectangularization. If it comes as a result of "freebies," that's one story, but the story is quite different if the rectangularization occurs as a result of extensive maintenance work on the machine that enables it to function without significant decline until it collapses in a heap. Thus, some of the factors contributing to rectangularization have unquestionably raised health care costs dramatically. The most noticeable is antibiotics, which have spared millions of people cheap early deaths in order to die costly later ones. I say that not in any denigration of antibiotics, they are absolutely miraculous advances that have improved the well-being of humanity. I am simply suggesting one should distinguish the issue of cost from the question of whether something is good, on balance, and worth having. In the same connection, a recent study done within the government suggested that if we could eliminate coronary artery disease overnight, health care costs would increase. Again, the reasons are similar, although the contrast between the cost of the cause of death in this case and the cost of eventual death from another cause is not as dramatic as in the case of antibiotics.

A second issue concerns a line late in the paper, "Given a present knowledge there is little prospect of the biological limit of life being extended." However, one would have said in 1940, given present knowledge, that such things as organ transplants were impossible because of the obviously known and virtually impossible problem of rejection. I'm not prepared to accept a "given present knowledge" assumption that puts aside the issue of biological life even supposing there is a fixed limit. We are entering a new age of research as a result of genetic investigations.

Dr. Robert Kane: A few months ago I was amused by an article in the Wall Street Journal which said that the only group that made worse predictions than economists were demographers. It seems to me that as we enter into this debate we are merging the worst of two worlds. One of the things that we need to take into consideration is that the data are insufficient to draw any conclusions, which means that the probability of prolonged discussion is increased. One of the things we can predict with certainty is that however bad the data were with regard to morbidity in this country, they will be worse. Last year a whole new system of payment was introduced to the hospitals which will change the way people record diseases. At the risk of being facetious, we can make dramatic changes in the prevalence of disease more by payment systems than we can by anything else, which would support the economic approach to health care.

On a more serious level, I think we need to be very careful about how we use definitions. Already this morning we have begun to drift a bit. Ms. Brody tried to bring us back this morning to talking about the difference between medical care and health care and the broader definition of what is meant by long term care and disability. We are beginning to confuse terms like morbidity and disability. They are really different kinds of things that are measured differently and counted differently and, indeed, may have a different etiology. As we began to look at policy questions, I think it is very important that we be sure that we know on what we are trying to make policies.

We need to clarify that in projecting our models for what the situation is going to be like in the future, we are dealing with a very dynamic situation and it is very dangerous to use cross-sectional data to extrapolate. It is erroneous to assume that the 85-year old 20 years from now will face the same financial problems that the 85-year old today faces. It is probably equally erroneous to assume that the 85-year old 20 years from now will be in the same morbidity or disability shape that the 85 year old of today is in. Now, the problem is that we don't know what the shape will be. The margin of error is likely to be at least as great for their health status as it is for their economic status. One needs to be very cautious in trying to interpret these rather naive, straight line extrapolations, whether they are made on the basis of economics or epidemiology.

The other important point that we can't neglect is the real contribution of epidemiology to this discussion: the obvious but often overlooked importance of the heterogeneity of the population and particularly the heterogeneity of the elderly population. We have a tendency to slip into discussing the elderly as though they were a homogeneous group. They are not anything more than the young or the middle-aged, or whatever sort of grouping terms we would like to use. We know that for subgroups of that population, medical care, especially medical care financing, is terribly important. It is differentially important for different people at different levels of risk.

Finally, I would like to remind us that we make different decisions when we talk about policy and when we talk about individual behaviors. It is important to remember that there are a number of people who have made very strong statements about the excess zeal of medical technologies and the need to constrain investments in this kind of activity. Then when they themselves enter the risk pool they make individual decisions about their own care that are exactly the opposite of the recommendations they made for policy in general. That is a part of human nature and we are going to have to accept it. I certainly plan to do exactly the same thing when my turn comes. I think we need to recognize that not everything is as rational as we would like to believe it is.

Dr. Steven Schroeder: I would like to note a different trend that is having the opposite effect of Dr. Fries theory when it comes to medical care consumption. If people have higher expectations of functions as they age, their threshold for seeking care is going to lower. They will, therefore, have earlier extraction of their cataracts, earlier plastic surgery, earlier treatment of their failing hearing, and so forth. While this may not change morbidity, it is a change in the threshold at which they want the morbidity improved. I see that as a major trend that counteracts the good news that Dr. Fries gave. It is still good news in terms of policy expectations, but is bad news in terms of health care costs.

Dr. Leon Eisenberg: There is a law I invented a number of years ago; namely that "nothing ever costs less." Any promise we issue of reduced costs is an invitation to disaster. My feeling about the argument Dr. Fries has presented is that it is irrelevant to health policy. Whether we believe there is a limit or not, we certainly will want to prevent or delay morbidity. However, none of us, including Dr. Fries, would expect that by the year 2000 we can reliably expect to lower health care costs because morbidity will have been compressed by that time.

I am persuaded that when it comes to understanding the genetic limits to any biological phenomenon, an opportunity to observe identical genomes in different environments is required. In the 1930s, Japanese growing up in Japan grew a full 2 inches less than Japanese growing up in California. If you had been studying genetic height potential of Japanese in Japan, you would have come to a very different conclusion than the one you would have drawn in California, even though the genetic mix was exactly the same. Today Japanese in Japan grow as much as Japanese in California, maybe even faster, because the economic differential has turned around. It turns out that eating has something to do with growing. There are a variety of other instances in which our conclusions about the potential of the genome are extremely dependent upon the environment in which the genome is found.

We must confront Dr. Leaf's point about the importance of preventive activities to which we are not only devoting very little and even penalizing the conscientious physician who attempts to conduct such activities. The U.S. reimbursement scheme must have been designed by somebody who is a friend of technology. I tell our medical students, "Before you ask the patient how he feels, think twice because he might tell you. If he tells you, it will take time, and if it takes time, your income will go down." If you are a gastroenterologist and you stick a tube into some orifice, regardless of what you see, you are reimbursed at six times the rate that you get if you spend time taking the history and doing a physical. Physicians' encouragement to stop smoking is said to be very ineffective, but conservative estimates are that five percent of patients counseled by physicians *do* discontinue smoking. If that is true, that's five percent of 60 million people, or three million people a year we might save if doctors bothered to become involved in prevention; but only a minority of them do.

We have to look at the kind of measures we use and the valuation we put on life. I have engaged in a futile correspondence for the last two years with the Centers for Disease Control in Atlanta. Those of you who read the *Morbidity and Mortality Weekly Reports* (MMWR) will have noticed that every month or so they publish a table entitled "Years of Life Lost in the U.S. Per Cause of Disease." If you read that table closely, you will see that the years of life lost are the difference between the age at which death occurred and *age 65*. Thus, deaths at 65 and deaths older than 65 *do not count as years of life lost*. The argument for this is that the table is intended to focus attention on preventable causes of disease in the young. It makes a difference. Their mode of calculation by the use of age 65 makes accidents the leading reason for loss of life. Heart disease drops to third on that list. When Dorothy Rice, Carl White and Jack Feldman did their calculation in the Institute of Medicine study using the current data for life expectancy, heart disease topped the list.

Thus, in the public health statistics we use, it makes a difference whether you think elder years are important. Certainly the moment you began to count income in deciding the value of a procedure, then you are not worth anything if you are over 65. You are not only not making money, but you are costing money because you are drawing from Social Security. You are worth less if you are black, you are worth less if you are a woman and you are a housewife. The moment you use the dollar as a way of measuring health outcomes you devaluate health and life. The last calculation I saw of the cost benefit of giving people 65 and over influenza vaccine is that there would be a net *cost* (rather than savings) of $100 a year per year of healthy life gained. Should we not give influenza vaccine to people 65 and older, because it is cheaper to let them die? I think not.

Ms. Elaine Brody: When we are talking about morbidity, as Bob Kane pointed out, we are talking about disability. When we are talking about health policy, we have to focus on disability and the cost to the system. I have been hoping that another kind of disability would be addressed by some of the people around the table, mental disability. Not only do we have an increasing number of older people who are experiencing Alzheimer's disorder or related diseases, but we have high rates of depression among the elderly. Of course, disability has been strongly implicated in the etiology of depression. We also have more people with developmental disabilities who are living into old age than ever before. I would like to broaden this discussion and hear from other people about the implications for health policy of mental as well as physical health, even though the two are very closely linked and can't be sorted out from one another in many instances.

Dr. Donald Young: When I first read Dr. Fries' paper I suffered from the advantage of knowing nothing about the subject. Now I suffer from the advantage of knowing more than I want to know. The question really is policy relevance. It has been suggested that the subject is not policy relevant. I think that whether it is or not, the information could conceivably be used in a political environment by those who wish to support their position. If you want to foster more resources into prevention and earlier interventions in life, you could certainly marshal arguments based on the paper, accurate or not. On the other hand, it could also be used on the opposite side. The question was raised about expenditures in the last years of life. That is a very significant policy issue and one that can be translated into immediate problems that I in my current job have to deal with. It centers around the question of why doctors and hospitals intervene the way they do. If there were a way of knowing that an individual patient was on the downslope of the rectangularization curve, I think that would be a very important piece of information. My initial response as a doctor is to say that I'll order a rectangularization level and after I have three of them, I'll know what treatment to pursue. If there was some way that you could gather that information, it could have significant practical implications. When one makes adjustments or changes in prices for certain levels of service or even when one looks at malpractice, if one knew where a patient was on the rectangularization curve, it would have immense importance. Those decisions are going to be made one way or another. Resources are going to be committed to intensive care units either increasingly or decreasingly. Therefore, any more we can learn and understand about it seems to me as a policy maker to be potentially very useful in clarifying my thinking.

Dr. Grant Rodkey: I think that Dr. Fries' model is very important and the concept is very important. I agree that whether it is true or not, it would be wonderful if it is. There is also a significant problem in the question or whether it makes any difference.

Emotional attitudes really drive our activities more than rational activities when we are making health policy at the extremes of life. The general attitude is to save money on health care, but when it comes to my care, money is no object. Dr. Stallones neatly stated it when he said he would regard his own death as unnatural. We can all relate to that.

Rebuttal

James F. Fries, MD

It has been a stimulating hour for me. I will review some of the points that I did not agree with. Dr. Hayflick expresses concern that if we focus on prevention, money will be siphoned away from medical research at the National Institutes of Health. I agree with him in that I think we spend a pathetically small amount on research in medicine. We are very irresponsible in sending products out into the marketplace that are not adequately tested. However, we need a complementary scientific establishment which involves epidemiology and some of the issues of the last hour, not any decrease in the biomedical program.

On the issue of long-term care, the demand is increasing, will increase further, and is a major national problem that needs planning. Not as urgently as Mr. Ball suggested, but it does need planning. The reason that it is a big problem is the number of people coming into the age group who sometimes require long-term care.

Prevention is another issue that arose during the papers and discussion. There are some other people whom I would call pessimists who argue that "You can't change human nature." You can't for example, get people to stop smoking. And if you can get them to stop smoking, what difference will it make? "Another disease will come along to take its place." Let's take physician cigarette smoking for example. In 1960, a reliable estimate of the proportion of physicians who smoked was 79 percent, compared to a population smoking rate of 58 percent. It is now six percent of physicians who smoke, and among our medical students only one percent smoke cigarettes. So, changes can occur and the changes can be striking.

I really don't want to go over the arguments that Dr. Hayflick raises in his paper about whether the life-span has or has not increased since three million years ago. It apparently did go up by a total of 10 years between three million and 100,000 years ago, which is a rate of seconds per century. I also agree with Dr.

Hayflick that there is no way that you can pick up very small changes in life extension. We do have enough data to show that the maximum lifespan has not been exceeded since 1928 in this country. There has not been a major change because the laws of large numbers would, in fact, have shown us this.

As Dr. Leaf pointed out it does not really matter anyway because whether the target is moving or not, the question is whether you are closing in on it. That is essentially the policy question. Whether it goes up seven months in a century, the optimistic estimate of the Bureau of the Census, or whether it is absolutely stationary is not crucial to the argument.

Natural death is not recorded because it is illegal to put it on death certificates. I also think the gene pollution argument is a minor one. We are going to see trivial impacts. Most people with such defects who are now surviving have relatively low reproductive capabilities.

I agree with almost everything Alex Leaf said. I want to add a couple of additional caveats. He said that I assumed that no new chronic diseases or few diseases like an AIDS epidemic would come along: that is true. I also am assuming no nuclear holocaust, and no biomedical breakthroughs. I don't know of any serious scientist who believes that if we are thinking of the next 25 years, that we are talking about changing the genetic clock of aging at the DNA level. If we developed the capability to do that, its social advisability would have to be very thoroughly debated; but it is not yet on the scientific horizon. And vitamin C, lydocaine intravenously, and jogging 200 miles a week are not going to change the life-span of the human species.

I agree with Dr. Stallones' comments almost in their entirety. I particularly wanted to echo his call for more research and data. Until we have the data and the data are of good quality, then we cannot draw the kinds of conclusions that we would like and we can't develop the rational policy we should follow.

I wanted to amplify Dr. Aaron's point to indicate that there are two scenarios that we can follow, and they depend in part upon where we place our resources. It is entirely possible to place resources after the illness occurs, and one can predict from the compression of morbidity model that you will pay even more money for even smaller increments of health if you do that. You could at least put some of the resources, perhaps 10 percent, into prevention and try to prolong the living part, rather than prolonging the dying portion of life.

There are a lot of power groups around and the political process is very difficult to predict. I have less confidence in the direction that the country will take, in terms of how to expend its resources in a wise way, than I do about the accuracy and nuances of the theory.

CHAPTER 3

Institutional versus Community Health Care of the Elderly: The Delicate Balance of Social Policy Position Paper

Elaine M. Brody, MSW

Notwithstanding the assigned title of this paper, institutional care and community care of the elderly are not in competition. To frame the issue as one *versus* the other obscures the real problems and ignores the solid body of information that has been developed during the past two decades. A balanced social policy should permit determination of the plan that is most appropriate to the needs and preferences of each individual and family at a particular time. To achieve that goal, it is necessary to develop and fund not only institutional care and in-home care, but also the other services and facilities that are essential components of the continuum of long-term support for the elderly.

Such concepts are not new, of course, but have permeated the literature for 15 years. Efforts to conceptualize the continuum of care and to identify its components were made as early as 1973,[1] and models of the continuum have been developed.

The Health Resources Administration defines long term care as:

> . . . those services designed to provide diagnostic, preventive, therapeutic, rehabilitative, supportive and maintenance services for individuals . . . who have chronic physical and/or mental impairments in a variety of institutional and nonin-

Women, Work, and Care of the Aged: Mental Health Effects, National Institute for Mental Health Grant #MH35252.

stitutional health care settings, including the home, with the
goal of promoting the optimum level of physical, social and
psychological functioning.[2]

The components of the long-term care continuum should be
available in sufficient quantity and quality to serve an elderly
population whose needs are heterogeneous to change over time. To
ensure the matching of individuals and families with the appropriate
service packages, methodologies have been developed that assess
the needs of elderly people.[3] Those assessments must be complemented by assessments of the capacities of their informal social
support systems (family and friends) to meet the needs identified,
and by linkages to connect the people concerned with formal
services (government and private agencies) that supplement the
available informal services.

Major streams of research and many program efforts have
attempted to identify the size and characteristics of the target
populations, to create and evaluate the different services needed,
and to compare the costs of those services. Other research has
examined the informal or family support system—the role it plays
vis-à-vis the formal system, the identity of the family caregivers,
and the effects they experience as a result of caregiving. In the
main, however, dollar cost studies and social cost studies have
proceeded independently of each other.

Progress toward creating an appropriate system of care is
hampered by constantly repeating stereotyped and incorrect notions.
Therefore, information will be summarized here that has a bearing
on the issue of institutional care vis-à-vis community care. The
interrelated questions to be considered in turn are as follows:

- Do institutions and community services serve the same popu-
lation?
- Is there a policy "bias" in favor of institutional care?
- Is home care cheaper than institutional care?
- Would expanding home care insure cost reductions?
- Should families increase their caregiving activities?

POPULATIONS SERVED

Do institutions and community based services (including home
health care) serve the same population? This question speaks
directly to the misconception that large proportions of institutional-

ized people need not be there. It has been established that older people in institutions differ significantly from the noninstitutionalized elderly in their demographic, health, and social characteristics.[4] The institutionalized elderly are a full decade older than the noninstitutionalized. Due both to the discrepancy in life expectancy between men and women and because men marry women younger than they are, older men are more likely than women to have a spouse on whom to depend and thus to avert or delay admission to nursing homes. As a result, women outnumber men in institutions in a ratio of about three to one.

Most residents of institutions have a mental problem; 50 to 60 percent have senile dementia (compared with 5–7 percent of the noninstitutionalized) and at least another 17 percent have a functional mental disorder. In comparison with the noninstitutionalized elderly, they also have many more disabling physical ailments which result in extremely poor functional capacity. For example, 86 percent of residents need help in bathing, 68 percent in dressing, 65 percent with mobility and 32 percent with eating; 45 percent are incontinent; 32 percent have impaired hearing, 26 percent have impaired speech; 34 percent have arthritis, and 11 percent have paralysis due to stroke (for more complete summary see 6).

Those data do not fully explain, however, why residents are in nursing homes since residents are outnumbered in a two to one ratio by equally disabled old people who are not in institutions.[7] Compared with the total elderly population, many fewer of the institutionalized are married (15 percent vs. 56 percent). Sixty percent of residents are widowed, 6 or 7 percent are separated or divorced, and 20 percent had never married. Fewer residents have at least one living adult child, 50 versus 82 percent of all older people; more of those children have only one child rather than two or more, and they have fewer daughters.[8] When seriously impaired older people live in the community, they live with their families.[9]

When the institutionalized elderly do have families, their family members often have incapacities that preclude extended or arduous caregiving. Surviving spouses of the institutionalized are likely to be in advanced age. Just as the elderly residents are a decade older than the non-institutionalized aged, their adult children are older, being in late middle age or even early old age. Catastrophic illnesses or deaths among these aging children often are the precipitants for institutionalization of the parent.[10] Though most residents have some family ties, 10 percent are without anyone at all to name as "next-of-kin"[4] and the family resources of others are very slender.

Many of the same individuals are part of both the nursing home population and the home care population. Long-term care has been described by S. Brody as consisting of long-term long term care (LTLTC) and short-term long term care (STLTC).[11,12] About half of those who are admitted to nursing homes in the course of a year stay less than three months. These are the short-term stayers, having been admitted for terminal care or for short-term rehabilitation or convalescence.[13] Some of those who are discharged alive become home care recipients. Residents who are the long-stayers most often are supported by Medicaid,[4] and people with dementia undoubtedly predominate among them.[13] The proportion of residents whose primary source of payment is Medicaid rises as the length of stay increases, in part reflecting the spend-down process.

Moreover, the needs of older people are not static, but change over time. While only 5 percent of the elderly are in institutions at any given time, 25 percent of all older people will spend some time in such a facility in the course of their lives. Moreover, because of their changing needs, there is an enormous amount of movement of older people between their own homes, hospitals, and STLTC before they become true LTLTC residents. Even then they often return to hospitals and then back either to the previous nursing home or to another.

In sum, the long-stay population in nursing homes is very different from the total elderly population. It does resemble a subgroup of disabled older people who are not institutionalized, but the latter have substantially more social supports in the form of family. It has been established that the vast majority of the institutionalized are appropriately placed in nursing homes. Every effort should be made to prevent admissions of those who do not require such care. However, because the needs of older people change over time, their status as short-term nursing home residents, long-term residents, hospital patients, and community residents shifts constantly. The effect of the prospective payment systems in hastening or preventing this movement is not yet known.

POLICY

Is there a policy "bias" in favor of institutional care? The oft-repeated phrase "bias in favor of institutional care" implies that institutional care has been funded adequately, even liberally, while home care has not. That phrase itself introduces a bias. It is certainly true that there are gross discrepancies in the dollar amounts spent for medical care, nursing home care, and in- home care. In fact, the ratio of expenditures for medically-oriented services to health/social services for the long-term support needs of the non-institutionalized elderly has been called "The Thirty-to-One Paradox."[14] But both community care *and* institutional care have been under-funded, as have other services and facilities on the continuum of care. *The real bias is against disabled old people who need long-term care of any kind, and against their families.*

The scarcity of home care services has been so thoroughly documented as to be notorious. Problems of scarcity and underfunding are compounded by the fragmentation of existing services and entitlements:

> Health services for the aged are multiple, parallel, overlapping, non-continuous and, at the very least, confusing to the elderly consumer. Rarely do they meet the collective criteria of availability, accessibility, affordability, adequacy and accountability or offer continuity of care in a holistically organized system. Planning for health services for the aged is similarly confused. Parallel systems of services have their own planning mechanisms. As a result, the various planning efforts overlap, contradict and are unrelated one to the other.
> Virtually all the services are funded by differing public money streams and have varied administrative arrangements, widely ranging eligibility requirements and different benefits for the same or similar services.[14]

A government task force on home health services concluded that under current legislation, home health services as provided by various agencies "defied coordination."[7]

A number of demonstrations have been mounted that attempt to overcome such problems through structural integration of services or mechanisms that integrate them (e.g., via "channeling" or case management). Findings of the demonstrations are not all in and, in any case, will be difficult to evaluate since they used different research designs, different data collection systems, and focused on different variables in assessing the impact of their programs (see 15 for review). In additions, they focus on different target populations and have different service configurations. All of them depend on waivers that will operate only until the demonstration funding runs out.

Despite calls for a family-focused social policy, there is almost a total lack of family-focused services to support and relieve overburdened family caregivers who are at risk of experiencing a negative impact on their mental and physical health. For example, temporary relief such as day care and respite care exist in some form in some places, but are not universally or adequately available. There is limited regular public or private funding for their consistent support; the programs that do exist are episodic, discontinuous, and vary greatly among the states.[16]

The size of the nursing home population has been depressed artificially by government policy. The United States has one of the lowest proportions of institutionalized older people in the developed countries. The growth rate in our bed supply has not kept pace with the growth in the number of heaviest users of nursing home care, those 85 years of age and over.[17] Cost-containment efforts such as moratoriums on construction, re-classification of patients to lower, less costly, levels of care, capping of reimbursement, and low, fixed-rate Medicaid reimbursement, offer strong incentives to deny admission to "heavy care" Medicaid eligible patients, most of whom undoubtedly suffer from Alzheimer's disease or a related disorder.[18]

In the past, such patients increased overall health costs because they were the ones most likely to back-up in costly hospital beds. Moreover, the Government Accounting Office (GAO) cites the finding of the Inspector General that some nursing homes discharge "undesirable" Medicaid patients to high-cost hospital beds.[19] It has been estimated that there are between one and nine million unnecessary hospital days annually[17] and that the Hospital Insurance Trust spends more than $1 billion a year in acute hospital fees for those waiting to enter nursing homes.[20] Prospective payments systems will close even that inappropriate, temporary avenue for care, but may open up STLTC. The net result is that those who need nursing home care the most may not be able to obtain it. The social/health costs to them, to their families, and ultimately to society have not been calculated.

In addition to under-bedding, the nature and quality of nursing home care has been so under-attended and under-financed as to be a national disgrace. Apart from the outright abuses that have been the subject of a plethora of Congressional hearings, books, and articles, basic health services in institutions are often grossly inadequate. Despite the multiple disabilities of residents noted above, the 1977 National Nursing Home Survey reported that among Medicare or Medicaid-certified Skilled Nursing Facilities (SNFs), 24.9 percent, 24.8 percent, and 27.1 percent routinely provided physical, occupational or speech and hearing therapies respectively.[21] Further, though 75 percent of the residents are dependent for one or more activities of daily living (ADL), in the previous year only 35 percent of them had received any therapy; 13.7 percent received physical therapy, 5.9 percent occupational therapy, and 0.9 percent speech or hearing therapy. As S. Brody points out, there is virtually no rehabilitation for long-stay patients.[22]

The most glaring inadequacies, however, are in the sphere of mental health care and social/recreational services that affect the quality of life. There are no federal standards for mental health care in nursing homes despite the fact that a minimum of 80 percent of the residents have a mental problem.[13] A survey by the American Psychiatric Association (APA) points out that the general practitioners who provide most of the medical care rarely call for consultations from psychiatrists who, in turn, are inexperienced in dealing with an aged population.[23] The Social Security Act's *Conditions of Participation* (405.1130 Social Services) give a token nod to social work and activity therapy, but do not require that such staff be professionally trained.

The Long Term Care Facility study[24] made a searing indictment of the lack of attention to psychosocial services in nursing homes. It pointed out that in most facilities there was a very limited understanding of the importance of psychosocial services. The goal of enriching the residents' daily environment was frequently cited in written policies, but rarely implemented in practice. Personnel were not oriented to psychosocial needs or rehabilitation concepts. Less than half of the patients had any psychosocial data at all on their charts. Less than half (49.2 percent) of the facilities had any social work staff and when they did, there were no requirements that they be professionally trained or full-time. About one-quarter of the facilities (26.3 percent) had a full-time social worker. A similar pattern obtained with respect to activities personnel, and psychologists are virtually absent.

The bulk of resident care in nursing homes is given by nonprofessional, untrained staff. Yet, the APA survey found that even in nursing homes certified for Medicare and Medicaid, the necessity for pre-training aides has been ignored for all practical purposes, despite some lip services in federal regulations. Tens of thousands of "patient care" personnel are largely, if not totally, ignorant of the requirements involved in caring for sick old people, and in-service programs have been of very limited scope.[23]

Given the inescapable fact that nursing home care in many facilities leaves much to be desired, it is a nonsequitor to say that institutional care should be eliminated or capped. Since such care is the incontrovertible need for an irreducible (but increasing) proportion of people, the goal should be to improve nursing homes so that their residents can exist at a decent level of health and well-being.

COSTS

Is home care cheaper than institutional care? The call for "alternatives to nursing home care" was spurred largely by the untested assumption that community care would cost less than institutional care and rationalized by the value that community care is better. However, the hard data have yielded some hard truths. As one review stated, " . . . the cost effectiveness of home care for many long-term care patients and the relationships of home care to reduced institutionalization rates has not been demonstrated either in the United States or abroad."[25] Recent demonstration projects have failed to yield consistent evidence of cost savings.[15] For older people as disabled as those in institutions, home care is at least as expensive and probably more expensive than institutional care (e.g., see 7, 26, 27).

While the best of the comparative cost studies include the costs of informal services in their computations, there are other costs that are generally not included. First, there is consensus that it is essential to mobilize and monitor the variety of home services that comprise effective service packages. The fragmentation of the mind-boggling array of formal entitlements and services (though inadequate) baffles even highly-skilled professionals. The task of gaining access to and mobilizing them, therefore, cannot be left to the consumers. As yet, there are no firm data on the administrative costs of that integrative function.

The need for outreach and coordination was well illustrated by the classic GAO study which documented the gross underutilization of programs by those who were eligible. For example, 77 percent of those eligible for food stamps, 52 percent of those eligible for SSI, and 29 percent of those eligible for Medicaid were not using those benefits, possibly because of unawareness of the services or hesitancy to use them.[7]

Second, studies of economic costs have not included either the social/health costs or the opportunity costs of caregiving to families. While a growing and consistent body of literature has documented the negative mental and physical effects many family caregivers experience (e.g., see 28, 29, 30, 31, 32), there is no information at all on the dollar health costs of those resultant problems to them or to the health systems.

In addition, there is a beginning awareness of other actual (until now invisible) dollar costs borne by caregiving families. Apart from data-based suggestions that caregiving *deters* labor-force participation,[33] there is early information to the effect that many women *leave* the labor force because of the needs of older relatives for care. In a Philadelphia Geriatric Center study, for example, 28 percent of a sample of nonworking, married daughters who were engaged in caregiving to elderly mothers had quit their jobs because of parent care.[34] Forty-two percent of that group had family incomes under $15,000 a year while only 115 of the other nonworking women and 6 percent of the working women in the study had such incomes.

Similar information about the relationship between care of the elderly and women in the work force is emerging from other nations (e.g., 35). One review of national data in Great Britain reported that the most common reason for women to have given up their jobs before retirement was to look after a sick relative and identifies those relatives as most likely to be parents and husbands over the age of 65.[36] It also found that about one-fifth of female workers who worked part-time did so on account of responsibility for an elderly or infirm person, and about 12 percent of female shift workers helped a dependent adult every day, usually their mothers or mothers-in-law.

In short, where severely disabled old people are concerned, there is no firm evidence that the dollar costs of community care are less than for nursing home care. That is not to say that costs should be the overriding determinent in the decision-making. Given the wish of older people to remain in their own homes if at all possible, adjusting the fulcrum of society's "delicate balancing" is a question of values.

EXPANSION OF HOME CARE

Would expanding home care insure cost reductions? This question, closely related to the one above, is best answered by quoting the title and summary of a recent GAO report: "The Elderly Should Benefit from Expanded Home Health Care But Increasing These Services Will Not Insure Cost Reductions."[37] The report states that:

> . . . when expanded home health care services were made available to the chronically ill elderly, longevity and client reported satisfaction were improved. These services, however did not reduce nursing home or hospital use or total service costs. . . . the critical policy issue is not whether expanded home care services are less costly than institutional care but, rather, how these services should be organized for maximum efficiency and effectiveness.

While expanded home care and other community-based services might decrease the use of nursing homes by some sub-populations of the elderly (those who are less disabled) *if* adequate sheltered housing and community services were available, the savings would be more than offset by at least two factors. First, the community services would be used not only by those now in nursing homes or those who would otherwise enter those facilities, but also by the two or three times as many chronically ill elderly in the community who are as disabled as the nursing home population. Second, the nursing home beds vacated would be filled by the increasing number of very old disabled people and by those who need and want such care[26] but who now cannot obtain it.

One careful review of cost-comparison projects concludes:

> On balance, the projects (community care) are not confirming a substantial cost-savings from such interventions uniformly across sites. Furthermore, studies that do report cost-savings often focus the cost analysis solely on Medicaid costs. These studies fail to consider certain public expenditures that are usually higher outside of the institution, specifically various welfare and social security payments, housing support, and social services programs. In summary, nursing home expenditures will rise significantly. Expanded programs of community services are highly desirable, but not as cost saving

measures, since services would undoubtedly be used by persons not presently receiving formal or covered long-term care as well as by persons presently covered in institutions. While the availability of noninstitutional services might well improve the living conditions of impaired individuals, it should be treated as a probably addition to—more than a substitute for—services currently covered by public programs.[26]

FAMILY CAREGIVING

Should families increase their caregiving activities? Due to the immense amount of knowledge that has been assembled, the responsible behavior of families in caring for the disabled aged is no longer at scientific issue. Nevertheless, its summarization is mandatory because the topic continues to be subject to widely held myths and misinformation.

Families of the disabled elderly have an excellent track record in caring for and about their elderly family members. Research findings are consistent in reporting that the vast majority (80–90 percent) of health and social services required by older people are provided by the "informal" system, not by the "formal" system of government and agencies. In addition, families provide a home for elderly people who cannot manage on their own. Elderly spouses go to extraordinary (even heroic) lengths to care for each other, often helped by adult children. Adult daughters (and to some extent daughters-in-law) are the principal caregivers to the spouse-less majority of very old people. (But only about 40 percent of all older people have a surviving daughter who is available for caregiving.)[38]

Families invented long term care, responding to the needs of older people sooner and more flexibly, willingly, and effectively than professionals and the formal system.[34] There has been an exponential increase in the demand for long term care because of:

1. the radical rise in the number and proportion of *very* old people (i.e., those who are most vulnerable to age-related disabilities), and
2. the fact that people live longer today after the onset of chronic disease and disability, with the number of years of active life expectancy decreasing with advancing old age.[39,40]

Those trends, combined with the falling birthrate, have resulted in a marked alteration in the ratio of those in need of care to the adult children who are available to provide it. Nevertheless, the evidence indicates that families have not reduced their caregiving activities. To the contrary, at present they provide more care and more difficult care to more older people over longer periods of time than ever was the case in the past.[34]

The vastly increased amount of care provided has not been without cost to the families providing it, however. Research findings are consistent: significant proportions of caregivers experience negative effects, largely in the realm of mental health but also in physical health and in terms of economic strain (see 34 for review). Despite fears to the contrary, the provision of formal services has been found to supplement (not substitute for) family services, and to strengthen their caregiving capacities.[29,41] More formal services simply mean fewer unmet needs but do not supersede family responsibility.[42] Not one research study or one of the recent demonstrations has found evidence of the withdrawal of family supports when formal supports were provided.[43]

The rapid entry of middle-aged women (the traditonal caregivers) into the work force prompted concern that their capacity to provide care might be reduced. Women do not work in order to shirk their other responsibilities; most who work do so because they and their families need the money. The evidence to date is that working women continue to meet their responsibilities to their families, their jobs, and their elderly parents; what they give up when confronted with competing demands for their time and energy is their own free time and opportunities for social and recreational activities.[29,44,45] The older caregiving women are (whether or not they work), the more arduous and time-consuming is the care they provide; they more often take the older person into their own homes, they more often are widowed, and their incomes are lower.[45]

Information is beginning to emerge to the effect that caregiving deters women's labor-force participation[33] and that some daughters leave the work force for parent care after prolonged periods of heavy caregiving that has deleterious effects on their health.[46] Reports from Australia[47] and the United Kingdom[36,48,49] also note the withdrawal of many women from the work force and the reduction in the working hours of others in order to care for older relatives.

It is important to note that "family responsibility" is not a global, undifferentiated concept. What older people want from their children is expressive support (affection, caring contacts, and the sense of having someone on whom to rely). They do not wish to share their children's households. They do not want to rely on their children for income. (Should we ask the grandparent generation to support the great-grandparent generation?) And the elderly do not equate filial "caring" with the doing of household chores or personal care.[34]

IMPLICATIONS FOR LONG TERM CARE

Scientists on both sides of the compression of morbidity controversy agree that the number of people in need of long-term care in the community or in institutions will increase at least for the next few decades.[40,50] The most vulnerable population (those over 85 years of age), for example, will double by the year 2000. Careful projections estimate that the number of nursing home residents will increase by 54 percent by 2000 and by 132 percent by 2030.[26] It was pointed out as long as 15 years ago that the needs of the elderly for help had gone beyond the "self solution" and the "kinship solution," so that societal solutions are required.[51]

Social policy in the United States has made virtually no response to the needs of families providing home care. Respite care and day care programs, for example, are scarce and not universally funded. Familial needs are virtually non-existent as determinants of eligibility for any service. And we do not hear of sabbaticals or flextime for caregivers who work.

Although other speakers at this conference will discuss patterns of care abroad, it is notable that the U.S. is one of the few industrialized nations which does not provide an attendance allowance; more than 60 nations do so under their social security programs.[25,52] Some countries provide social security credits for the years caregivers remain at home, Norway gives pensions to those who have taken care of an elderly or disabled person and grants caregiving wage earners the right to shorter working hours, and in Sweden and the U.K. supportive services are more.[52] Foreign programs consistently use cash allowances rather than the U.S. pattern of in-kind services. One expert argues that cash payments are preferable for a variety of reasons, among which is that "Attendance allowances, by putting decision-making back into the hands of . . . elderly persons, may further reduce dependency and may help to eliminate the harmful stereotypes which diminish their role as normal members of society."[25]

In the United States, patterns of services vary regionally. Though such patterns should depend to some extent on differences in the local ecology and the populations at risk, the states have shown that they cannot be left to their own devices if there is to be equity. For example, the states vary widely, even wildly, in how much they spend for nursing home service for each state elderly resident, in the percentage of their Medicaid programs spent on SNF and ICF services, in their bed/population ratios, in the growth of nursing home expenditures and in reimbursement rates for SNFs and ICFs.[17] The same diverse patterns among the states list in their provision of community care services.

In sum, social policy at present is callous and inequitable rather than delicate and balanced. It can only be reiterated that the task ahead is to develop the services and facilities that appear on the theoretical continuum of care, filling in its gaps by inventing new services and facilities, and seeing to it that they are adequate quantitatively and qualitatively. Special attention should be paid to fiscal and service supports to help the family in its efforts to care for the aged. Current attempts to encourage non-use of the formal system, underpinned by a sanctimonious call for families to return to "old" family values and to increase their caregiving activities, represent an abdication of social responsibility. Sufficient knowledge is available about what is needed to enable public policy to put that knowledge to work. Decisions to do so or not to do so depend on society's values.

REFERENCES

1. Brody, S. J. Comprehensive health care of the elderly: An analysis. *The Gerontologist*, 13(4):412–18, 1973.

2. Health Resources Administration, Division of Long-Term Care. *The Future of Long-Term Care in the United States—The Report of the Task Force*, Washington, D.C.: U.S. Government Printing Office, 1977.

3. Lawton, M. P., Moss, M., Fulcomer, M. C., and Kleban, M. H. A research- and science-oriented multilevel assessment instrument. *Journal of Gerontology*, 37:91–9, 1982.

4. U.S. Bureau of the Census. *1976 Survey of Institutionalized Persons*, Current Population Reports, Special Studies, Series P-23, No. 69, Washington, D.C.: U.S. Government Printing Office, 1978.

5. Brody, E. M. The formal support network: Congregate treatment setting for residents with senescent brain dysfunction. In: Miller, N. E., and Cohen, G. D. (editors), *Clinical Aspects of Alzheimer's Disease and Senile Dementia*. New York: Raven Press, 1981, 301–31.

6. Lawton, M. P. *Environment and Aging.* Monterey, California: Brooks/Cole Publishing Co., 1980, Table 5-3, p. 110.

7. Comptroller General of the United States. *Report to Congress on Home Health—The Need for a National Policy to Better Provide for the Elderly,* Washington, D.C.: U.S. General Accounting Office, HRD-78-19, 1977.

8. Soldo, B. J. The determinants of temporal variations in living arrangements among the elderly: 1960–1970. Doctoral Dissertation, Duke University, 1977.

9. Brody, S. J., Poulshock, S. W., and Masciocchi, C. F. The family care unit: A major consideration in the long-term support system. *The Gerontologist, 18*:556–61, 1978.

10. Brody, E. M., The aging family. *The Gerontologist,* 6:201–06, 1966.

11. Brody, S. J., and Magel, J. DRG: The second revolution, Health care for the elderly. *Journal of the American Geriatrics Society, 32*(9):676–79, 1984.

12. Brody, S. J. Planning for long-term care—implications of the Medicare prospective system. In: *Issues in Planning for Long Term Care,* National Council on Health Planning and Development, Washington, D.C.: U.S. Government Printing Office, 1984.

13. U.S. National Center for Health Statistics. *The National Nursing Home Survey: 1977 Summary for the United States,* Washington, D.C.: U.S. DHEW, PHS, 1979.

14. Brody, S. J. The thirty-to-one paradox: Health needs and medical solutions. *National Journal,* 11:1869–73, 1979.

15. Zawadski, R. T. (Guest Editor). Community-based systems of long term care. *Home Health Care Services Quarterly,* 3&4:209–28, 1983.

16. Meltzer, J. W. *Respite Care: An Emerging Family Support Service.* Washington, D.C.: The Center for the Study of Social Policy, 1982.

17. U.S. General Accounting Office, *Medicaid and Nursing Home Care: Cost Increases and the Need for Services are Creating Problems for the States and the Elderly.* Washington, D.C.: U.S. Government Printing Office, 1983.

18. Brody, E. M., Lawton, M. P., and Liebowitz, B. Senile dementia: Public policy and adequate institutional care. *American Journal of Public Health, 74*:1381–83, 1984.

19. U.S. Office of the Inspector General. *Restricted Patient Admittance to Nursing Homes: An Assessment of Hospital Back-Up,* Secretarial Report. Washington, D.C.: U.S. Government Printing Office, 1980, p. 7.

20. Vladeck, B. Interview. *Older American Reports,* 7 (Nov.):7, 1983.

21. U.S. National Center for Health Statistics. *Advance Data, An Overview of Nursing Home Characteristics: Provisional Data from the 1977 National Nursing Home Survey.* PHS NO. 35, Washington, D.C.: U.S. Department of Health, Education, and Welfare, 1978.

22. Brody, S. J. Rehabilitation in nursing homes. In: Schneider, E. L., et al. (editors), *The Teaching Nursing Home: A New Approach to Geriatric Research, Education, and Clinical Care.* New York: Raven Press, 1985, 147–156.

23. Glasscote, R. M. *Old Folks at Homes: A Field Study of Nursing and Board and Care Homes.* Washington, D.C.: American Psychiatric Association and the National Association for Mental Health, Joint Information Service, 1976.

24. U.S. Department of Health, Education and Welfare, Office of Nursing Home Affairs. *Long-Term Care Facility Improvement Study, Introductory Report.* Washington, D.C.: U.S. Government Printing Office, 1975.

25. Grana, J. M. Disability allowances for long-term care in Western Europe and the United States. *International Social Security Review, February 1983, 207–21.*

26. Fox, P. D., and Clauser, S. B. Trends in nursing home expenditures: Implications for aging policy. *Health Care Financing Review,* Fall 1980, 65–70.

27. Palmer, H. C. The alternatives question. In: Vogel, R. J. and Palmer, H. C. (editors). *Long-Term Care Perspectives from Research and Demonstrations.* Washington, D.C.: Health Care Financing Administration, U.S. DHHS, 1983, 255–305.

28. Sainsbury, P. and Grad de Alercon, J. The effects of community care in the family of the geriatric patient. *Journal of Geriatric Psychiatry,* 4:1, 23–41, 1970.

29. Horowitz, A. *The Role of Families in Providing Long-term Care to the Frail and*

Chronically Ill Elderly Living in the Community. Final Report submitted to the Health Care Financing Administration, U.S. DHHS, 1982.

30. Gurland, B., Dean, L., Gurland, R., and Cook, D. Personal time dependency in the elderly of New York City: Findings from the U.S.-U.K. cross-national geriatric community study. In: *Dependency in the Elderly of New York City*, New York: Community Council of Greater New York, 1978, 9–45.

31. Hoenig, J. and Hamilton, M. Elderly patients and the burden on the household. *Psychiatra et Neurologia*, 152:281–93, 1966.

32. George, L. K. *The Dynamics of Caregiver Burden*. Final Report submitted to the American Association of Retired Persons Andrus Foundation, 1984.

33. Soldo, B. J., and Myllyluoma, J. Caregivers who live with dependent elderly. *The Gerontologist*, 23:605–11, 1983.

34. Brody, E. M., Johnsen, P. T., and Fulcomer, M. C. What should adult children do for elderly parents? Opinions and preferences of three generations of women. *Journal of Gerontology*, 39:736–46, 1984.

35. Hunt, A. *The Elderly at Home*. London: Office of Population Censuses and Surveys, Her Majesty's Stationery Office, 1978.

36. Rossiter, C., and Wicks, M. *Crisis or Challenge? Family Care, Elderly People, and Social Policy*, Occasional Paper No. 8, Study Commission on the Family, London, 1982.

37. U.S. General Accounting Office. *The Elderly Should Benefit from Expanded Home Health Care But Increasing These Services Will Not Insure Cost Reductions*. Washington, D.C.: U.S. General Accounting Office, 1982.

38. Soldo, B. J. *Supply of Informal Care Services: Variations and Effects on Services Utilization Patterns*. Report for contract #HHS-100-80-0158, DHHS, Center for Population Research, Georgetown University, Washington, D.C., 1982.

39. Katz, S., Branch, L. G., Branson, M. H., Papsidero, J. A., Beck, J. C., and Greer, D. S. Active life expectancy. *The New England Journal of Medicine*, 309:1218–24, 1983.

40. Schneider, E. L., and Brody, J. A. Aging, natural death, and the compression of morbidity: Another view. *The New England Journal of Medicine*, 309:854–856, 1983.

41. Zimmer, A. H., and Sainer, J. S. Strengthening the family as an informal support for their aged: Implications for social policy and planning. Paper presented at the 31st Annual Scientific meeting of the Gerontological Society, Dallas, Texas, 1978.

42. Sherwood, S., Morris, S., and Morris, J. N. Relationships between formal and informal service provision to frail elders. Paper presented at 37th Annual Scientific Meeting of The Gerontological Society of America, San Antonio, Texas, 1984.

43. Zawadski, R. T. Research in the demonstrations: Findings and issues. In: Zawadski, R. T. (Guest Editor). *Community-Based Systems of Long Term Care, Home Health Care Services Quarterly*, 3&4:209–28, 1983.

44. Cantor, M. H. Strain among caregivers: A study of experience in the United States. *The Gerontologist, 23*:597–604, 1983.

45. Lang, A., and Brody, E. M. Characteristics of middle-aged daughters and help to their elderly mothers. *Journal of Marriage and the Family*, 45:193–202, 1983.

46. Brody, E. M., Kleban, M. H., Johnsen, P. T., and Hoffman, C. Women who help elderly mothers: Do work and parent care compete? Paper presented at the 37th Annual Meeting of The Gerontological Society of America, San Antonio, Texas, 1984.

47. Kinnear, D., and Graycar, A. *Family Care of Elderly People: Australian Perspectives*. SWRC Reports and Proceedings No. 23, Wales: Social Welfare Research Centre, University of New South Wales, 1982.

48. Jones, D., Victor, C., and Vetter, N. Careers of the elderly in the community. *Journal of the Royal College of General Practitioners*, 33:707–10, 1983.

49. Nissel, M. The family costs of looking after handicapped elderly relatives. *Aging and Society*, 4:185–204, 1984.

50. Fries, J. F. The compression of Morbidity: Miscellaneous comments about a theme. *The Gerontologist*, 24:354–59, 1984.

51. Blenkner, M., Normal dependencies of aging. In Kalish, R. (ed.), *The Dependencies of Old People, Occasional Papers in Gerontology*, #6, Institute of Gerontology, University of Michigan, 1969, 27–39.

52. Gibson, M. J. Women and Aging. Paper presented at International Symposium on Aging, Georgian Court College, Lakewood, NJ, October 19, 1984.

Institutional versus Community Health Care of the Elderly:
The Delicate Balance of Social Policy
A General Policy Perspective

Eugene A. Stead, Jr., MD

It is easy to be a good citizen until one reaches the age where dependency overtakes us. We have not yet found an easy or graceful way for most of us to leave the stage on which we performed adequately as independent persons. Ms. Brody has presented the problems in an excellent fashion and all her remarks fit with my own observations.

The question is what to do in the situation. I know of no way to make dependency as attractive as independence. The devotion of all our resources to the care of the dependent elderly would not make old age as attractive as youth.

We have to face a most difficult issue: What level of care do we want to give to what groups of persons? Professionals in aging have rarely faced this problem directly. They want more of everything and would have the surroundings and personal services equal to that of the independent population.

We have accepted that comatose persons who have dead brains may be declared dead even though circulation and respiration can be maintained. Will we, in time accept dementia as slow dying, and when it disconnects the patient from his/her surroundings, will we make no attempt to prolong life? In a demented person, what is the purpose of the medical procedures, the administration of food and water, the use of antibiotics, the daily vitamins, the polypharmacy? It is not to help the patient enjoy life. Too much of the brain is dead. We care for the partly-dead person because we have not developed an ethical or religious system that allows us comfortably to "call it quits." We are afraid that we will become dehumanized if we don't postpone death. The care is for the living and not for the dying. We face the same issue with birth control and abortion. The egg, sperm, and embryo never complain. It is feelings of the persons who live which are at stake.

When I have cockroaches in my living quarters, candy in every nook and corner, and a refrigerator filled with rancid food, and have stopped bathing, I won't care. My children will be appalled and want to instigate change. They are afraid I'll break my hip and die before I'm found. If I'm institutionalized, what is the minimal acceptable care that society can offer me?

The same ethical considerations and the same feelings of frustration at having no workable ethical frame of reference confront us as we care for patients who have only one chance in 100 of being restored to a life they can enjoy with expensive medical technology. In the old days it was simpler. In 1930, Dean Wilburt Davison, a renowned pediatrician, came to the medically-underserved southeast. He was in great demand as a consultant who could work out a care plan for demented children who placed heavy demands on the family and community. The consultation had some aspects of a festive occasion. When Dean Davison got down to business, he requested everyone except members of the family to leave. He then determined who was going to contribute personal services or money for support of the child. He asked all other family members to leave. The final hard choices were then made by persons who had to implement them from their own resources.

In our day, the family is not dependent on their own resources. They have a variety of community, state, and federal resources to cushion them. Insurance coverage, Medicare, Medicaid, and state and community agencies dilute the feelings of personal responsibility. If we let patients finish the act of dying without intervention, we must ask ourselves: Are we letting demented persons die because we don't want to pay more taxes? Are our actions moving us to tolerate a new holocaust because there is no ethical basis for non-intervention?

It is interesting that we have devised cultural and ethical systems that allow us to kill millions of healthy persons without feelings of guilt. We have a name for that system. We call it war. Until we have a philosophical and ethical system which accepts death as a part of life and acknowledges that the last part of living is the first phase of dying, we will make no progress. How will we develop an ethical base for new types of behavior? I assume that it will come about by forces tangential to problems we are discussing today.

Two changes in our culture have occurred by a tangential approach. Knowledge that cancer is caused by exposure of our bodies to a variety of chemicals has changed much of our behavior. You no longer have to put out ashtrays when doctors congregate in large groups. Workers in chemical plants are forcing management to adopt new methods of reducing exposures. Years ago no one thought that prevention of cancer would be possible and that prevention would produce major changes in our lives. Cancer in many situations is now recognized as the work of humans on biological systems. It is no longer an act of God.

The study of the reproductive cycle and the acceptance of womens' rights has resulted in striking changes in living patterns. Thirty years ago no one would have believed that such striking changes in sexual mores would have occurred by the year 1985. In those days we did not recognize "spouse equivalents."

Eventually, a new generation will come to believe that there are limits to the amount of money and services they are willing to expend for persons who have suffered "brain death" which prevents them from relating in any way to their environment. The concept of partial brain death and ways to deal with it will emerge. By one device or another, a system of behavior compatible with this belief will evolve, and society will permit the partially dead to complete the act of dying in peace.

Many families and doctors have allowed death to come quietly and painlessly to patients with terminal cancer. Patients permanently out of touch with their environment may be allowed to die from infections if they have expressed this desire in a living will, or if the family requests the witholding of anti-microbial drugs.

We need to take a new small step and define the boundaries of partial brain death which permits some demented persons to die as they would have died in the home many years ago. In those days food and drink were offered, but no actions were taken if the patient did not eat or drink.

It will take time and thought to define the syndrome of partial brain death which allows the withholding of antibiotics and of feeding, by spoons, by tubes, and by intravenous fluids. There is no hurry; it took several years to define total brain death and to make organs available for transplantation from a person with a dead brain to a living recipient.

We do not want to move quickly or become involved in legal issues. We simply wish to define the state of partial brain death which allows families not to force food and drink on persons whose brains will never allow them to relate in any meaningful way to his environment. This is a small step, but one that would relieve the suffering of many families.

Meanwhile we struggle with the economics of home and institutional care. I have no objection, because we must fill in time while forces we have not yet anticipated mold our attitudes.

Institutional versus Community Health Care of the Elderly:
The Delicate Balance of Social Policy
A National Policy Perspective

Carroll L. Estes, PhD

Elaine Brody presents an accurate and intelligent assessment of social policy in relation to home care and the important role of family caregivers. She argues for a balanced social policy—that is, a rational continuum of care model which would encompass appropriate levels of quality care all along the way. As she states at the outset, institutional and home health services are not in competition with one another, but rather are a part of a continuum of care. She argues that such a dichotomy of institutional versus home care is incorrect because it sets our conceptualization on the wrong track. She is at her strongest in arguing:

- that the "real bias is against disabled old people who need long-term care of any kind and against their families" (1, p. 7);
- that families and informal caregivers provide most of the care and that there is no evidence that this caregiving is diminishing; and
- that the issue of long term care is well beyond "self-solution" or the "kinship solution."

The major portion of Ms. Brody's paper discusses the dominant stereotypes and incorrect notions pertaining to institutional vs. community-based services, largely the cost-quality debate. Ms. Brody, then concludes her paper with attention to the task ahead— "to develop the services and facilities that appear on the theoretical continuum of care . . . filling its gaps by inventing new services and facilities," noting that "sufficient knowledge is available about what is needed to enable public policy to put that knowledge to work" (p. 21).

Both empirical and political issues are raised. One empirical issue relates to Ms. Brody's argument that those who need nursing home care most may not be able to obtain it. An empirical issue that is raised concerns the availability of needed nursing home beds or supply. From research at the Aging Health Policy Center and studies conducted as part of the Institute of Medicine's current committee on nursing home regulation,[2] we know that:

- Nursing home demand is increasing because of population growth among the elderly and particularly among those age 85 and over, who are the greatest users of service; although the number of nursing home beds has been increasing steadily in the U.S., this growth rate has not kept pace with the increases in the aged population;
- Factors associated with the recent reduction in the growth rate of nursing home beds include high interest rates, high construction costs and difficulty in obtaining financing, (e.g., Certificate of Need (CON) policies and the differential between the state Medicaid and the private rates);
- Approximately 19 states have been identified as having an undersupply of nursing home beds;[3,4,5] and nursing home bed supply has been shown to vary considerably across states (e.g., from a low of 22 beds per 1,000 aged population in Arizona to a high of 89 beds in Wisconsin in 1983).

In spite of the nursing home supply situation, a major problem that Ms. Brody addresses is the unavailability of nursing home beds to those who need them. An important dimension of this problem concerns how the existing beds are used. Evidence suggests that inappropriate utilization continues to be a problem, although some recent data indicate that the residents in nursing homes are more severely impaired than in the past.

The point of my disagreement with Ms. Brody's argument is her assertion that the availability of nursing home placements is at least partly a problem of "under-bedding." Whether or not demand exceeds the supply of nursing home beds, the *problem of access* has *remained*—that is, access for certain populations remains a problem both in states that have been identified as "oversupply" and "undersupply" states in terms of nursing home beds.[4] Access to nursing home beds is limited, particularly for those who are on Medicaid because the reimbursement rates are sometimes substantially below the rates paid by private payers. Access is also limited for those with the greatest physical and mental impairments because these individuals are more costly to provide care for (2, pp. 51–53).

In sum, Brody is correct that states vary, in some cases even "wildly," in nursing home bed supply. The problem of access will not (and, I believe, should not) be resolved by creating more nursing home beds. Increasing bed supply, under current policy, will *not* solve the problem for those most in need of those beds—the very sick, the "old old," those who are female and poor. Present incentives, we all know, encourage quite the opposite. The problem with nursing home beds is more one of *access* for the public-pay heavy care patient than one of supply.

The dangers of expanding nursing home supply through new construction include not only the cost (estimated at $20,000 per bed), but also, as Vladeck[6] and Harrington[7] have argued that new beds will do nothing to alter the inappropriate placement problem, while a self-fulfilling prophecy may result, i.e., the new supply will create its own demand.

Nursing home access at appropriate levels of care could be addressed by several options:[2]

- federal or state policies to prevent facilities from refusing to accept public pay patients (as seven states, including New Jersey have done);[8]
- all-payer regulation for nursing homes to discourage discrimination between public and private-pay patients;
- state contracting for specified beds in nursing homes to guarantee Medicaid patient access; case-mix reimbursement (based on patient characteristics and resources required to provide care); and hospital based swing-beds, for Brody's short-term long term care patient.[*]

I do not believe that our limited resources should be placed on new nursing home beds, but on income-related options and com-

---

[*]This recommendation is similar to Vladeck's and Harrington's to achieve more appropriate utilization of services for different levels of care, while restricting nursing home bed supply to those most in need.

munity based services that can provide alternatives to that institutionalization.

A second empirical issue concerns the continuum of care, which
Ms. Brody correctly identifies as a major and critical policy
direction for the future. Regrettably, recent research conducted by
the Aging Health Policy Center indicates that—contrary to moving
toward the goal of a continuum—we are rapidly and progressively
moving *away from* this goal.[9]

First, there have been reductions in federal outlays both in social
service and health programs, with social services incurring much
larger cuts than health care programs, if Medicare and Medicaid are
included.[10] Compounding these reductions are other trends, notably:

- a pervasive competitive ideology;
- deregulation;
- hospital cost containment policies, such as Diagnosis-Related
  Group (DRGs) hospital reimbursement policies;
- tax policies encouraging the entry of proprietaries in the social
  and home health domains that have traditionally been the
  province of the non-profit sector, and concern with reducing the
  federal deficit by reducing domestic spending.

Our research on community-based health and social services in
32 communities and eight states* is documenting a subtle, but
profound restructuring of the community delivery system.[11] This is
characterized by the vertical and horizontal integration of systems of
care in ways that particularly affect small nonprofit community
health and social service agencies that have traditionally served as
the bedrock on the delivery system.

The proprietory sector is growing in market influence in home
health and nutrition and beginning to move into other areas such as
adult day care. Competitive bidding requirements (partly as a result
of deregulation) and competition with for-profits are forcing non-
profit services agencies not only to bid for short-term contracts

---

*The sample of nonprofit health and social service agencies is comprised of 335 such
organizations representing: home health, homemaker's chore, adult day health, senior centers
and nutrition agencies; community health centers, community mental health centers and
information and referral agencies. Telephone surveys were conducted in both 1983 and
1984.[12]

(threatening their fragile financing and inhibiting long range planning), but also to bid on single reimbursable services—abandoning what they report as the important, more comprehensive service array that their agencies had been providing (e.g., transportation, information and referral, homemaker). In a word, services are becoming "unbundled," or disaggregated and sold separately. Increasingly, it would appear that only those services that can be reimbursed can be offered. The potential result is a growing privatization and fragmentation of community services. Particularly challenged is the ability of community agencies to continue serving low (or no) reimbursement Medicaid and other low income clients.

In addition, the social service system is being "medicalized," as the hospital has moved to the home as a result of hospital cost containment policies such as the Medicare DRG policy.

The restructuring of community services appears to be creating a new dichotomy between medicalized in-home services for the frail elderly (which are growing), and community-based social services (which are shrinking). The concept of the "no care zone" has been introduced,[12] and the marginal but ambulatory frail and non-frail elderly are at risk of being pushed out of the system.

Where does this situation bring us in the context of the political dimension? Retrenchment in federal spending, the federal deficit, and the ideology of competition have unintentionally pushed us *away from*, and undermined, the hopes for a rational continuum of care. Any expansive reading of the federal role in health has been "chilled" at least as it concerns a national force for planning or financing an integrated system of access and service availability across the states.

National policy goals such as access to health care for the poor are being supplanted by autonomous and variable state policy choices. Our research documents that there is less, rather than more, consistency or uniformity of long-term care and health policy across the different states.[13]

The "New Federalism" now places human service demands on the most fiscally vulnerable and politically variable state and local levels of decision making. Decisions about long-term care and health services for the poor, in particular, are thus located precisely where pressures to control social expenses are greatest. This is occurring in the face of Brody's observation that "states have shown that they cannot be left to their own devices if there is to be equity."

In long term care, federal policy is most notable for its absence, or alternatively, for the fact that it is 50 states' policies. The key issues concerning health and the elderly must be understood. They are income and housing, hospital, physician, and nursing home care, and community-based health and social services. The continuance and extension of the present disarticulation of federal, state and local policy will only assure a more fragmented and more costly health care "solution." A long range and intergenerational agenda is needed to achieve an equitable and efficient use of the nation's resources in health. This cannot be achieved without a vital federal role. National policies are required to provide the framework for both public and private action in order to continue to improve the health of the nation at a price we can all afford.

REFERENCES

1. Brody, E. M. Institutional versus Community Health Care of the Elderly: The Delicate Balance of Social Policy. In: Andreoli, K.G., Musser, L.A., Reiser, S.J. (editors). Health Care for the Elderly: Regional Responses to National Policy Issues. New York: The Haworth Press, 1986.

2. Harrington, C. and Grant, L. A. *Nursing Home Bed Supply, Access, and Quality of Care*. San Francisco: Aging Health Policy Center, University of California, submitted for publication 1985.

3. Swan, J. H. and Harrington, C. Estimating undersupply of nursing home beds in the states. In: Estes, C. L., et al. (editors). *Correlates of Long Term Care Expenditures and Utilization in 50 States: Final Report*. San Francisco: Aging Health Policy Center, University of California, 1985.

4. Harrington, C. and Swan, J. H. Medicaid nursing home reimbursement policies, rates, and expenditures. *Health Care Financing Review*, 6(1):39–49, 1984.

5. Harrington, C., and Swan, J. H. Medicaid nursing home expenditures. In: Estes, C. L., et al. (editors). *Correlates of Long Term Care Expenditures and Utilization in 50 States: Final Report*. San Francisco: Aging Health Policy Center, University of California, 1985.

6. Vladeck, B. *Unloving Care: The Nursing Home Tragedy*. New York: Basic Books, 1980.

7. Harrington, C. Public policy and the nursing home industry. *International Journal of Health Services*, 14(3):481–90, 1984.

8. National Citizen's Coalition for Nursing Home Reform (NCCNHR). *Medicaid Discrimination in Long Term Care*. Washington, D.C.: NCCNHR, 1981.

9. Estes, C. L., and Lee, P. R. Medicare and Long Term Care. Paper presented to the American Association for the Advancement of Science, Los Angeles, California, May 29, 1985.

10. Salamon, L., and Abramson, A. J. "Nonprofits and the federal budget: Deeper cuts ahead." *Foundation News*, 26(2):48–54, 1985.

11. Wood, J. B., Fox, P. J., Estes, C. L., Lee, P. R., and Mahoney, C. W. *Public Policy, the Private Nonprofit Sector and the Delivery of Community-based Long Term Care Services for the Elderly: Executive Summary*. San Francisco: Aging Health Policy Center, University of California, 1985.

12. Wood, J. B., Estes, C. L., Lee, P. R., and Fox, P. J., *Public Policy, the Private*

Nonprofit Sector and the Delivery of Community Based Long Term Care Services for the Elderly: Final Report. San Francisco: Aging Health Policy Center, University of California, 1983.

13. Estes, C. L., Lee, P. R., and Newcomer, R. J. and Associates. *Correlates of Long Term Care Expenditures and Utilization in 50 States: Final Report*. San Francisco: Aging Health Policy Center, University of California, 1985.

Institutional versus Community Health Care of the Elderly:
The Delicate Balance of Social Policy
A Regional Policy Perspective

Karl L. Shaner, DrPH

I was traveling in West Texas and I happened to be leaving the town of Pecos at the same time as the afternoon school bus. This was before the advent of the 55 mph speed limit and, since I was driving a small car, I tucked in behind the bus to catch a "draft." We drove along for more than 40 minutes at about 65 mph before the bus stopped for the *first* time to let out a small boy. Since I passed the bus then, I don't know how much further the second stop was.

The point of this story is that there are large parts of Texas and many other Southwestern states in which the distribution of the population makes the delivery of even the most vital services a difficult and expensive task, especially such services that are not mandated by law.

With regard to community services for the elderly, there are obviously demographic limits to the feasibility of some services. Just as health maintenance organization (HMO) planners presently believe that a population base of at least 100,000 is necessary to sustain a viable HMO, I am sure that there are basic criteria in terms of numbers and concentration of elderly persons for the provision of organized "community" services for the elderly. The existence of such limits on organized services dictates that certain community services for the elderly might not be feasible in many smaller towns in Texas, unless they are heavily and continuously subsidized. The prospect for such subsidies is not bright.

We should not, however, despair for the welfare of the elderly residents of such locales. It is my estimation that, in the great majority of such situations, the elderly in these smaller towns are receiving a wide range of assistance and care from relatives, neighbors, and other volunteers in the community, but that these services are not *organized* in the administrative sense. It is the administrative organization and funding of community services for the elderly that appears to be the fundamental problem for discussion.

Ms. Brody has made an excellent case for more adequate organization and funding of community services through examination of the results of the programs and funding mechanisms of several countries and proposals for programs in the United States. The need for such services and programs is difficult to deny. I would, however, raise one issue before joining in praise of the aims of such proposals.

If such programs are to be supported by governmental resources (i.e., taxes), be they state or federal, then it follows that a relatively high degree of organizational and procedural structure must be imposed on them. If service providers are obliged to conform to these organizational and procedural requirements in order to obtain funding, the result may well be that, while the services are uniform, there may be little innovation or adaptation to local needs. We are presently in a time of significant transition—if not revolution—in our health and human services systems and, in the long term we will be better served by encouraging *local* and *voluntary* approaches to the provision of community services for the elderly rather than seeking the "assistance" and the constraints of governmental solutions. I would admit that governmental solutions might guarantee the access of a majority of the elderly to a specified, basic level or range of services; but the imposition of arbitrary structure in a time of transition may not contribute to the development of more innovative or locally appropriate solutions. The attainment of a certain degree of imposed order may indeed facilitate planning, but it does not promote innovation or progress.

My appeal for local initiative and responsibility is consistent with the social attitudes of many Texans who usually have more faith and reliance on their own abilities than in those of government, especially a distant government. Texans tend to believe that problems and solutions have similar locations. For example, if the origins or causes of problems are local, the most effective solutions may also be local. Admitting some responsibility for a problem usually encourages taking some responsibility for the solution. I am suggesting that a potential solution to the funding of some services to the future elderly may lie in that ultimate "local" level—the individual.

To illustrate the logic behind my suggestion, I would like to digress once again. When the Pilgrims came to these shores 360 years ago, they believed that if you became sick, it was because you had done something "wrong." They believed that sickness was a punishment for sin and that good health was evidence of good moral behavior. Then, with the development of the germ theory of disease in the 1800s, this burden of guilt was lifted from the sick. We learned that germs were everywhere and that everyone was exposed to them—sickness was a random event and not caused by the "victim." The whole foundation of health insurance is based on this notion of protection from random events that are not within the control of the individual being insured. During the past 20 years, however, we have begun to more clearly understand the health consequences of our behavior. Today, about two-thirds of the hospital admissions of individuals over 65 are the direct result of such personal, discretionary behavior as cigarette smoking, abuse of alcohol, lack of exercise, poor nutrition, and poor stress management. While this knowledge does little for those current elderly who suffer these conditions, these lessons should not be lost on those who still have the opportunity to choose more healthful behaviors.

Demands on the working age population for massive funding of programs for the elderly are not likely to be answered positively in the near future. We know that the next 30 years will bring an increase in the over 65 population and a decline in the numbers of those under 65. While we must find near-term solutions drawing on public support for the needs of the current elderly, we are not condemned to following those same solutions to their ultimate collapse in the long-term. In this regard, I would like to suggest that certain health and social services for the elderly in the future be funded by mechanisms that, first, rely upon individual responsibility and, second, establish an economic relationship between the behavioral causes of disease and their consequences.

With regard to individual responsibility, there is a concept that has been receiving some discussion recently that might permit individuals during their working lives to provide more adequately for health and related service during their later years. The idea has been given the acronym MIRA—Medical Individual Reimbursement Accounts. With the authorization of federal legislation, such accounts might be built with tax-free contributions during the working years and then drawn upon for health and related services during retirement. Such a mechanism would encourage individuals to take some responsibility for their future anticipated needs based on their own health behavior.

For the second mechanism, I would suggest placing appropriate "user" taxes on items and activities that have negative health consequences. Based on economic analyses, taxes might be assessed on tobacco, alcohol, and other substances, such as sugar and animal fats, that have known, causal relationships to specific diseases and conditions, and then directly funding prevention and treatment programs with those dedicated revenues. This solution places the burden of funding the consequences of negative health behaviors on those who choose those behaviors. If such a burden provides an incentive for some to choose more healthy behaviors, then they will benefit along with others.

My objective is not to attempt to mandate that individuals change their behavior, but to require each person to participate in the future costs of their current behavior as it relates to health consequences.

Institutional versus Community Health Care of the Elderly: The Delicate Balance of Social Policy Panel Discussion

Dr. Eli Ginzberg: I don't think it is correct to say that our society has made no progress with the problem of long term care. I would argue, unequivocally, that the increasing affluence of the society has basically provided a lot of income for most of the middle class. They don't perceive the lack of long term care provisions as a major threat, and that is one of the reasons that there is so little political pressure to do much about long term care. Further, we are not a society sensitive to the questions of income or distributional equity and, clearly, since we don't handle even acute care very well for the poor, we don't want to get involved in long term care for the poor. We stumbled into Medicaid, which was not conceived initially to take most of its money to provide long term care for the poor. Our society is very restive about moving on this front, because it got itself into a position that it does not like.

In addition, the quality of much of long term care for the poor is very questionable. We don't look with any enthusiasm to expanding it, and we don't have the slightest intention of coming up with resources to raise the quality and quantity of such opportunities for the poor. I would say, therefore, that everything that I have heard today is both reasonable and totally irrelevant, in that it is not a part of a real ongoing social agenda. I think that the resistances that we have seen are completely consistent with our general behavior. I don't think we are going to get ahead in this game unless we put our discussions about Medicare, Medicaid, and the elderly in a larger framework to understand the margins of this society at this time in different states. Otherwise, you just have wish lists.

Dr. Leon Eisenberg: One issue that Ms. Brody's paper illustrates, and it comes up repeatedly, is that the federal government is concerned about public monies that appear in the bills for health care, but not about private monies. In principle, if we were to move from the present system to a national health insurance plan, costs wouldn't rise, assuming that things were reasonably well regulated, but the money would appear on the federal tab, be visible, and be a concern to everyone. If the man in the White House says that families should take more responsibility for elderly parents, what he is saying is that the cost will not be a drain on the public treasury. But it's real money, or its equivalent in time. It is, as Ms. Brody pointed out, the cost to families, the opportunity costs of work forgone, the mental health stress, and all the rest, that are never taken into account.

When the clothing manufacturers in the South claim that they cannot afford to reduce the cotton fiber level in the air, they are saying that the cost of byssinosis should be borne by the workers, not by the manufacturer. The community says it does not want prices to go up and the prices would have to go up to make employment safe. We shift the costs back onto those least able to speak for themselves. Here, the effort is to shove it back into the family sector, despite the fact that the family is carrying much of the burden under present circumstances. That's my first point. How do we get a social cost accounting system?

I disagree with Dr. Shaner. Of course, someone who smokes is not being "forced to." However, when you examine at the extraordinary differences in smoking rates by social class and by education, there is something about prolonged schooling that leads people who have had that higher education to smoke less. If we had a society in which advertising were removed so that there was not external duress, if we had a society in which stress related to jobs was distributed equitably, then we could say that people who smoke are responsible for their smoking; then we could imagine a system of incentives and punishments that could be equitably applied. At the moment, to hold people responsible for their eating or smoking behavior in the face of all the television advertising for eating exactly the wrong thing, all of what tobacco companies do, the subsidies the government gives, etc., seems to me to put disproportionate emphasis on the behavior of the individual. The individual is controlled by membership in a given culture group; that is not a matter of choice; what you are born into is associated with different life chances. It would seem to me to be a very grave error to take an individually-directed strategy, rather than a social strategy. When it comes to taxing, changing subsidies, then I would support many of Dr. Shaner's proposals.

Mr. Robert Ball: I would like to raise a question about the first point that Eli Ginzberg made as to whether people are really concerned about long term care. I think he is probably right about the lack of a measurable pressure on this issue. The reason may be misinformation rather than that people have enough of their own resources to handle the problem. I have two pieces of evidence. One is a study conducted for the American Association of Retired Persons which found that a very high proportion of their members, when asked whether they would be protected against long term care costs, said yes, Medicare would take care of it or Medicare and their medigap policy would take care of it. The second piece of evidence is even more convincing to me. I am on a Commission on College Retirement, with several college presidents, financial officers, and professors. They were amazed when they learned that Medicare and medigap policies do not cover the kind of thing that we are talking about, and they have become quite interested in designing something that would be a regular part of retirement protection.

Dr. James Fries: I have a couple of comments about the themes that we have been discussing. With overall budgetary pressures, it is hard to put in new programs or even get yourself taken seriously when talking about new programs, unless you say where the money is going to come from and what is going to be cut out. I have some favorite suggestions of my own as to where the money can potentially come from.

By my calculations, about 18 percent of total lifetime medical costs occur in the last year of life. Victor Fuchs has done a very interesting analysis with Medicare data in which he removed the effect of the last year of life by adjusting for it. By doing that, the increase in expense with age was completely eliminated. As a matter of fact, there was actually less money being expended for the 75 to 85 year olds. So we clearly have a lot of, by definition, futile expenditures of funds in the last year of life. The public clearly indicates in every poll and by the living will movement, that it wants less technology, not more, at the deathbed. I would suggest that these expenditures represent a source of funds for much more productive things, such as those that Ms. Brody has been talking about.

·The second funding issue is that of finding the funds for prevention.

That may end up being a private sector job over the next decade because there are two major parts of the private sector that are fairly eager to get in the business: corporations and health insurance companies. Both are beginning to see ways of decreasing immediate cash expenditures if they can change the health behaviors causing some of those expenses.

Dr. Henry Aaron: I want to raise the question of what it means from a policy standpoint to say that X percent of health expenditures occur in the last year of life, or X percent of Medicare expenditures occur in the last year of life. We don't know with certainty at the time that expenditures are being made, that it is the last year of life. I am sure that we are all aware through personal experiences or anecdote, that expenditures are lavished or wasted on people at a point where informed physicians would agree that the chance of survival, beyond a very brief period, is close to nil. Each of us has our feelings about the propriety or impropriety of using resources in that way. We are talking about expenditures that are made in cases where there is a finite probability of survival, you are rolling the dice a lot of times, and a number of those people die. What's the policy significance of knowing that 18 percent of lifetime medical costs occur in the last year of life?

Dr. James Haughton: Ms. Brody's paper begins with the statement that institutional care and home health care for the elderly are not in competition. I would be willing to believe that, if I saw any evidence that there was a mechanism in place for rational decisions about who went to insitutions. Twenty-three years ago, when I was Medical Director of the Welfare Department in New York City, I inherited about 9,000 older people in 90 nursing homes. In visiting those nursing homes, I found that many of the people who were there did not seem to need to be in an institution. What I learned was that most of those patients came from public hospitals, where the residents decided they did not want that "old crock" on their ward anymore. So they applied for home care, nursing home care, chronic disease hospital care, foster home care, and whichever one came first, that's where the patient went. It had nothing to do with the patient's needs.

At that time, we got the state's permission to contract with a health maintenance organization and many patients went home. The fact was that those nursing home patients had reached the point where they no longer needed hospital care, but they did still need medical care, and when there was no mechanism for providing medical care in the nursing home, they stayed there indefinitely. Provided with the means for medical care in the nursing home, patients improved significantly and returned to their own homes in many instances. That did not empty out nursing homes, but it did mean that a number of people for whom the city was paying high nursing home rates were able to go to another level of care that was less costly.

Three years later, I became Commissioner of Hospitals in New York. We had twenty-two hospitals, almost all of which had home care programs. We found that because we were using medical residents in the home care program, many people who needed home care could not get into it because residents did not like home calls. When we replaced those residents with salaried attending physicians, our home care census went up, and when Medicare went into being in 1966, we were able to negotiate a $4 a day per diem rate for nursing home care.

Five years later, I moved to Chicago and found that the medical residents of Cook County Hospital, of which I was Director, were doing the same thing in getting patients into Oak Forest Hospital, a chronic care facility. Nothing to do with the patients' needs, just trying to get them out of the acute care bed. When we hired full time attending physicians to care for the patients in that chronic facility, we were able to discharge many of those patients back to their families, as long as we promised them that if that older person became ill again we would immediately return them to the institution. We would allow them to return at least once a year for ten days for social admission to give that family a rest and we were able to keep people in the community.

No, it will not empty the long term institutions, but a substantial portion of funds that could be used for social alternatives are being squandered in institutions, because we have not found the way to link them to other alternatives so people can pass to the right level.

Dr. Mathy Mezey: We have noticed in the Robert Wood Johnson Teaching Nursing Home Programs, a difference between "short term-long term care" patients and "long term-long term care" patients. There is some reason to question whether the short term patients are really short term care or whether they are short term care patients on their way to becoming long term care patients. One of the reasons that we don't know what is happening with this group of patients is because you essentially have service delivery by source of payment. The sources of payment between hospital, nursing home, and home/ambulatory care are discrepant and often work at cross purposes. The nursing home side is primarily private pay and Medicaid, while hospital and home/ambulatory care are private pay and Medicare. There is continuous cost shifting such that someone may need and qualify for long term care but the differing payment sources delay how long it takes for them actually get in to the system.

One final comment. One of the reasons for the myth that the middle aged are unconcerned about nursing home and long term care is that there is no focal point around which they can coalesce and express their concerns. Currently, each individual, spouse, child, and so forth, attempts to determine what needs to be done for the aged relative. Each person accesses services as best they can and in whatever way they can. By the time the family member becomes aware of the deficiences in the system, the person who was the focus of their concern has often died. Middle-aged children and caregivers have yet to develop an effective forum through which to voice their collective concerns about the long term care system.

Dr. Robert Kane: I think Eli Ginzberg is wrong. The middle class does care about long term care, not so much about their own long term care, as their parents'. The more cocktail parties you go to and identify yourself as somebody who works in the field, the more individuals who have previously denigrated the field of geriatrics or gerontology suddenly come up to you with a particular problem they have in managing their own parents. In making health policy, one needs to focus on other generations for whom we feel responsible.

One of the differences that you encounter between discussions about acute care and long term care is the belief that acute care basically is worth the gamble and the investment most of the time, because you can tell definitely when that last dollar is being spent on a lost cause. The burden of proof for long term care seems to be on the other side. The sense is "What's the difference? Let's do it the cheapest way we can because what we are really trying to do is maintenance."

The number of well-documented experiences, like Dr. Haughton's, that suggest that one can do something meaningful with these individuals, is very sketchy. There are few good studies in the literature that demonstrate the efficacy of intervention. The truth is, a great deal can be done for those individuals, whether in a medical model, as Dr. Haughton suggests, or in a more universal model, as some of the other more traditional geriatric/gerontological models suggest. There are ample data suggesting that interventions probably are more cost effective for that population than they are for much of what we do in the area of acute care. We have not really developed that information in a way that it has been widely disseminated and, therefore, we tend to think about long term care as a low-return investment.

The other problem that we have is the perception of the nursing home as a prison. When a person goes into a nursing home they essentially lose the same civil liberties as when they are admitted to prison. We have not been creative in the way we have organized long term care. We have not thought about separating out the various functions that are performed under that rubric, and allowing people who are, by necessity, placed into these long term institutions to retain the right to services in the community. One could, in fact, reorganize much of long term care by looking at the nursing home as an entry point, and focus services around it. Home care could be delivered from the nursing home; don't make them competitive, merge them.

It is this narrow focus of long term care, much of it driven by the financing system, more of it driven by our lack of initiative, that has allowed us to back into this kind of policy of hopelessness. We should redefine long term care in more creative ways.

Dr. Charles Gaitz: We are confusing long term care with the places where long term care may be available. If we separate the sites of care and think more in terms of what else is involved in long term care, our thinking will be a lot clearer.

I would like to give you one anecdote about this matter of whether the middle class is or is not interested in long term care. The American Psychiatric Association now has a Council on Aging and, of course, we have been much concerned with the issues of whether old people are getting their share of mental health services, especially in nursing homes. We got the American Association of Retired Persons (AARP) to put a notice in their bulletin asking their readers to tell us about their experiences with nursing homes. We had been told that requests like this often yielded barrels full of letters. We only got a handful of responses. The issue of nursing homes and psychiatric services was not important relatively when compared with the concern of the AARP member about whether or not there would be a means test for Social Security or Medicare.

I think it is a relative issue and I am inclined to agree with Dr. Ginzberg that there is much apathy, and I agree with Dr. Kane that it is largely related to a denial that this is really a problem that is going to hit me. When it finally does hit me or when my parent finally gets old enough, then I will begin thinking about it.

Dr. Eli Ginzberg: Let me put a New York City experience on the table to illustrate a middle class response. The city now has a home care program under Medicaid in which we spend half a billion dollars a year to keep 40,000 people at home. These people on average, receive 51 hours of paid outside help per week. The state finally put a ceiling on this program because it was costing so much money. What we don't know how to do with home care, long term care, home care and all of its manifestations, is how to combine public and private monies. So I think the taxpaying public and a lot of other people have dug their heels in. If people require 51 hours of paid help, then you really should consider putting them into a nursing home, not all of them, but many of them. Upjohn figured out, with their long experience, that once you need to buy more than something like 20-25 hours of help a week to keep somebody at home, it gets to be too expensive to keep them at home.

I think we are at Stage One of designing an "admixture" of flows of funds that would make this possible, including the fact that we have not even begun on the insurance side to know any way at all of putting in some money early and then taking care of it in a better way. Therefore, I am forced to say the really affluent middle class is not at all worried; the middle-middle class that is not so affluent, gets very upset when they run into a problem. As for the poor, we just dig in our heels and say no more facilities for them because it is too costly.

Rebuttal

Elaine M. Brody, MSW

I want to express my gratitude to Dr. Shaner, who may have changed my whole attitude toward life. Since I was a small child, I had the notion that if I got sick it was something that I had done wrong. My mother drilled that into us over and over again. If it was winter time, she would say I did not button up enough; if it was summer time, I had gotten overheated playing basketball; nowadays, it's I'm working too hard or run around too much on airplanes. Now when I go home, I'll be able to tell her about the germ theory. You have relieved my guilt and I do thank you.

Dr. Haughton, with all due respect, I have to say that the name of the game has changed since years ago when we were first interested in institutionalizing old people. I have been in this business at least thirty years. When I first started, there were lots of old people in our facility who did not need to be there at all because they could be categorized as the so-called "healthy, but indigent aged." They had no place to live and would starve if they lived outside, but they were not ill people.

I think the human being in the U.S. who has done more to keep old people out of institutions than anybody else is Bob Ball, because as income support, Social Security and the other forms of support took hold, more people were able to live outside. I am not talking about an adequate income, but they were not starving. I remember as a young social worker, going to homes of people who did not have enough to eat, were buying the well-publicized dog food, but did not have a radio. Many of those old people found their way into our homes for the aged. The situation shifted very dramatically because at the same time that the income supports were enabling well old people to stay in the community, we began to feel the very dramatic impact of the increase of very old people.

Nowadays, we don't get well old people in nursing homes; most are very deteriorated, very old, most with some form of Alzheimer's disease. The people who come to nursing homes need round-the-clock surveillance, their families can no longer manage it. They need changing because of incontinence; they need to be watched lest they wander out without clothes on; they need to be cleaned up when they smear their feces on the walls, and so on. This is the population whom we are dealing with in nursing homes, and I submit that for many of these people, there is no alternative but nursing home care. I don't want one older person who could live outside to come into a nursing home.

Now, I am not selling nursing home care because there are many sub-populations of older people. In addition to the 1200 people who live on our campus at the Philadelphia Geriatric Center in our residential facilities, we serve thousands more with the other services. The day care, the respite care for family caregivers, consultation and diagnostic services, home care of all kinds, services that meet the needs of different populations of old people.

There is an additional reason why people are not interested in the problem of long term care: it does not have the glamour of the acute care on which the American public is hooked. You know there is nothing as dramatic as these fancy diagnostic tests. People are constantly hoping for magic and willing to spend or have the community spend money for those things that may make a magical cure. Long term care does not have that kind of glamour and, therefore, it is harder to sell. I think it is true, however, that the middle class and all classes of people are becoming more attuned to it. About half of all middle generation women at some point have to care for an elder parent. Dr. Ethel Shanas once told me that the conversation in the beauty parlor used to be about how to take care of your children; now it is how to take care of your parents. Certainly this is true. Everybody gets tuned into it but people don't expect a problem, which is another reason why they are not as interested in it. What we hear over and over again is, "I didn't expect it to come to this. This is something that happens to other people and other families, but not to us."

As far as short term-long term care, there is a great deal of movement between short term care and long term care. Older peoples' capacities change over time and the kind of service they get is often dictated by the stream of reimbursement that is available, rather than their particular needs. Older people move about five times as often before they go into a nursing home as the total population.

With respect to swing beds in a hospital, I have a very strong opinion on that. I think it is important for hospitals to get into what are called the "step-down" services, now that we have the prospective payment systems and hospitals are discharging older people sooner than they did before. I don't think we should make the assumption that because older people are staying in hospitals a shorter period of time, that it is bad for them. What is important is that they get the care they need after they leave. My bias is that, while it may be legitimate and appropriate for hospitals to get into short term care, it is not their business to get into long term care. They are not oriented to it, attuned to it, and it does not need the kind of high tech medicine that we have become accustomed to in the acute care setting. Certainly older people in institutions need meticulous medical care. People with Alzheimer's disease are likely to have many other diagnoses, but the amount of time that they spend in getting actual face-to-face doctor care or technical nursing is infinitesimal; one study found one percent of their time. The rest of the time they need good social care and personal care. I am not in favor of long term care under hospital auspices, although I am in favor of the short term care.

With respect to housing and life care communities. A lot of people are very much in favor of life care communities and so am I, but they don't serve the total elderly population. As for any other aspect of services to the aged, each has a specific target population and there is no one service or one kind of facility that is going to serve all of these subgroups of a very heterogenous population. Some people think that people can be insured against long term care, and that is economically and actuarially possible. Certainly, housing with services is tremendously important for older people who don't need nursing home care but need some form of service in a housing arrangement; meal services, accessibility of medical services, etc.

What the Government Accounting Office study and lots of other studies have shown is that for severely impaired older people, community care is more expensive than nursing home care. However, I don't think that the economic cost should be the only determinant of the plan for older people. People have preferences and different needs, and the question is, what's appropriate in those terms. If you take two elderly ladies with similar diagnoses and similar incapacities, living in third floor rear walk-ups, one may be a fiercely independent type who says she wants to stay there until the day she dies, and should, if that's what she wants, while the other is fearful and anxious, and prefers to live in a more sheltered setting, and she should, if she wants to. I think values should be controlling. We should respect the rights of people to determine where they want to be.

On the issue of dependency and independency, we usually think of dependency as the giving of services and help to people who can't make it on their own. Some services help people to become independent. If you give somebody who can't walk a crutch and that enables them to walk by themselves, then giving them the service makes them independent. We have to keep in mind when we are dealing with older people who in general have not gotten rehabilitation services. Believe me, when an older person is living with a family the ability to walk, even the small increments in function, can make a major difference in that family.

I will end on a value note, because there have been hints about the controversy relating to allocation of resources among the generations. That is a very dangerous kind of controversy. If we know anything at this stage of our development, we know that what affects one member of the family affects them all. To use an economic illustration, before Social Security, more than half of older people were totally dependent on their families for income. With the advent of income supports, that figure has dropped to 1.5 percent. No longer do middle aged people have to choose between sending a child to camp or college and putting bread in the mouths of older people. The well-being of the generations is really interlocked. We should keep that in mind, plus the fact that we are the older people of the future, some of us not too far away from it. We have to look to the future and not try to set one generation against the other.

CHAPTER 4

The Impact Prospective Payment Will Have on De-Institutionalizing Health Care for the Elderly Position Paper

Donald A. Young, MD

In moving from cost-based reimbursement to the setting of a price in advance for the care of a hospital inpatient, the Medicare prospective payment system (PPS) radically changes the financial incentives related to clinical care. Since its beginning in 1966, Medicare paid for inpatient hospital service through a retrospective, cost-based system. This system contributed greatly to the tremendous increase in hospital costs and Medicare expenditures over the past 18 years by paying, after the fact, for whatever costs were incurred by a hospital caring for Medicare patients. There were few incentives built into the system to encourage hospital management to seek alternative and most cost effective systems of care.

The major goal of prospective payment is to reverse the incentives of a cost-based system and replace them with a system which rewards efficiency by allowing hospitals to make a profit when their costs fall below the prospective payment amount. The system encourages efficiency and productivity in the delivery of inpatient hospital services and has controls built in to maintain quality of care and to foster continued improvements in health services through scientific and technological advances.

PPS offers strong incentives to hospitals to alter their admission patterns, to decrease the volume of services provided an individual patient, and to shift services from an inpatient to an outpatient setting. Although it is too early in the history of PPS to draw firm conclusions, the incentives appear to be creating the desired results.

Hospital length of stay is declining for all groups, but especially for the Medicare population. Hospital admissions are also declining in the general population and are stable or slightly decreased for the Medicare program. Anecdotal evidence indicates that the mix of services provided to inpatients is also changing, with a shift to outpatient settings. Related to shifts in sites of service delivery, hospitals are accelerating the diversification of services they offer: in some cases by converting acute care to long term care beds or offering home health care services, in others to competing directly with other providers in the community such as ambulatory surgical centers, pharmacies or medical equipment suppliers.

The financial incentives in PPS complement the significant changes in the organization and delivery of health care as well as the changing public beliefs and values regarding health care. The impact of the changes on the American population, including the elderly, will be significant. I will examine this impact in the framework of a set of social forces converging and impacting on a rapidly-evolving health care delivery system.

The social forces include: first, very significant technological changes, including new capabilities to provide services in non-institutional settings. Second, the emergence of health care cost-containment as a public policy. And, third, a desire to change the role of the federal government by shifting the locus of decision-making to a more local level through policies which promote competition and more effectively utilize traditional market mecha-nisms in decisions regarding the allocation of resources to individual patients. The prospective payment system is one of the federal reforms. A payment amount is set in advance for a package of services and the hospital management and staff make individual allocation decisions.

It is necessary to set some limits and provide some definitions for the discussion. First, there are many prospective payment mechanisms and systems used by the Medicare program and other third party payers. These have differing policies and incentives. The emphasis here will be on the Medicare prospective payment system for inpatient hospital services. Second, the "elderly" will be defined as the Medicare population eligible for hospital benefits by reason of age. I will not discuss the elderly poor as a specific subpopulation, but acknowledge that a special set of problems related to health care and institutionalization for this group require further examination. Third, "institution" has many meanings and in considering "deinstitutionalizing health care" I will refer to the common meaning of a building or place, usually of confinement, unless otherwise noted. Finally, "health care" is variously used to describe a place or structure, a process or an outcome. As will be developed, the centerpiece of the American "health care" system has been the hospital, an institution in all meanings of the word devoted to furnishing acute medical care services. I will examine structures (institutions) and processes (also, frequently institutions), but will point to outcome as the critical measure of health care.

SETTING THE STAGE

There is general consensus that the Medicare program has accomplished the goals set for it in 1965. The great majority of the elderly, poor and non-poor, have a regular source of mainstream medical care and their health status has improved each year. The success of the Medicare program in achieving access to care and the costs of the success, however, is in part responsible for the perceived crisis in Medicare funding that propelled the legislation leading to PPS through the Congress.

From the time of its inception, Medicare focused on the hospital in the development of its benefit structure and payment policies. In 1965, the choice appeared simple and logical. The hospital was the institution, in all meanings of the word, of greatest importance to the Medicare age population, and the funding provided by Medicare allowed the institution to grow and thrive. Prospective payment and health policy today challenge the choice of the hospital as the fundamental health care institution. Nevertheless, the technologically-intensive medical model of health care has brought spectacular achievements, including artificial hearts, organ transplants, and extraordinary diagnostic, monitoring and therapeutic capabilities.

While some technological advances were moving forward as a result of the system of cost-based hospital payment, other technological advances lead to a growing number of questions about the wisdom of the choice of the hospital as the centerpiece of the health care system. Advances in anesthesiology and surgical practice led a few pioneers to begin performing surgery in ambulatory settings which were, at times, far removed from the hospital. While ambulatory surgery was initially decried by some as a catastrophe waiting to occur, it is now a well-accepted method of practice. You do not need a hospital to have your cataract removed or your "trick knee" fixed. Deinstitutionalization of health care for the elderly was moving into place, at significantly less cost, and with equally satisfying patient outcomes.

Numerous other examples can be given of technological change that allowed movement of services from the hospital to other settings. Parenteral nutrition, intravenous antibiotic therapy, terminal care for cancer patients, complex laboratory and other diagnostic and therapeutic services previously available only in the hospital are now available in the home or community.

The change in institutional focus has not been without its turmoil, however. The fear of a deterioration in quality of care continues to be voiced. The hospital has a critical mass of highly specialized and qualified staff with the newest and most expensive equipment. The hospital and many of its staff are subject to qualification and certification standards that do not exist in many non-hospital settings. There is no convincing evidence, however, that the movement of services to the home or community has had an adverse impact on health outcome. But it may be too early to tell.

Payment policy for the Medicare program has lagged behind changes in the organization and delivery of services. It was relatively late in the movement of surgical services to ambulatory settings that Medicare legislation was changed to allow payment for the facility component of the services. The policies now in place are regarded by many as flawed. The problem resides in part in the Medicare program's traditional approach to defining benefits in terms of the institution as a "place." The hospital is a place with one set of payment and benefit policies, the skilled nursing facility is a place with its own policies, the ambulatory surgical center is a place with very different policies. Cutting across the benefits defined by a place, are the benefits furnished by an individual such as a physician or a physical therapist. The problem is that Medicare is neatly divided into Part A and Part B, with differing policies for differing institutions and individuals. The health services world is not so neatly divided. As alternative approaches to delivery of health care emerge, and the prospective payment system encourages these alternatives, the disjointedness of this policy will become increasingly obvious. The flaws in payment for hospital care, renal dialysis services, and ambulatory surgery are examples of the difficulties in developing sound policy. The process of deinstitutionalization and the resulting disjointed policy significantly affects the elderly. At some point a fundamental restructuring of benefits will be necessary.

Benefit and payment policy for non-institutional services has not kept pace with changes in the sites of service delivery, because of fears that alternative delivery sites will lead to expanded Medicare benefits and increased expenditures. The issue centers on the difference between unit cost and aggregate cost. If services furnished in the home or in the community substitute for traditional institutional services with a comparable outcome, they are likely to decrease total costs. At times, however, they do not substitute, but are added on. In addition, many individuals do not use services furnished only in an institution, but when the services become available in the community, with Medicare funding, many individuals begin to consume them. Recent discussions concerning the Medicare home health benefit and Congressional interest in this benefit illustrate the problem.

Finally, the Medicare program has moved slowly and hesitantly from the traditional medical model to incorporate relevant social needs in its benefit structure. The difficulties associated with implementing the Medicare hospice benefit is an example. Whether the development of alternative delivery systems with reasonable payment policies will meet the problem of linking medical and social needs remains to be seen. There are encouraging signs, however. The Health Care Financing Administration, after significant debate, has agreed to examine the concept of a "social health maintenance organization," and research is underway.

THE PRESENT

Medicare policy change in recent years has been driven largely by the concern with costs of services and expenditures. It is unlikely that the Medicare prospective payment system would have been enacted in 1983 in the absence of a perceived cost crisis. Since the great majority of Medicare's expenditures are directly or indirectly related to hospital care, it is logical in setting a public policy of cost containment to look first to the hospital. As early as 1972, the Congress recognized the inflationary incentives of cost-reimbursement and authorized the Secretary of the Department of Health and Human Services to set limits on the costs reimbursed under

Medicare, to produce a more efficient delivery of services (the Section 223 limits). Because of the difficulties associated with controlling costs in an area as diverse, complex and socially valued as hospital care, the 223 limits covered only routine hospital care, i.e., room and board and nursing care. Ancillary services such as x-ray and laboratory services, drugs and intensive care units, were not subject to the cost limits because of the lack of a suitable methodology for setting total limits in a manner that was both equitable and cost-efficient.

The Tax Equity and Fiscal Responsibility Act of 1982 (TEFRA) placed additional important controls on hospital cost reimbursement under Medicare, paving the path to prospective payment. These new controls were possible because of the development of diagnosis related groups (DRGs) and their use in measuring the mix of patients in a hospital in terms of the use of hospital resources. For the first time, the payment system provided some incentive payment for hospitals that keep their costs below a target as well as penalties for those that exceeded their target.

Other cost saving measures for the Medicare program were enacted by Congress as part of a new budget reconcilliation process in each year from 1980 through 1984, and more are promised for 1985. It was in these years that new policies were established for ambulatory surgery, the hospice program, and some changes made or proposed for home health care.

It is interesting to note that the focus was primarily on institutional benefits and payment policy, not on the elderly as individuals or on the Medicare benefit structure as a comprehensive whole.

It is difficult to forecast with any degree of accuracy the aggregate impact of the changing policies, including PPS, on the health care of the elderly. Some generalizations can be made, however. First is the clear trend to deinstitutionalization, if institution is defined as a building or place of confinement. The recognition and acceptance of service delivery in ambulatory surgical centers, by a hospice, or in the home is a significant break with the past. Society's institutional view of the hospital as an established and structural pattern of behavior that is accepted as a fundamental part of a culture, may be undergoing a fundamental change. If so, the change in social beliefs and values may have a far greater impact on health care for the elderly than prospective payment. PPS merely adds financial incentives which are congruent with the set of changing values. Hospitals, as established patterns of behavior, places of confinement, and buildings, are, in some cases, leading the change as they move from being organizations devoted to the promotion of inpatient, acute medical care model to more diversified, "vertically integrated" providers of a much broader array of health care services. The hospital as an institution is itself "de-institutionalizing."

What impact will the de-institutionalization process have on health care for the elderly? At this point it is necessary to refine the notion of health care. In 1965 when Medicare was enacted, health care was thought of primarily as access to the process of care. And that process was furnished generally by hospitals and doctors. The structures and the processes of medicine have changed and it is necessary to examine health care as an outcome. Health care services are available in many alternative settings and arrangements. Cost containment as public policy will continue for the present to encourage the least costly setting, either by direct policy change or by the structure of payment incentives as the PPS. The change in public values is leading to the choice of non-institutional settings and health care services. The impact of these choices on health care cannot, therefore, be measured in terms of institutional structure or process. It is fallacious to conclude, as we have had a tendency to in the past, that the elderly have the desired health care merely because their hospital or their community has transplant facilities, long term care beds, or the newest development in computer-assisted diagnostic imaging capabilities. The impact must be measured in terms of health outcomes.

The geriatric imperative in health care becomes the geriatric imperative in quality of living. Quality of living blends medical with broader social needs, needs of the elderly as well as needs of the family and the larger community. Quality of living also involves individual value systems. In the United States, a heart attack results in a hospital stay with intense technological intrusion. In England, the heart attack may be treated at home. For the patient with cancer, the place for death until recently was the hospital. Increasingly, the choice is hospice care; and hospice service focuses on the family as well as the individual. What is the impact of the choice of the home or the hospital on the quality of living? Much remains to be learned before the question can be answered, but the answer will not be found if institutionalization/de-institutionalization are the only variables examined.

THE IMMEDIATE FUTURE

A public policy of health care cost containment will continue in the immediate future, as will the Medicare prospective payment system. Public interest in cost control, new technological capabilities, and changing social beliefs and values will promote the continued diversification of hospitals and development of non-institutional patterns of health care services delivery. Individuals, including the elderly, will have a broader array of choices to meet their individual values and needs, but the choices will likely be within "packages," with a price set for a package of services. Federal policy makers will continue to be involved in packaging and pricing, but choices of alternatives among and within packages will be made at more local levels, as they are with PPS. HMOs and payment by capitation were the first major moves in this direction. The Medicare prospective payment system follows the pattern in a somewhat different format. The system, however, is limited by its focus on inpatient hospital services. Nevertheless, PPS contains strong financial incentives which will affect health care services far beyond the walls of a hospital. In addition, there is interest in adding additonal services to the PPS package, including skilled nursing facility services, home health services and physician services.

The continuing shift of health care services from the traditional inpatient institutional setting to alternative settings will lead to a whole new set of issues related to distribution, access, quality of care and health outcome. Predictions of dire consequences and expectations for declining levels of quality of care continue to accompany the implementation of the prospective payment system. Many of these appear to be based on the association of health care with the structure and process rather than the outcome of the care. Similar predictions and expectations were associated with the early years of the movement to ambulatory surgery. A conclusive assessment of the impact of prospective payment on the elderly must include an assessment of the much broader social move to de-institutionalization as well as the use of appropriate measures of health outcome and quality of living.

CONCLUSION

The Medicare prospective payment system sets a price in advance for a package or services furnished during an inpatient hospital stay.

The focus of PPS is the hospital, but the impact extends well beyond the inpatient setting. PPS is merely one of many continuing changes in the organization, delivery and financing of health care for the elderly. The impact prospective payment will have on de-institutionalizing health care for the elderly will be determined by social values and choices related to continued technological and scientific advances, the willingness to change beliefs, the amount of money we are willing to spend, and the value assigned by the individual to the outcome of the health care services received. PPS should share only partial credit for the success or partial blame for failures related to the changing institutional order. Partial solutions have been found for old problems. New problems are sure to emerge.

The Impact Prospective Payment Will Have on De-Institutionalizing Health Care for the Elderly A General Policy Perspective

Grant V. Rodkey, MD

On behalf of the American Medical Association I would like to express appreciation for the opportunity to participate in this conference and to respond to Doctor Donald Young's paper. Dr. Young has chosen the acute care hospital as the institutional focus of his remarks. This is appropriate, but we recognize that the effects of de-institutionalizing services rendered in acute care hospitals will create significant social changes, including modifying some other institutions.

It is helpful to review the salient factors which led to the enactment of Medicare Prospective Payment System legislation in 1983. These include the Hill-Burton Act and federal health-manpower policies, which have served to double the annual number of medical students graduating each year, and essentially double the numbers of U.S. practicing physicians over the past twenty years.

When Medicare was enacted in 1965, it was modeled conceptually on the pattern of the leading private health care insurer, Blue Cross-Blue Shield. It was divided into Part A, which reimbursed hospitals on an open-ended cost-based formula, and Part B, which reimbursed physicians on a formula related to charge-based data which, in fact, was obfuscatory and encouraged cost-inflation. Benefits to patients for hospital services featured first-dollar coverage, payment for acute hospital services, no catastrophic illness coverage and very restricted benefits for nursing home or other long term care.

Thus, both private and public health insurance programs encouraged access, utilization, and supply in health services and fueled the inflationary cost spiral from 6.0 percent of Gross National Product in 1965 to 10.5 percent in 1982. While the program conveyed many health benefits to its covered population and provided a significant stimulus for technological advancement as Dr. Young has noted, there was still a pervasive mismatch between Medicare's coverage of short-term acute illness and the essential need of the elderly population for insurance against the costs of catastrophic illness and long term care. However, it was only the cost of health care that was addressed by the Tax Equity and Fiscal Responsibility Act of 1982, which created prospective payment for acute care hospitals on the basis of diagnosis-related groups (DRGs).

Stripped to its essentials, the Prospective Payment System (PPS) introduces powerful financial incentives for the hospital to restrict the cost and quantity of its services to individual Medicare beneficiaries. The Congress, recognizing the potential of this sytem for adverse effects upon health care of the elderly, also established the Utilization and Quality Control Peer Review Organization (PRO) program and the Prospective Payment Assessment Commission (PROPAC)—of which Dr. Young is the Executive Director—to monitor the system's effects upon the quality of health care services.

Unfortunately, the regulations and implementation of the PRO program thus far appear to emphasize restrictions on utilization or site of services as opposed to quality of services to beneficiaries. Thus, in Massachusetts the PRO has defined 155 procedures for which payment will be made only if they are performed in an outpatient setting. These include some rather substantial treatments which entail significant inconvenience and discomfort and some increased risk to elderly, frail people. These represent restrictions in previously available benefits. However, it is too early in the program to have a clear impression of their effects.

Undoubtedly, it is also too early for PROPAC to have clear evidence of the trends to health care generated by these dramatic changes. Dr. Young's emphasis upon the analysis of health care outcomes as a criterion is laudable, but thus far this has proved to be something of a "quicksand" in objective evaluation. Most observers conclude by recommending more intensive research into the matter.

The American Medical Association is working with John Hopkins University to develop a series of research proposals to study long term effects of PPS on the quality of health care for the elderly. In the meantime, we established a monitoring system in June, 1984 soliciting information directly from physicians who observe the program in operation. Several hundred written reports have been received, most focusing upon the quality of care issue. Of the respondees, 37 percent indicated that quality had not been adversely affected in their hospitals, while 63 percent reported that quality had deteriorated or would deteriorate with continuation of the program. Areas of most concern relate to premature discharges, growing numbers of readmissions for the same or related problems, and administrative restrictions upon the site of service or allowed ancillary services.

The United States House of Representatives Select Committee on Aging and its Task Force on the Rural Elderly met on February 26, 1985 to consider some of the effects of PPS. Their survey of all state nursing home ombudsmen (75 percent response) reported that following findings:

1. 77 percent of respondents said patients are being discharged "sicker or much sicker" than before PPS.
2. Over 71 percent indicated that "more or many more" people need skilled nursing care since PPS.
3. Over 50 percent of respondents stated that existing skilled nursing care is *not* adequate to meet the needs of discharged patients in *rural* areas: 1/3 said care was inadequate in urban areas.
4. 10 percent of the respondents indicated that existing services are less adequate in rural than urban settings for each of the following areas: intermediate nursing home care, home health and homemaker services.
5. 59 percent indicated that nursing homes did not have adequate personnel to provide care in rural areas before PPS and 67 percent after PPS. In urban areas 49 percent responded that personnel were inadequate before PPS and fifty-six percent after PPS.

In addition, the Committee heard testimony that rural hospitals are especially hard-hit by the PPS reimbursement formula and by reason of small size, unable to absorb the excessive cost of outlier cases. Thus, many rural hospitals are on the list of endangered species.

The United States General Accounting Office, in a report to the Honorable John Heinz, Chairman of the Senate Special Committee on Aging dated February 21, 1985, raised questions as to whether beneficiaries have been adequately informed as to the restrictions in their covered services and whether Medicare is appropriately administering coverage determinations. They confirmed that the average length of stay per PPS discharge declined to 7.5 days in fiscal year 1984 from 9.5 days in fiscal year 1983. Hospitals, nursing homes, home health care providers and discharge planners all agreed that patients are discharged in poorer states of health than prior to PPS, requiring more visits per case, multiple visits per week and more need for specialized services. A marked increase in skilled nursing facilities in many areas is precluded by a shortage of available beds—due in part to inadequate formulas for Medicaid reimbursement for nursing home services. In some areas, nursing homes are reluctant to admit Medicare patients because of the limited term of insurance coverage. Beneficiaries are confused and upset at changes in their Medicare benefits and how PPS has affected them. Whether the total costs to the system have been lessened or not by PPS, the costs as well as inconveniences to beneficiaries have been increased by the system.

Thus, although it is too early to have definite data, and although we must applaud any reduction in waste, inappropriate or inefficient utilization of hospital services accomplished by PPS, enough warning flags are already up to suggest that "de-institutionalizing health care for the elderly" from acute care hospitals will have an adverse effect upon the quality of their care if we do not assure that their needs are met in the community.

In fact, squeezing the providers of their payments and the beneficiaries of their services will accomplish neither the goals of quality of health care or fiscal stability for the Medicare program. What is needed is a restructuring of the program to align realistically incentives, benefits, resources, services, and demography to fit the health care and social needs of our elderly citizens with their varying states of health and senescence. The American Medical Association is conducting an active program of review of Medicare based on guidelines designed to accomplish these objectives.[4,5] We welcome the support and participation of other advocates for quality health care on a sound fiscal basis for elderly Americans.

REFERENCES

1. Task Force on the Rural Elderly, House Select Committee on Aging. Results of Survey to State Nursing Home Ombudsmen. Reported to the Joint Meeting of the Committee. United States House of Representatives, February 26, 1985.

2. White, Ben C. Statement to The Joint Meeting of The Select Committee on Aging and the Task Force on Rural Elderly, February 26, 1985.

3. Chelimsky, Eleanor. Report to the Honorable John Heinz, Chairman, Special Committee on Aging, United States Senate, February 21, 1985.

4. American Medical Association. Report on the Medicare Program: Board of Trustees, II. Adopted by the House of Delegates of The American Medical Association, June 17-21, 1984.

5. American Medical Association. Report on the Medicare Program: II; Report of the Board of Trustees adopted by the House of Delegates, American Medical Association, December 2-5, 1984.

The Impact Prospective Payment Will Have on De-Institutionalizing Health Care for the Elderly
A National Policy Perspective

Eli Ginzberg, PhD

Dr. Young's contribution, which is well focused, clearly written, and direct, makes the following principal points:

- The DRG system will probably prove successful in controlling costs and speeding alternatives to inpatient hospital treatment.
- The U.S. is moving away from the acute care hospital as the center of its health care system.
- More emphasis on ambulatory care treatment modalities need not lead to a deterioration in quality.
- The system of payment for health care in terms of "locations" is faulty and should be replaced by a shift toward patient needs and outcomes.
- In the case of the elderly, the medical and social issues (quality of life) are, or should be, closely linked, and Medicare is finally beginning to underwrite some experimental programs in this arena.
- Government (and insurance) must aim to restrict benefits so that they are substitutive and cost-efficient, not additive and cost increasing.

Let me first comment briefly on each of the above generalizations that I have extracted from Dr. Young's paper and then add a few more wide-ranging considerations. I do not believe that the DRGs will turn out to be a viable, effective long term system, either for Medicare alone or for all payers. The early successes—and I agree that the results to date are generally favorable—reflect the slack in the system which made it possible for both government and

175

hospitals to make initial gains. But after the system has been ratcheted down and most of the slack eliminated, I expect all sorts of trouble, from multiple admissions to DRG creep. No economist, not even a skeptical economist like me, can be readily persuaded that price-fixing for 469 categories is viable over time.

I agree with Dr. Young that the centrality of the acute care hospital that has dominated the U.S. medical care system over the last decades is being successfully challenged by a public that is opting increasingly for alternative treatment sites. To put it bluntly, the hospital industry has peaked.

Considering the high rate of infections among hospitalized patients, there is much to be said in support of Dr. Young's view that more treatment in ambulatory settings should not necessarily lead to a reduction in the quality of care. But let's not be too quick to cheer. The appalling results with the deinstitutionalization of mental patients should serve as one warning. Peer control in well-run hospitals cannot by reproduced in physicians' offices to which many diagnostic and therapeutic procedures are being ''unbundled.'' There is no reason that a sizable surgi-center should not be able to maintain quality control, but there are many reasons that quality control in solo or small group practices will prove difficult, if not impossible.

On many counts I agree with Dr. Young's critique of the difficulties that Medicare got itself into by setting different levels of reimbursement by ''locations,'' inpatient, skilled nursing home, etc., and by providers. But beyond noting the difficulties, he does little to point directions as to where solutions might be found.

So too, about his comments on the desirability of looking more closely at the medical and social services that the elderly require. I agree that in life the overlap is great. Many of the frail elderly need more personal than health care. But having said that, what does one do about the merger of Social Security benefits with Medicare, Medicaid etc.? Dr. Young provides us no clue.

The distinction that Dr. Young makes between add-on services and substitutive services is surely valid. Once again, however, beyond noting the importance of the distinction and warning that government and insurance must guard against indiscriminate add-ons, Dr. Young leaves us without specific guidance.

Now that I have commented on each of Dr. Young's theses, I am somewhat restive that my remarks may be overcritical. Dr. Young has illuminated several aspects of health care for the elderly incisively and perceptively and I suspect that I demand too much in searching for the next step beyond analysis—for policy recommendations.

In any case I will now put myself on the spot and single out a limited number of policy directions that are suggested by Dr. Young's effort. I indicated my strong suspicions that the DRG system would fall apart, sooner or later, even if it were expanded to include all patients. What follows? I postulate that we will not *really* contain total health care costs and that in the process of attempting constraints on inpatient treatment, the following are likely consequences: less effective treatment of complex cases because of efforts to save on diagnostic expenses and to shorten hospital stays; a marked unsettling of graduate medical education; and an abandonment of low income neighborhoods where marginal hospitals will close. There is nothing favorable in this forecast.

Our society will be forced to face up to the complex questions of care for terminal patients. Sensible resolutions will not come easily.

While the per unit costs of ambulatory surgery will be lower, total social costs are likely during the long intervening period to be higher beacuse of the difficulty of shrinking inpatient capacity commensurately and concurrently.

To restructure benefits with the patient at the center of the system rather than via locations and providers is easier said than done. To do so effectively probably would require the installation of a modified or total national health care system, something that does not appear to be on the horizon—nor should its arrival be hastened.

There may be an opportunity sometime in the future, but not very soon, to think about a partial integration of Social Security, Medicare, insurance, IRAs, etc., to provide a broader revenue base with which to meet the "total" needs of the elderly. But I would not assume that much progress will be made in the near or middle term.

Increased emphasis on "health outcomes" is an attractive slogan. It may even be a useful criterion whereby to gauge new investments in health care. I have long believed that the "system" will be constrained only when the public, including the elderly, come to recognize that medical treatment has the capability of causing harm as well as contributing to their well-being and that, in any case, death is inevitable, the continued progress of medicine notwithstanding.

The foregoing comments were based on a close reading of Dr. Young's prepared paper. During his oral presentation he raised some additional points and expanded on his original formulations. I will respond briefly upon the more important "new" issues.

DRGs are a classificatory schema and are not to be confused with PPS which is the basically new approach in federal reimbursement policy. I consider this distinction important.

It remains to be seen whether reducing hospital stays by one day impairs quality, is neutral, or possibly improves quality. It is hard to believe that with the incentives favoring early discharge some or many relatively sick patients will not be forced out before they have reached an optimal point in their recovery.

One of the big gains from DRGs/PPS Dr. Young points to is that decision-making is being forced out of Washington to the field (hospitals and physicians). The "manipulation" of the basic rates, however, will rest with Washington, and hence much of the action will continue to be centered there.

It is necessary to distinguish "need" from "waste." Surely the two often overlap. But we have few criteria that can distinguish between them and still less help to design social interventions that can be used to eliminate waste. Consider the difficulties of eliminating "excess" beds and personnel.

The federal government will not solve the financing of long term care. I agree that this is a reasonable prognosis but I would expect some expanded role for the federal government if the public is determined to put in place some new and expanded efforts to help the elderly obtain long term care. The recent voucher option for Medicare enrollees indicates to me that the federal government cannot remain frozen and do nothing if the pressure mounts.

The Impact Prospective Payment Will Have on De-Institutionalizing Health Care for the Elderly Panel Discussion

Dr. Steven Schroeder: It's been fun over the last year to watch the anticipation generated by prospective payment. The literature included many comments on how it was not going to work. Hospitals would "game it"; they'd "code-up" (the so-called "DRG-creep"); and they'd readmit patients. Dr. Ginzberg seems, part of the time, to be one of those people who feel it's not going to work. On the other side, there are people like Dr. Rodkey who say it is going to work too well, get people out of the hospital, de-institutionalize them, and hurt the public sector.

So far, the data seem to show that prospective payment is working; average length of stay is down; hospital capacity oversupply is more manifest; readmissions have not gone up; and the "creep" appears to be a one-time phenomenon in terms of coding. The question is, is it working by cutting down on hospital care that should not have been there in the first place, which would be good, or is it getting some people out who need to be in the hospital and harming quality of care? I think it's probably doing both, and that's something that should be watched very carefully. The possible good news, if it is working, is that the outcomes may add pressure to long term care issues for which there has not been enough pressure. It may actually stimulate the development of long term care facilities and capability, and add to that political consciousness and lobbying effort that Dr. Young pointed out was not sufficiently visible. I think it is going to work, although perhaps not sufficiently for everyone, and I think we have seen an end to double digit medical cost inflation for a while.

Dr. Knight Steel: I think this discussion of DRGs and whatever it is that will replace them, is the pivotal issue in the future of geriatrics. In Boston, we have 1000 people with a mean age of 80, who are cared for in their homes. I can tell you, even without data, which aren't all in, that certainly the feeling is that these people are sicker. I don't think there's much doubt about that.

I was wondering if the General Accounting Office or the American Medical Association have examined whether there is an improvement in care, as well as a deterioration of care, with the diminishing length of stay. There is some reason to believe that that might be true.

It is also important to raise the issue of whether DRGs will affect the way care is delivered because of the concomitant introduction to the health care system of the for-profit industry. If ever there was a way of finding your niche and caring for a select group of people or a select group of diseases, this is it. We are seeing this in some parts of the country, or will be shortly.

I wonder is Dr. Young would comment on whether he feels that prospective payment, good or bad, is tantamount to rationing. Older persons clearly will fare less well than younger people under most diagnoses, even granting that there is some fudge factor in there.

They will have an increased length of stay, and hospitals, to control their losses, will clearly limit the number of potential outliers, so rationing will occur. If that is true, there won't be any way of finding that information because the DRGs will only see "those people who actually enter the system," so you may actually lose people from the system altogether who would require care and previously did receive care, but won't now. If you then add "bundling" to the system, it's quite possible that we'll have not only rationing, but discrimination, because if you include both out-of-hospital and in-hospital care under a fixed fee, physicians will begin to discriminate against people who require more time, translated into money.

Dr. Robert Kane: First, I would like to clarify some terminology that we tend to use loosely. I have been carefully counseled by my colleagues that DRGs are a classification system and PPS is a payment system. What we are talking about is PPS, not DRGs, and that makes a real difference in terms of how you view the system and what you view it as doing.

I want to comment on some points raised by several of the speakers and commentators. The first one is the danger of the temptation to

view the prospective payment system as an opportunity for geriatricians or long term care enthusiasts, by seeing it as a technique for
promoting linkage. What we are really seeing in the PPS is a
resurrection of the Medicare philosophy of 1965. There is a
rediscovery of the Extended Care Facility; we have not quite gotten
around to calling them ECFs again, but we are coming full circle to
calling something "long term care" that really is "post-hospital
care." Long term care is something different. There are some
arguments for wanting to get into the rich trough of the heavy dollar
investment in acute care and see if we can't siphon off some of that
into the long term care establishment. However, it is a little bit like
the lamb of long term care lying down with the lion of the hospital
and it is usually the lamb that remains sleepless. I am not sure that
this necessarily is the kind of bedfellow that one would most want
to seek out. I think that one would want to be very wary of hospitals
that suddenly get interested in long term care.

The second question, which I will address to Dr. Young, really has
to do with what PPS, whether we think it's working or not, tells us
about the American health care system. Prospective payment has
made formal a transition in our basic value structure that has been
occurring informally for a long time. It has removed the hospital
from its previous sacrosanct position as a special institution gov-
erned by different kinds of rules, help up for different kind of
accountability, and said essentially, "You're a business and all we
have to do now is haggle about price. We know what you do, we
know what you are, and now we are getting down to some basics."

The third point has to do with this question about the effects of PPS
on quality of care. One of the things that has disappointed me a great
deal, is that people who have begun to study quality of care with
regard to PPS have done it as though they could simply take quality
of care technology and plug it in, forgetting that PPS is a program
designed for a Medicare population. It seems to me that if we are
going to talk about quality of care for a Medicare population, we are
looking at a population who are different because, among other
things, they are older, and indeed one would expect a differential
effect on different subsets of that population. All of the attributes of
the heterogeneity of that population really come to the fore. One is
going to miss the disadvantageous effects of PPS on quality unless
one looks at those groups who are truly at high risk, about 20
percent of the Medicare population.

The fourth point is an observation about what I think is happening as I talk to people who run organizations under what they think is PPS. That is what I call "Management by the Mean." The PPS system is essentially set up to balance DRGs against some kind of geometric mean for length of stay. If you talk to the managers, however, they view the mean as the maximum. They manage so that anybody who stays over the mean is an over-stayer. You don't have to be too much of a statistician to recognize that this approach is going to have perverse effects on your whole management strategy, if you are using averages as an upper bound. The capacity to either inadvertently or deliberately misunderstand the basis by which the program is being proposed suggests that it is not going to be effective, or at least, it is going to have some perverse effects as well as potentially beneficial effects on the system.

Dr. Henry Aaron. A number of us have heard Stuart Altman, chairman of PROPAC, talk about DRGs. One of the lines that Stu uses, which I think is exactly right, is that we have broken the old mold of cost-based reimbursement, and while DRGs are not free of flaws by any means, we are not going to go back to cost-based reimbursement. If you rule that out, then the question is, what sort of an evolutionary pattern are we going to follow? I think Dr. Schroeder is right that DRGs have worked; they certainly haven't produced the outpouring of pernicious responses to the real incentives within the system that economists like me and a lot of other folks anticipated. It is also true that non-Medicare hospital costs have exhibited similar trends, as one or more of the papers have pointed out. I think the real question is, where do we go from here and what is the implication?

Dr. Steel raised the question of whether there will be rationing. It doesn't take a deep thinker to hypothesize, and I feel it's highly likely, that in the initial stages we're going to squeeze out activities that are relatively low priority. There may be some loss of benefits initially, but not much. Eventually the waste is going to be gone and the question will be, will the slowdown in the rate of growth be sustainable over the long haul? It is at that point, after waste has been eliminated, you get into the question of whether rationing is going to be necessary. If it occurs, we have to keep in mind that we are talking about cost controls. If there is rationing, I think it is likely to take the form of changing the character and intensity of care rather than discouraging admissions.

I think Dr. Kane's remark about composition is very important in that one should expect the consequences of DRGs to be quite different for different groups. Just because we have not seen the incentive effects that economists and some physicians predicted early on, I am not prepared yet to give up on those forecasts, because at least so far, DRGs have not been very binding for a lot of hospitals. If you get them a quiet room where they know that nobody except you is going to hear them, a lot of hospital administrators will admit that they have been doing very nicely under the DRG system so far. I think that we are going to have to wait until the pressure is a lot more intense before we can be confident about the incentive effect.

Dr. Phoebe Liebig. I wish I could be as sanguine as Dr. Young and Dr. Schroeder that somehow de-institutionalization will lead to a greater array of services. I cite one example in California. We de-institutionalized people out of state mental hospitals. One of the things that is increasingly clearer, eight to 10 years later, is that communities did not provide services for those people. For instance, where Bob Kane and I live, there is a great hue and cry that all these people are out there sleeping in our parks and on the streets. To me, just because de-institutionalization occurs does not mean that services are going to be available.

Ms. Elaine Brody: I am speaking neither in favor nor against DRGs. I don't think the evidence is all in, and that has been made amply clear up to this point. It is certainly true, and I haven't heard anybody speak to this point yet, that hospitals all over the country are developing what are called the "step-down services." They are going into the foster home care business, day care, short term rehabilitation, convalescent care, and so on. How many hospitals are doing this, I don't think is known, but at the least it is having the effect of compelling hospitals, or encouraging hospitals, into developing these kinds of services. I think the evidence won't be in for a long time as to the overall impact, but we have to recognize that that is indeed happening. Some of that cost shifting is indeed going on.

Dr. Leon Eisenberg: A number of the speakers have implied that through DRGs or prospective payment control we will squeeze waste out of the system; if so, who could object? My concern is that present systems do not differentiate between needed care and unneeded care. There is a good deal of evidence that many patterns of care in common use cannot be justified on the basis of available data. The variation in rates for prostatectomy, hysterectomy, and so on down the line, indicate that doctors don't have a factual base on which to go when making their decisions. Jack Wennberg's studies show that when you look at countries that have no fee-for-service reimbursement, you still see these small area variations in rates for procedures; so it is not just doctors' pecuniary benefit that causes these differences. In fact, John Bunker showed that doctors use worthless procedures on their families even more than on their patients. It's possible that doctors hate their families, but I think the truth of the matter must be that we don't have the information base to make sound decisions.

It would be much more sensible, from my point of view, to devise a system which attempts to control overuse in various communities, as Wennberg has shown can be done in the case of tonsillectomy, and Vayda and his colleague showed can be done for hysterectomies, by getting medical bodies to examine disproportionate rates and bring them down. Thus, one, in fact, saves money by stopping unnecessary surgery rather than capping all surgery. The only way that we can assume that Medicare clients will benefit from caps is if we assume medical care is bad for you and, therefore, if they have less, they are better off than the rich. Since the rich won't decide on that basis, I'd like the poor to have the same option. I don't see any evidence for the assumption that putting caps on these costs will drive out poor care differentially. What it is going to do is deny access differentially, not because that is the purpose of it, but because that is the consequence of such a system.

Finally, the huge growth of the for-profit industry seems to me a disaster. It represents the very worst features of the medical care industry as it has been, but more so. The General Accounting Office studied the consequences, for all third-party payers, of the acquisition by one large hospital chain of a smaller chain. The large one bought the small one, with some 54 hospitals, at a price of approximately $1 billion. In the year following the transfer of ownership from one group to the other, the results for third-party payers was a $50 million increase in the cost of care delivered by those hospitals. They weren't any newer or better; they just cost more. How did that happen? A hospital more than 20 years old no longer has any depreciation value. When it is bought, it suddenly acquires a new value and depreciation starts over. In the second place, it is bought with borrowed money, which costs interest; and the interest is passed on to the third party payer. Chains are simply parasites on the system. The money they earn comes out of cost that should have gone into care for patients. There is no evidence that they are more efficient. All of the studies that have been done show no better efficiency in the delivery of care; the only thing they are better at is charging and collecting.

Dr. Stanley Reiser: I think Dr. Young made an important point in his paper when he discussed how the prospective payment system and DRG system were part of a larger trend to change the place of the hospital in American medical care, and to create new incentives to investigate new forms of care delivery outside of hospitals. I think this would have happened without DRGs and PPS; movement of technology would be a force that would create this anyway. However, this has accelerated the movement. I think we are facing an era, no matter what happens to PPS and DRGs, when we are going to have to deal with the development of new health care systems not solely centralized in a hospital. That being the case, the elderly play a particularly important role in this.

Dr. Liebig's comments that the system of de-institutionalization resulted in a disaster for the mentally ill, are very important and I don't think we really have addressed that yet. The examples we have of de-institutionalization have been very bad. What leads us to believe that we are going to do any better with the larger number of people that will be affected by this de-institutionalization? One example of the issues that we have to start thinking about relates to the way in which we design and build houses. For example, the round door knob is a very difficult mode of technology for anyone with arthritis to deal with, and yet, we continue to build houses with round door knobs. The Europeans build houses with handles which makes it much easier for the disabled or the elderly to deal with living at home. So it's not enough to create new loci of care outside of the hospital. Not only do we have to rethink the ways we deal with medical care, but we must rethink the ways we design the environment of living so that those who are being forced to maintain their lives more independently can be helped by the way we create an environment.

Dr. Robert Kane: I have a propensity to compare nursing homes with prisons because there's a lot of interesting data on expenditures for those two groups. It turns out that in the prison population, it is much more effective to assign every inmate a guard 24-hours-a-day than it is to operate the institution. It would be cheaper to take all the people in prison and assign them round-the-clock coverage on a one-to-one basis. How we look at this system really depends very much on what we are willing to invest in terms of care. In the nursing home situation, it is entirely the opposite. We did a mini-survey in Los Angeles in which we looked at the cost of taking care of primates in the Los Angeles Zoo, of inmates in Los Angeles city jails, and of elderly in average nursing homes in Los Angeles, and discovered that the nursing home was the cheapest of the three; primates were in the middle.

When we talk about how you design environments, it really goes back to the question of what basic values we assign to the care of these individuals, and harkens back to the discussion that we had earlier about how we view these people in this society and what is the obligation to society to make them more functional. I'm not sure that Europeans use handles because they are concerned about arthritics. But there are things that the Europeans have done that suggest that they do think about people in a very different way. For example, Dutch money is encoded in braille so blind people can tell the denominations. I don't know whether that means the people are more likely to cheat Dutch people if they didn't encode it, but I suspect it's the small things that count. There are in the Paris subway system these delightful seats that are set aside for veterans and old ladies, where you are not supposed to sit. I always find a good seat there so I know about how comfortable they are. There are societies that have set aside certain aspects, at least tokens of their belief of where these people fit into their value system. It is much harder to find that kind of even tokenism in the American society.

Mr. Bob Ball: I want to address the concern of Bob Kane and Elaine Brody about hospitals getting into the step-down services or moving into nursing home care, and so on. I just wanted to recall for them the way we thought of this in the very early days of Medicare, which was the opposite. We had hoped that a large number of hospitals would take on the responsibility of having an actual connection, not just a paper one, with the extended care facility because we thought there would be better attention to quality medical care that way, rather than leaving everything to the predominately profit-making nursing homes, which at the time, and I don't know that it's really changed very much, were not very good. Why do you feel that in hospitals, where occupancy is low and buildings are available, moving some of those beds into a dedicated nursing home situation under the hospital's auspices, along with other step-down services, would not be a good thing to do?

Ms. Elaine Brody: I didn't express negative views about hospitals getting into the short-term, long-term care business. I think it is appropriate for hospitals to give short term care that is of lesser intensity than care in the acute hospital setting and, perhaps, play a case-management role, and I'm deliberately not saying discharge planning, in the short term interval after hospitalization. What I feel very strongly against is hospitals getting into long term care, into the business of running nursing homes and community care support systems that are ongoing over long periods of time. For one thing, they are not equipped and don't have the expertise or the mandate to go on managing "cases" years after a patient has been discharged.

With respect to nursing home care *per se,* long term care is a totally different animal than that the acute care model is equipped to deal with. A long stay institution is a living arrangement. People live there for the rest of their lives, and it has to address itself to creating a living environment rather than a following the medical model blindly. I think that if hospitals began to run long stay institutions, it's quite natural that this will continue the trend that always occurred for the long stay facility, to take on the character of an acute care hospital. This is inappropriate where the rhythm of life is dictated by the crisis and cure atmosphere and where the technical personnel are paramount.

Dr. Robert Kane: I have great concern about hospitals doing case-management. You cannot have the case manager also being a major provider of services; you don't give very unbiased case-management when you do that. My second point is if there were a device to take hospital beds out of hospital service, it will probably be worth it even though there may be some other price to pay to accomplish it. The swing bed concept is not a satisfactory method because it does not take them out of the pool on a permanent basis.

Third, I think the ethos of the hospital is really counterproductive to the ethos of long term care. One simply has to go through the British system to see it in stark contrast. If you go to a British geriatric ward in a hospital, it is all starched, prim and proper; if someone urinates on the floor, the nurse comes over and cleans it up right away. When you go into a British accommodations, which is their nursing home run by the social system, what you see is a home-like environment which is really run on a different set of values. The beds do not have hospital corners on them, the patients are not necessarily as neat as they are when they're cared for by ward sisters. Many of the ethics that have predominated in both nursing and medicine don't apply or can be applied differently when you begin to integrate into a picture that looks at a total lifestyle question.

Finally, I think that the real question about hospitals is that they are big spenders. It makes me very nervous to think about how a hospital is going to gear down suddenly to run on a tight budget. It may be that they can adapt to a different lifestyle, but I have seen very few of them do it. I think one really is going to the wrong group to try and find an economical solution to the problem. They are too used to flying first class and we are talking about a tourist operation.

Ms. Elaine Brody: I don't like the word "tourist operation"; long term care could be a first class operation, but it is a different operation altogether. It need not be as nearly as costly as hospital care. When one-third of long stay patients stay more than three years in a nursing home, and another third stay from one to three years, you don't want to turn them into full-time, professional patients. They should be residents and have an integration of the different kinds of services.

Rebuttal

Donald A. Young, MD

This has been a very interesting and good discussion, and it certainly fits with what my opening comments were: there are extraordinary changes taking place in the world today and extraordinary changes in health policy. It is obvious that each of us around the room lead different lives, and when we look out our windows we see different worlds. One of the problems that I think I have to confront with policy in Washington is reminding myself constantly that the view from the Federal window is very different from that in other parts of the world. On the other hand, the same applies to all of you.

My assignment was to discuss the impact of prospective payment on de-institutionalizing health services for the elderly. It was not a justification for, or a defense of, the Medicare prospective payment system. It so happens that I worked for the Health Care Financing Administration and that my staff wrote the regulations for the Medicare prospective payment system. Therefore, I was very used to defending them in my prior life. I feel no need to defend them in my current life and I hope, Dr. Ginzberg did not read my paper as a defense of the Medicare prospective payment system.

Let me turn to the issue of nosology/nomenclature. Bob Kane's advisors at the Rand Corporation are indeed accurate when they point out the difference between PPS and DRGs. I did not make the point today because I was limited in time. I make it repeatedly as I speak to groups. The Medicare prospective payment system enacted in October, 1983, has two separate and very different characteristics, that must be kept apart to clarify thinking. One is prospective payment, where a price is set in advance for a package of services. It does not matter how you define that package, there are a set of very strong incentives merely by setting the price in advance. The second is the way in which the services are packaged, the tool. That happens to be diagnosis-related groups, DRGs. I dealt with the

189

issues of incentives of prospective payment and I did not get into the issues of DRGs. It's important to make that distinction.

Dr. Rodkey, I agree with you as a physician and as the Executive Director of the Commission, that the issue of quality of care may be the central issue for examination. On the other hand, it does not serve me well to receive a report that says, 63 percent of physicians think that quality of care has decreased or may decrease under PPS. That is not very useful to me as a policymaker. I think that we must find a way to look at quality. If you look at our annual report, which was submitted to the Secretary two weeks ago, we do not have a definition of quality of care because we could not come up with one. The Rand Corporation has a contract to look at this issue for the Health Care Financing Administration, and we will be looking at it as well. It is a critical issue; I simply don't know how to define it, let alone to measure it, but I stressed over and over again in my paper, the difference between process of care, structure, and outcome. I think that the issue of quality has to be looked at as an outcome issue.

Clearly, people who are leaving hospitals today are sicker. They're leaving, on the average, a day earlier. Is that bad? Do you measure quality at the point the patient leaves the hospital or some other point? A lot of work has yet to be done. I agree that benefits will need to be restructured. Were we to sit down and chat about it, however, I may not agree with you on how they should be restructured. There appears to be widespread belief among the discussants here that the Medicare program must restructure its benefits at some point; the A/B dichotomy has simply worn out.

I felt a touch of nihilism on Eli Ginzberg's part about public policy in the health care system today. The most important point where I may disagree with you is that a public policy of cost containment is with us. Disliking it doesn't help a great deal; it is with us. At the point that prospective payment with the DRGs were put in place, it went through the Congress like lightning. Actually, it had been on the public agenda for a long time. The reason it went through as quickly as it did, is that prospective payment and the policies associated with it were far less onerous to the hospital industry than the Tax Equity and Fiscal Responsibility Act. I am not defending DRGs as a case mix measurement tool or prospective payment, I am pointing out that the public policy of cost containment is here. I happen to share Steven Schroeder's assessment, however, that the policy is a reasonably good one. It was not intended to be a panacea to the health care costs of this country, and I hope I didn't state that in my paper.

On the issue of ambulatory surgery, there are good data that prospective fees have not, so far, decreased the quality of care. I share your concern, however, about the movement out of the hospital and point out in my paper that hospitals have conditions of participation, certification standards for employees, and critical masses of people looking over each others' shoulders. Once you get out into that community, the one-man ambulatory surgical center or any of the alternatives, you will not have that. I agree that issue has to be examined and that is part of the quality issue that I talked about earlier.

On the issue of integrating medical and social programs and services, I also agree that it is extraordinarily complex. There are movements into that: the hospice program, social HMO research, etc. Medicaid home and community-based waivers in many states do link medical services with social services. It is a beginning.

Finally, on the issue of substitution and additions, I was not saying that you have to only have substitution, not additions. I was saying that the public policy today is one of cost containment. It will be very hard to sell to Congress, impossible to sell to the Administration, new benefits that are added one. All you have to do is review the last two years in Congress. I hope you did not attribute that to my personal views, I was being reportorial.

The GAO study that got wide press from Senator Heinz was not a study. It is cause for concern, but not empirical evidence that the Medicare prospective payment is having an adverse impact. There remains a question, on which the GAO study sheds very little light. Yes, people leaving the hospital are sicker, but is that bad?

Is prospective payment tantamount to rationing? I have a whole lecture I give on that subject. I start by pointing out I do not care for that word. It is misleading in many cases, at least it does not let me think clearly. Is there a limit on resources and allocation of resources? Absolutely. Will that limit be more severe under prospective payment? I think so. The Medicare program has never paid for eyeglasses. Isn't that rationing? The Medicare program has never paid for dental care; it has paid for a very limited numbers of devices in the home. The problem of allocation of limited resources related to health care services has been with us forever, probably always will be. That doesn't mean we should not continue to work on it. Prospective payment in this resource allocation decision does something that is very different. It shifts decisions from a bureaucrat working in an office in Baltimore to a hospital's medical staff. At the local hospital level, it is that shifting that is creating as much consternation and instability as anywhere else. They want it back in the hands of that bureaucrat where they can second-guess it when they don't like it.

The issue of what PPS tells us about the American health care system, that Bob Kane raised, is an important one. Congress has asked us to submit a report next February on that very subject of where the hospital fits as a centerpiece in our society. I won't pursue it further at this point.

The mean length of stay issue raised is a technical one. It's worse even than was suggested because indeed some hospital administrators appear to be saying "the government told me to get you out in 3.6 days and it is now 3.6 days." We have examined a couple of DRGs where that issue has been raised with us. It turns out that those lengths of stay are reasonable and appropriate in some kind of a skewed or normal distribution.

Dr. Aaron raised the question of where we go from here. I am sure where we are going. There will be a period of stability. The Medicare prospective payment system clearly needs areas of maintenance and we are setting about doing those, working with HCFA. I also agree with the comment that now is not the time to look for adverse impacts from the system because hospitals are doing well, they have apparently been able to engage in moderate efficiencies. Aggregate expenditures are down on the hospital side and I gather that the rest of part A and part B are not up in a commensurate manner. Hospitals have not been squeezed yet and it may be very premature, as we said before, to say that things are okay. However, they are engaging, apparently, in efficiency/productivity behavior without significant impacts.

Finally, the question of de-institutionalization was raised. Dr. Liebig said she wished that she was as sanguine as Dr. Schroeder and I, that de-institutionalization would lead to a greater array of services. I hope I did not say that. It is important to distinguish between the availability and financing of services. I did say that there were extraordinary things happening with the availability of services. Will what is happening now lead to greater financing for the services that are de-institutionalized? The bottom line projection for the next year or two or three is probably no, because we have an administration and a Congress that is not going to expand benefits.

Therefore, the services may be there or they may be capable of going there. There will not be financing through the Medicare program for them and I doubt there'll be through the "Blues" or commercial insurance.

Dr. Eisenberg raised a series of questions and made some comments as well. The implication that prospective payment will squeeze waste out of the system and leave all the good behind, I cannot argue with. Anytime that you have a system that is as diverse and shifts the locus of decision, how do you know what's waste? I also agree and have been a follower of Jack Wennberg's work for a very long time. What is medical necessity? What is waste and what is need? I don't know the answer to that. I know that when I was in practice I engaged in certain behaviors related to taking care of patients that now don't seem to have been right. I kept heart attack patients in hospitals for 21 days, now it's 14 days. Was I wasteful? Was that unnecessary or unneeded? We just need to know an immense amount more. My only concern about some of the research that Jack Wennberg is doing and working with Bob Brook on, is that when we don't know enough, is getting doctors together to decide how to do it the right way? I'm very much in favor of democracy, but I'm not absolutely sure in the care of the individual patient whether a democratic vote is the way to go. If you have a procedure that is done 20 percent in one place and 60 percent in another, and doctors agree that 50 percent is right, that does not make 50 percent any more right than 60 percent or 20 percent. On the other hand, I don't know the answers to those questions. I think that they are very important ones and we need to do a great deal more.

On the issue of proprietaries, there was discussion of reevaluation of assets or accelerated depreciation. Let me point out that under prospective payment, proprietaries are now paid the identical amount as non-proprietaries. Under DRGs, they get the same amount. The question is, do they skim or do they have different case mix? And there is a separate capital policy, which I will not go into.

CHAPTER 5

Educating Practitioners
for the Care of the Elderly:
The Teaching Nursing Home?
Position Paper

Phoebe S. Liebig, PhD

This paper examines the place of the nursing home in the education of practitioners to care for the elderly. These issues emerge in the context of a general discussion about how and where health professions education should take place,[1,2] and the goals of education in geriatrics and gerontology.[3,4]

Three publicly and privately funded programs, while markedly different from each other, now carry the title of "teaching nursing home" (TNH). And most recently, another federally-funded program has been announced by the National Institute of Mental Health, which bears a striking resemblance to the TNH program of the National Institute on Aging, although it lacks the TNH designation.[5] Similarly, recent state legislation has identified the TNH as a vital aspect of geriatric education.[6] Thus, the increasing visibility of TNH or TNH-like programs warrants examination.

Practitioners requiring education for care of the elderly include physicians, nurses, dentists, pharmacists, allied and public health personnel, social workers, clinical psychologists, physician assistants, optometrists, gerontologists, podiatrists and health care administrators.[3] There are numerous para-professionals also involved in institutional and noninstitutional care of the elderly, such as hospital and home aides. Their important roles in care of the elderly are increasingly recognized by state-mandated training and by reports on education in aging.[3]

The concept of using nursing homes for instructional purposes has been around for nearly two decades. Training in aging for current practitioners employed in the nursing home has been mandated by various states since the mid-1970s. Starting in the late 1960s and early 1970s, various levels of personnel (e.g., administrators, nurses aides) were given short-term training in care of the elderly. In 1973, through the Community Health Service program, a number of programs were inaugurated to train activity directors, RNs, a wide range of professional and auxiliary personnel, physicians in their role as medical directors, and boards of trustees. Colleges and universities played a role in these programs and in similar short-term training experiences for nursing home personnel. While nursing schools and associates were involved, their medical counterparts and other health professional groups were rarely so.

Over the years, both direct onsite and offsite training plus "train the trainers" formats have been used, with professional associations, accreditation bodies or legislative bodies providing the impetus for such training. Additionally, summer workshops have been conducted for practitioners not employed in nursing homes with onsite instruction provided by nursing home personnel. Thus, existing practitioners have been receiving training in nursing home-based elder care for some time; however, the training has tended to be non-systematic, and has been plagued by a number of problems such as intermittent funding, lack of training in rural areas, and rapid turnover of nursing staff.

Nursing homes themselves have been isolated from community-based practitioners and generally have not served as an education resource for local health personnel. Many small nursing homes find it sufficiently difficult, both programmatically and economically, to provide inservice training. Similarly, even the large nursing home chains have not seen this extramural educational function as an important mission, at least not until recently. The educational linkage with the community, however, seems to be developing, spearheaded by Beverly Enterprises and Hillhaven, and facilitated by such groups as the American Association of Homes for the Aged. Even with these present efforts, it is clear that the training of practitioners in providing care for the elderly in the nursing home, specifically, and in long-term care facilities, in general, requires major improvements, both quantitatively and qualitatively.

ARGUMENTS FOR THE EDUCATIONAL NURSING HOME

Within the past five to ten years, the focus on nursing homes as an education resource has switched to the training of future practitioners. This shift has been made particularly visible through the flurry of comments about the training of future physicians in the nursing home setting. While the "educational nursing home" has been used since the early 1970s by a number of health professions programs including pharmacy, dentistry, psychology, dietetics, nursing, and health services administration,[7,8] only a handful of medical education programs utilized nursing homes as clinical training sites. The Mount Sinai program established in 1972 by Dr. Leslie Libow was unique for many years.[9]

The teaching of geriatric care must include experiences in every type of environment in which older persons are likely to need care,[10] especially those settings that provide medical and social services often required by that population. Because the nursing home is such a setting, it has been recommended that nursing homes and other long-term care facilities be included as clinical sites for the teaching of geriatric medicine.[11] While some question the wisdom of overemphasizing use of the educational nursing home,[12,13] there is general agreement on its utilization as a geriatric training site.

Rationales advanced for the utilization of nursing homes for education include:

Demographic

The nursing home will continue to be the locus of care for a large number of elderly patients. Student learning is enhanced in the nursing home setting because trainees need not compete with hordes of faculty, house staff and other students as is the case in more classical training sites.[14] The nursing home setting also lacks the press of continually arriving, acutely ill patients, and involves a smaller patient load, so there is more time available to focus on ongoing problems.[14,15]

Generalizability of Chronic Care Management

Kane[16] has suggested that the nursing home provides a setting for the teaching of chronic disease and an opportunity to emphasize basic points generalizable to all phases of medical care. The nursing home is seen as a goldmine of clinical problems. Students encounter a wide variety of problems and are provided with good examples of diseases of all types in advanced and chronic phases with complications.[16,17,18] It provides the best model for attending to the patient's functional status and an opportunity to focus on the outcomes of care through the development of a long term plan, its evaluation and subsequent adjustment.[16] In addition, the nursing home setting presents a situation in which students become aware of the importance of patient compliance and the need to develop expertise to maximize it. (Although Kane doesn't mention it, presumably students also become aware of the negative impacts that institutionalization can have on compliance and motivation for self-care.)

Skills Development

The educational nursing home experience allows faculty and students to work with both highly skilled and relatively unskilled health care professionals and to become sensitive to the importance of the latter group for patient well-being.[19] The educational nursing home can provide experiences not only for becoming aware of the potential of other health care team members,[20] but for adopting a systematic approach to choosing and involving other health professionals.[10] The development of student research skills is also facilitated.

The nursing home provides a wide array of opportunities for student research;[17] however, there are constraints on that opportunity because clinical research is easiest with a particular disease,[20] rather than with several concurrent diseases in one individual. Other skills whose development are facilitated in the educational nursing home are the ability to create and implement a problem-oriented medical record,[21] improved history taking and physical examination techniques,[19,22] improved means of communication with the severely impaired so as to learn what goals are realistically acceptable to the patient and his/her family,[14] the development of treatment modalities that are less dependent on the hardware of medical technology[15,23] and the encouragement of decision-making with limited resources.[17] (Although the virtues of relying less on high technology are extolled, the need for high touch or what might be termed "skinware" is sadly lacking. The art of compassion and the necessary capacity and ability to convey it are missing from the skill armamentarium.)

Health Care System and Community Resources

The nursing home setting is also seen as a rich environment to learn about community resources and to identify gaps in the health care system.[16] Geriatric care occurs in a variety of settings, including multi-purpose senior centers, day centers and other well-elderly programs, community screening and counseling services, old-age homes and home care programs.[13] The future health care practitioner must not only learn about what these services provide, but also must become skilled in the mobilization and management of community resources[13] and, if necessary, development of those resources that may be lacking.[10]

Ethics

The educational nursing home is also seen as a place to learn about the humanities of medicine,[24] to grapple with ethical issues of health care delivery, and to develop a new or different set of values and attitudes towards the delivery of care to the elderly. The nursing home presents more problems requiring ethical considerations than other health care settings, especially because the quality of life can be a different issue for an institutionalized patient who may have limited goals and very constricted lifestyles,[14,15] compared with the non-institutionalized patient. Issues of informed consent are heightened in this setting.[16,25]

The Nursing Home as the Geriatric Care Institution

A final rationale is based on the perception that the nursing home is *the* institutional base for geriatric care. Geriatric care is generally taught in such a fragmented way that there needs to be a place where the fragments of geriatric theory and practice can be integrated. The acute-care hospital is a poor setting for such integration;[9] the nursing home is far more appropriate. The nursing home setting provides a model for teaching that medicine cures little except acute infections,[19] that both care and cure are relevant in treating older patients,[26] that with respect to functional improvements to be achieved, small is beautiful, and that quality health care can be delivered outside the acute-care tertiary hospital.[14]

ARGUMENTS AGAINST
THE EDUCATIONAL NURSING HOME

A number of writers have commented on the problems of using nursing homes for instructional purposes, ranging from philosophical perspectives to practical concerns. Some have identified generic problems such as their negative image, the atypical characteristics of nursing home patients relative to the elderly population as a whole, or the lack of attention to mental health care. Others have focused on realistic considerations such as the problem of most nursing homes being inappropriate for instructional purposes, the lack of charismatic and committed teachers, or the often crushing logistics of developing university-nursing home affiliations, especially with proprietary facilities. Again, while most of these analyses have sprung from concerns relative to medical education, they are equally applicable to the education of all health professionals. Similarly, while these positions have been delineated relative to the educational nursing home, many are equally relevant for the TNH.

Negative Image of the Nursing Home

Generally speaking, "nursing home" has extremely negative connotations: its general image is as a warehouse for the elderly, a place to die. The fact that 20 to 25 percent of persons aged 65 or older die in nursing homes[27] lends greater credence to the nursing home as the end of the line. The cultural gap between the elderly and many health practitioners, especially physicians[16,28] can be exacerbated in the nursing home setting because of negative stereotypes.

These negative views of nursing homes and of aging in general are also held by many faculty members. The need for change in these faculty attitudes is a prerequisite for developing practitioners who will care for the elderly.[29] Student attitudes can also be negatively effected and dampened by the exposure to nursing home patients.[12,30] Trainees can become overwhelmed by the problems presented as being untreatable,[16] and the failure of nursing home patients to get well can be a source of frustration and negativity. If a positive experience can be developed, however, the apparent initial disadvantage can be turned around.[16] Additionally, multiple exposures over the entire period of training can be instrumental in inculcating more positive attitudes.[22] It is clear, however, that unless positive experiences can be appropriately structured, negative and hostile attitudes towards older people may be strengthened, especially if the student encounter is with very sick individuals for a very short period of time.

Nursing Home Population Characteristics

One argument against over-reliance on the use of nursing homes for the training of future practitioners stems from the perception that nursing home patients tend to be atypical, compared with the majority of the elderly who, although they may have the same range of chronic disease, remain in the community. The aged nursing home patient, who over time may represent 20 to 38 percent of all persons 65 and over,[16,31] does not have the key functional or social strengths of the community-based elderly.[9] By relying heavily or exclusively on the nursing home patient for teaching about geriatric care, the stereotype of all elderly being sick and debilitated is strengthened. The concepts of well elderly or the chronically ill, but independently functioning aged can easily get lost.

Nursing home patients differ markedly from the rest of the elderly population in a number of significant ways. They are disproportionately white and female[17] and while the heterogeneity of nursing home populations has been identified,[17,31,32,33] on the average they tend to be far sicker, especially since the implementation of DRGs,[34] and often suffer from severe mental deterioration. Additionally, because of Medicaid spend-down requirements, many nursing home patients are severely economically disadvantaged compared to the rest of the older population. Additionally, the "oldest old" make up a sizeable proportion of nursing home residents, many of whom have been abandoned by their families,[16] a phenomenon not experienced by the majority of the elderly,[33] Veterans Administration (VA) nursing homes, which often serve as educational facilities, are also atypical because they serve predominantly males.[35]

A counterargument has been advanced that, while the nursing home population is unrepresentative of the elderly just as the hospital population is, there are good reasons for using both. A faculty mentor can demonstrate by example that a demented, debilitated older person is a human being, often dear to someone, who deserves the same respect and care as a more functional individual.[36] Similarly, if the nursing home is a setting where a sizeable proportion of the elderly will receive care at some time in their lives, that setting is sufficiently typical to warrant training being conducted there.

Lack of Mental Health Care

Although mental health services for the elderly are lacking in most settings,[37] their absence in nursing homes is severe and especially problematic when it is recognized that many admissions are for mental problems.[33] Psychosocial services and the necessary staff to provide them are generally unavailable. The hospital-like characteristics of the nursing home lend themselves to a strictly medical focus and to the primacy of physicians,[33] most of whom have little or no training in mental health care. Care of the chronically ill, however, entails attending to social and emotional needs. Therefore, there is a need to teach a psychological/social/ medical/environmental model of care and treatment, as well as a need to conduct research on psychosocial issues such as family relationships of people in nursing homes.[33] The majority of nursing homes, especially the ubiquitous intermediate care home of 30 to 50 beds that has been proposed as a model of the educational nursing home,[16] are simply not capable of supporting these kinds of efforts.

Philosophies of Care

Another issue that has been raised is the incompatibility of the traditional nursing home philosophy with the acute-care philosophy.[23,26,33] Not only does this presage problems of developing closer links between those two institutions ("mainstreaming"), but it also calls into question whether the possible irreconcilability of the goals of the two institutions will become a problem for students who are trying to integrate their geriatric training experience conducted at both kinds of sites. The dominant nursing home philosophy is to make the patient comfortable, to limit invasive measures and allow a peaceful death, if non-heroic methods prove inadequate.[12] The competent management of disease in the acute care hospital does not insure and, indeed, may differ from competent management in the nursing home.[23] One danger may be the "medicalizing" of the nursing home care,[38] with an emphasis on undertaking therapeutic measures which are incompatible with the philosophy and pace of nursing home care. A net result of "mainstreaming," therefore, may be the teaching of old models (viz., the medical model) in a new setting.[39]

One practical consideration relative to the philosophy and pace of care and the use of the educational nursing home is the length of time spent in rotations or assignments to the facility. While nursing homes provide an opportunity to track the incremental changes in functional ability so characteristic of the older person, those changes may require a long period of supervision, observation and care.[40] The majority of student assignments to nursing homes are generally two weeks in length or shorter, which provide limited opportunities for becoming aware and appreciative of these slight changes. Students need a program which will permit them to follow patients on a long-term basis in order to establish a relationship with them and to supply patient education information.[41] It has been suggested that longitudinal exposure over the entire period of early professional education at various times and various levels of sophistication may ameliorate this problem.[22] Otherwise, the involvement of the student is little more than a visit to the zoo,[28] and is not likely to lead to the necessary attitude that the emphasis on diagnosis and cure, so prevalent in the medical model of care, must give way to assessment and functional improvement.

Lack of Adequately Trained Faculty

Perhaps one of the most telling arguments against utilization of the educational nursing home, at least for the present, is the lack of faculty who have been adequately trained in nursing home care and the philosophy of long-term care; few have had direct patient care responsibilities in the nursing home.[26] While there is a dearth of trained faculty from all disciplines in geriatric care,[3] this lack is particularly evident in the area of nursing home care. While the greatest focus has been on the training of physicians who will be academic role models,[13] especially in long-term care, it is clear that the majority of academic health professionals have spent little time in nursing homes and other long-term care facilities and that they, in particular, require this kind of training. Although a member of privately and publicly funded programs have been created to fill these gaps in faculty training, it is clear that even after a decade or more of educational activities, there is still a crying need for trained faculty,[3] especially those who are knowledgeable about long-term care. In short, all the skills that students can learn via the nursing home experience must first be learned by faculty.

Cost of Affiliations

The interinstitutional arrangements needed to establish effective clinical sites are very time-consuming, and involve important accommodations by both academics and the clinical facility.[42] This is particularly true of affiliations with an unfamiliar type of facility with the novel philosophy of care that the nursing home may represent. The teaching hospital, the university-dominated model of care, may not be generalizable to the educational nursing home.[34] Additionally, the type of nursing home affiliation chosen by some schools or departments at a single university may be less appropriate for other academic units, thus necessitating multiple affiliation agreements and greater expenditures of time for negotiation. Similarly, many health professions programs are based on the academic year, yet nursing home care requires year-round care and, therefore, continuous faculty involvement.

Legal Problems

Kapp has identified a number of legal problems arising from academic affiliations with nursing homes.[25] Because students are viewed as unlicensed laypersons, they must have supervision and control exercised by an appropriately licensed or certified professional. While reimbursement policies may require that a physician be the supervisor, licensing requirements and/or departmental guidelines may require that a preceptor from a non-reimbursable discipline be in charge of that supervision. Providing appropriate supervision, especially for a wide range of health disciplines, is one of the most difficult challenges facing the establishment of linkages between health professions educational programs and long-term patient care, especially as the nature of those linkages may vary depending upon the particular health profession(s) involved.[25,43] Informed consent of patients requires that they be apprised about the identity and role of students involved in their care, not only in terms of the procedures to be performed but also who will do them. With institutionalized patients, especially those who are mentally impaired, guidelines for informed consent and confidentiality must be strictly adhered to. Other legal liabilities may arise for the nursing home and its professional staff for negligent conduct on the part of students.[25]

To avoid these problems, the nursing home must have a policy and procedures manual setting forth how the administration and professional staff of the facility delegate authority to and exercise supervisory control over subordinates, including students.[25] Similarly, the educational institution must develop guidelines concerning supervisory expectations for its paid and voluntary faculty,[25] especially nursing home personnel who have joint appointments.

OPTIMAL ENVIRONMENTAL CHARACTERISTICS

In order to present an optimal educational experience, one that is free of the majority of disadvantages and maximizes advantages cited previously, the educational nursing home should have at least 100 patients. This minimum size, enhanced by "open" admissions policies, will insure sufficient diversity in the patient population.[44] An overdose of any one kind of patient, but especially demented patients, can be deleterious to appropriate learning.[23] The small size of homes suggested by Kane as the model educational nursing home would not provide the necessary breadth of experience.[16] Smaller nursing homes, to become candidates for educational nursing homes, would have to form networks of facilities to attract university affiliations.[44] It is not surprising that the most successful educational nursing homes appear to be those facilities with 250–300 patients,[9,45] that admit patients for a variety of problems and incorporate several levels of care.[10,16]

To establish a positive teaching model, there must be a sufficiently high level of care.[16] Staff performance levels must be of a caliber to promote student learning about the value of the team approach and para-professional care. Similarly, several levels of care will enable the student to follow patient progress (or regression) to different levels of functioning, including return to the community. To enhance student comprehension of geriatric care appropriately, something approaching Libow's multi-level system must be in place.[9,10,46] The ideal training situation would include a nursing home facility with a rehabilitation unit, an acute care facility, and ambulatory clinic, day hospital and home visit program;[46,47] but few nursing homes have this wide range of services.

Similarly, the facility must have extramural linkages with the community, including a wide range of agencies and organizations. Too often the nursing home is isolated from the mainstream of professional groups and from the community at large.[26] The care of the elderly involves social and welfare agencies in addition to medical care organizations[46] and these must be marshalled and managed for the benefit of the patient.[13] Thus, the facility must be located in a geographically appropriate way for easy access. Additionally, the candidate educational nursing home should have programs providing interaction with both professional and lay communities.[44]

To enhance the learning of students, there must be present endogenous staff who recognize the need for education activities, are good instructors, and are not threatened by medical center and university-based faculty.[44] Additionally, there needs to be a commitment by the Board of Trustees or owner and the medical director to the educational enterprise, and a willingness to confront the problems and opportunities created by the presence of students. It is especially important that the medical director act as a positive force. It is also vital that students not be regarded as a substitute for quality staff that the facility may have problems in recruiting.[12]

The physical plant must be appropriately designed and attractive. Poor facilities reinforce for the student the belief that people living in nursing homes are not worthy of care.[44] The site must also be a therapeutic environment, with attention paid to the mental health of the patients.[33] In addition, there must be sufficient physical space in the nursing home for teaching and research activities. If unoccupied space is not available, then existing space must be converted for those activities, representing an opportunity cost to the facility.

Finally, the financial status of the home is also important. There needs to be stable funding for patient care, teaching activities and research.[44] Often patient care funds cannot underwrite the university related activities. Thus, affiliation with all nursing homes may be a problem. Proprietary homes can present special problems because their market place incentives may not be compatible with the university's objectives of teaching and research.[16] Because of this, most affiliated nursing homes are non-profit.[9] Yet, the majority of nursing homes in the United States are proprietary homes which may be unwilling to absorb the costs incurred by taking on a new set of activities that are not directly care-related.

THE TNH—THE ACADEMIC OR MULTIPURPOSE NURSING HOME

Not until Butler's seminal article appeared in 1981 was the concept of the formal or "official" TNH proposed[48] and widely identified. While earlier discussions of the educational nursing home had described those training experiences in relationship to a variety of health professions, the TNH was consciously put forth as a model, especially for medicine. Butler, then Director of the National Institute on Aging (NIA), identified the TNH as the organizational focus for geriatric research and training parallel to the role played by the teaching hospital (TH) in enhancing medical research and education. He clearly envisioned TNHs as becoming models for more than 18,000 nursing homes and several thousand home-health services based in or associated with nursing homes.[48] (For a more recent, contrary view see Schneider[18] who specifies that TNHs are not intended to be such a model; however, it is possible that he may be speaking specifically to the NIA's TNH program, described in the next section of this paper.)

In affiliation with schools of nursing and social services, the TNH concept envisioned the adoption of medical schools of several goals: (1) to foster systematic clinical investigations of disease processes and develop diagnostic techniques and treatment methods adopted for the elderly; (2) to train geriatricians, physicians in traditional specialties, geriatric and other nurses and other needed professionals; (3) to establish a research base to improve care of the elderly in nursing homes and physicians' practices; (4) to design community services and clinical strategies to postpone or prevent institutionalization and to promote rehabilitation of elderly patients; and, (5) to devise and demonstrate cost-effective strategies for care of the elderly.[48] The TNH concept set forth in the Butler article has become the basic blueprint for all subsequent discussions, as well as for specifically labelled TNH programs. Contrasted with most earlier discussions on nursing home utilization, with the exception of Kane,[16] Butler's focus was heavily on the role of research in mainstreaming geriatrics into the intellectual framework of American medicine.

Butler's concept emphasized training, with a heavy, if not almost exclusive, focus on medicine. In connection with the TNH, there would be required lectures and courses for medical students in their clinical years and for students in nursing, pharmacy, social work, and the therapies. He also envisioned required rotations for house staff and for medical and other health-related students in TNHs, with provision for grand and bedside rounds for several medical specialties and dentistry. Preservice and inservice training for nurses aides was also to be part of the TNH's educational activities.[48] Last year, Butler expanded inservice training to include a broader group of nursing home personnel.[45]

Through the TNH, Butler expected medical school traditionalism to be altered and major reforms precipitated: improved public image and quality of nursing home care and enhanced ability of nursing homes to attract and retain professionals. He has recently acknowledged that rather than use the expression "teaching nursing home," it might have been better to have spoken of an academic nursing home—that is, a nursing home with the classic academic goals of teaching, service, and research.[45]

Comparisons of the Conventional Home and the TNH Model

In contrast with expectations of the conventional home where disability and palliative care are taken for granted, the TNH undertakes vigorous assessment and diagnosis and active treatment where appropriate, with the goal of changing patient care routine. The goals of the conventional home may similarly be contrasted with those of the TNH: care with an emphasis on immediate, good results versus research which may be without immediate practical applications. The profit orientation of the characteristic nursing home is in contrast to the TNH commitment to the use of space and staff to develop models of care with associated costs. Additionally, nursing homes usually have fixed levels of care while the TNH has different protocols that cut across care levels. Finally, in the conventional nursing home, nursing is the dominant discipline, whereas, in the TNH, medicine is dominant, with social work and physical therapy included more fully.[49]

EXISTING TNH PROGRAMS

Currently, three formal TNH programs exist (that is, programs with the label of TNH), one funded by the National Institute on Aging, another by the Robert Wood Johnson Foundation and a third by Beverly Enterprises. "Unlabelled" funded programs that have used the nursing home as a training site include the Geriatric Nurse Practitioner program funded by the Kellogg Foundation, the Robert Wood Johnson Foundation's Clinical Nurse Scholars program, and training funded by the Veterans Administration and by the Division of Nursing of the Public Health Service. Some (e.g., Kellogg) have specified the use of the nursing home as a program component, while others have assumed its incorporation or have left its inclusion to the discretion of the awardee.

The National Institute on Aging (NIA) TNH Program

The NIA TNH award, first announced in November 1981, was designed as a specialized center grant to support research by a small, select number of academic medical centers and nursing homes on geriatric health problems particularly prominent in the nursing home setting and among geriatric outpatients, rather than in acute care hospitals. Another goal of the program has been to develop research on current and new therapies and health maintenance strategies in acute care hospital, geriatric outpatient and nursing home settings.

The program's title was intended to emphasize the analogy between the teaching hospital as a setting for research in acute care settings and the "teaching nursing home" as one site to develop research in long term care settings.[50] Thus, while support is provided for research projects developed by members of the participating components (staff of teaching hospital, medical and nursing schools, and nursing home) and for core activities, personnel and facilities to facilitate that research, teaching, training, or service activities per se are not supported by this program. Unlike the more recent NIA Alzheimer's Disease Research Center program, there is not even a stated expectation that education is to be an integral part of what is actually a program project grant.[51] Among the requirements of the program is the obligatory participation of schools of medicine and nursing. That of other health professionals (i.e., pharmacy, public health, dentistry, allied health and social work) and of graduate department in the biological, behavioral and social sciences, is seen as desirable, but not mandatory.

As of 1985, six awards have been made. A brief questionnaire was distributed by the author to each NIA TNH requesting information concerning their educational activities. Of the four responding institutions, one indicated that because the title of the program is a misnomer and there are no funds for specifically educational purposes, health sciences students are not directly associated with the project. Another institution indicated that their program was not primarily intended to educate health professionals. The two other responding institutions stated that students from medicine and nursing are indeed involved in their TNH programs on an elective basis; one indicated the participation of physician assistant/nurse practitioner students as well; at both institutions, the trainee level most often emphasized is the undergraduate medical student. One program also emphasized the training of fellows, and the other, of RNs. Both also stated that instructional activities included clinical care, research, and didactic instruction, with the first two predominating; in addition, one specified inservice training activities. Finally, both programs indicated that they had characteristically used the nursing home setting for instructional purposes for several years prior to receipt of the award.

Information concerning a fifth TNH program has been supplied in a recent article in *The Gerontologist*.[49] Aronson describes implementation of the TNH not only as a research endeavor, but also as part of a spectrum of activities required to impart knowledge about the continuum of care in geriatric medicine. The Hopkins' TNH program perhaps best illustrates the emerging model that Butler had in mind when he wrote his 1981 article,[48] especially as it related to education. Research in gerontology/geriatrics has been given visibility; hence, student interest has been raised. Student teaching is supported by faculty volunteer effort, with the principal incentives and rewards deriving from the stimulation of, and pleasure in, instruction. Support for the teaching of residents and fellows comes from patient care funds and also from faculty volunteer efforts.[52] Thus, the approach used to develop teaching hospitals as a means of training physicians appears to be successful transferred to the nursing home.[48]

Because of the newness of the NIA TNH program, it is premature to try to determine the extent to which its long range objectives of improving the quality of patient care or of mainstreaming the nursing home into the medical care system have been achieved. Given the program's structure, it is not easy to determine its effects on educating practitioners for care of the elderly. Some training-related questions can be raised about several aspects of the program: the status of educational activities in the TNH program, the transfer of information from the TNH to long-term care practice,[49] the visibility of the TNH nursing homes as role models for other nursing homes,[48] and the involvement of various disciplines.

First of all, the research focus of the TNH, accompanied by the lack of funds for educational activities, relegates education for current and future practitioners for care of the elderly to a secondary or byproduct status. The approach seems to corroborate the view that teaching stands low on the totem pole of medical school incentives.[1] While the need for quality clinical research in the nursing home setting as a basis for future training can be viewed as a laudable objective, the current incentives for the program do not lend themselves specifically to the inclusion of educational activities. Rather, it is necessary to rely upon education being an outcome of other programs and activities of the host academic medical center.

For example, the characteristics and quality of the six awardees make it highly likely that both basic and clinical research training are ongoing activities; however, direct care of the elderly is not the primary objective of such training. Similarly, the extent of clinical training for future practitioners in the nursing home setting seems to be dependent on its characteristic use by the univeristy (e.g., Hopkins and University of California, San Diego), on the interpretation (or reporting) by the awardee as to whether health science students are or should be involved (e.g., Harvard and Case Western Reserve), or whether other training programs for similar purposes exist at the same institution (e.g., Case Western).

Given the strengths of the six participating institutions in medical research and education in aging, the NIA can be seen to have been strategic in funding those academic medical centers where existing educational programs would be benefited, sooner or later. The NIA strategy to involve academic medical centers in geriatrics through research also wisely takes into account the academic reward structure for research grant acquisition and subsequent publications. Thus, this long-range tactic should result in the *eventual* incorporation of geriatrics/gerontology into the educational program of at least the medical and nursing programs of the recipient institutions.

But in the short run, education for care of the elderly receives less effort and direct attention than in the Robert Wood Johnson TNH program or in a number of medical and other health professions school programs which are using the nursing home for training, but without outside funding.

The extent of and/or improvement in inservice education reported by two of the TNH programs is unclear. An additional imponderable is whether that presumably increased education is based directly on the results of TNH research or is simply a spillover product of the university faculty being in residence. In view of the customary time lag between research findings and their incorporation into practice, the needed interface between research and practice is not likely to be achieved unless a mechanism, such as directly related inservice training, is created for the transfer of information from the TNH programs, programs to long-term care practice. The very small number of TNH no matter how prestigious, mitigates against broad transfer. Aronson's suggestion of developing links with other projects whose focus differs from that of the NIA program may be worth exploring to insure this needed transfer.[49]

Also at issue is whether or not the TNH program can be a role model for thousands of nursing homes. Although there has been some disagreement about the appropriateness of this role,[18,48] if the teaching hospital analogy holds true, then a long range outcome of the TNH should be its leadership in the nursing home industry and a consequent improvement in the level of care. Again, the TNH programs are so few in number (and likely to remain so) and so different from the average nursing home in size of patient population and other characteristics, that it is hard to anticipate their having much impact any time soon. Focused dissemination programs would enable the TNH programs to act as role models for nursing homes nationwide more rapidly. However, dissemination to professional and local communities was listed as an optional activity in the first announcement[50] and did not appear as a criterion for review and evaluation in the second.[51] In addition, without extramural dissemination to those responsible for education of future health care providers and to practicing health care providers, the TNH impact is likely to be limited.

A final concern about the NIA's TNH program revolves around its disciplinary focus. With the exception of the Albert Einstein program, only the two obligatory disciplines seems to be involved, and even with that program it is unclear as to whether the disciplines enumerated represent faculty participation in addition to that of students. If the multidisciplinary/interdisciplinary team approach is the appropriate model fo quality care for the elderly, then the NIA's approach of designating other disciplines as only "desirable" is not particularly supportive of that care concept. While it makes sense to try to bring medicine and nursing together in a research program, the other discplines, especially dentistry, social work, pharmacy and allied health, have a great deal to contribute beyond the acute-care model where the medical and nursing disciplines are key. Unless the TNH requirements change markedly, it is unlikely that other disciplines will become part of the program in the near future. Students who may be trained at the TNH site will thus not be exposed to interdisciplinary team care there and presumably will have to learn about it elsewhere, either as a function of the host institution having other training sites where this emphasis exists or as part of their on-the-job training upon completion of the formal education.

Robert Wood Johnson Foundation (RWJ) TNH Program

The RWJ TNH program, cosponsored by the American Academy of Nursing, was announced in mid-1981 and awards were made in late February 1982; thus, the implementation of this program predates that of the NIA's. The program was designed to bring nursing homes into the mainstream of nursing and medical care and related professional activities.[53] By helping university schools of nursing establish clinical affiliations with nursing homes to undertake clinical service, education and research within the homes and in their surrounding communities, the program has sought to improve the long-term health care of the elderly. Analogous to the university-affiliated teaching hospital, it is anticipated that the TNHs can become models for 18,000 nursing homes and several thousand home-health services. It is expected that these demonstrations will offer a testing ground for professional care and management innovations that will influence national policy decisions. Because nurses are responsible for the bulk of care in nursing homes,[54] the target institution is the school of nursing rather than the school of medicine, as is the case with the teaching hospital. Indeed, the homes are seen as a yet unchallenged territory where nurses can exercise their underdeveloped potential to assume autonomous and collaborative roles in clinical management and leadership positions.[32,38] In addition to enabling the homes to develop a a primary base for clinical faculty to provide care, conduct research and undertake outreach activities serving elderly living in the community, they are to facilitate the education of nurses, physicians and other health care professionals for care of the elderly and to conduct training programs for staff of the affiliated and other nursing homes. A specific area of need to be addressed is the education of more nurses in gerontology, especially at the graduate level as clinicians and faculty,[54] to bring about an upgrading or educational preparation of nurses in leadership positions.

This very specific disciplinary focus of the RWJ program is seen even more clearly in recent articles about the program objectives and progressed thus far in achieving the desired outcomes.[32,55] Awardees are to provide clinical training to undergraduate and graduate nursing students to increase the pool of nurses interested in working in nursing homes, and to facilitate the use of the home as a clinical training site for other health sciences disciplines. Recipients are also to offer continuing education opportunities to nurses employed by the home to enhance their opportunities for career advancement, and to provide training to update the clinical skills of nursing home personnel.[38] An anticipated outcome of this skill improvement is more competitive salaries and benefits for nursing home nurses.[53]

The eleven participating sites consist of six public and six private educational institutions, with one site including two schools. They are located in the District of Columbia and eight states. It is likely that this number will remain constant because, at least for the forseeable future, the Foundation does not expect to fund similar efforts (private communication). In comparison with schools of nursing nationally, participating schools have tended to be considerably larger in numbers of both faculty and undergraduate nursing student body, but only slightly larger in numbers of master's level nursing students.[55]

Similarly, the twelve participating nursing homes are generally non-proprietary and/or public institutions and tend to be larger than the national average: none have fewer than 100 beds, have 24-hour RN coverage, while 73 percent of nursing homes nationally do not, and the level of nursing staff also appears to be higher. One-third had personnel with school of nursing appointments prior to the beginning of the TNH program. Since the inception of the program, the number of joint appointments has increased substantially.[55]

From the foregoing, it is clear that the quality of educational programs for both future and current practitioners conducted by the recipients is likely to be considerably higher than in non-TNH program schools and their affiliated sites, especially if the quality of clinical research is high. Although specific details are lacking, other educational activities reported include the TNH sites developing as regional centers for gerontogical research and education, with several offering courses preparing nursing home staff for ANA certification in gerontological nursing and nurse's aide certification programs. Training of students in medicine, dentistry, social work and many other health professions is an ongoing component of the program.[55] The numbers and level of students involved, however, are not specified. It is also not clear whether this activity occurs in all recipient sites or whether this training is a direct result of the TNH program.

Of perhaps more long-range impact on education for both nursing and non-nursing future practitioners is the observation that TNH-funded initiatives have increased nursing school visibility within the university. Nursing school personnel are assuming important positions on university-wide gerontological programming committees. In addition, gerontological offerings in several of the participating schools have been strengthened through their ability to compete successfully for federally funded training and faculty development programs.[55]

Some of the same questions raised concerning the viability and appropriateness of the NIA's program for the education of practitioners for care of the elderly can be raised about the RWJ program. This is especially true of its disciplinary focus. Despite the assertion that the TNHs will improve education and research opportunities for all health professionals,[38] that outcome is probably a very long range one, as it is clear that the primary disciplinary focus of this program is nursing.

Long-term care institutions (viz. nursing homes) are seen as the purview of the nurse, with the physician acting in a consultant role.[38] Current reports on this TNH program do not indicate the participation of faculty from other discplines and only sketchy accounts exist about multidisciplinary student involvement. Clearly, the multidisciplinary team approach is not emphasized in this program. This unidisciplinary focus seems asynchronous with one of the major models and tenets of long-term care, the multidisciplinary/interdisciplinary team approach.

A parallel issue related to model-building revolved around the strengthening of the already dominant role of nurses in nursing homes. It can be asked if a truly new educational model is being developed or whether this reflects the orientation of a particular profession[39] and its need for developing a stronger educational program within its own boundaries. This exclusive approach, however, may be justified on the grounds of improved patient care in a fairly immediate fashion. This is in contrast with research programs designed to entice medicine, pharmacy and dentistry into geriatrics gradually, with improvements in patient care developing over the long haul.

The major issue related to model-building and replication stems from the atypical characteristics of the participating schools and nursing homes, as well as the lack of certain dissemination activities. Not every nursing program combined with an affiliated nursing home will be positioned to implement a TNH program. Clearly, the greater capabilities of the awardees are not resident in, or available to, many nursing programs. Thus, we are faced with the not uncommon dilemma of transferring the experience of centers of excellence to those far less fortunate. However, it is a dilemma that is preferable to live with than its alternative!

Also, other than the expectation (and in some cases, implementation) that RWJ TNH institutions will act as regional resources to other nursing homes, there seems to be no defined role for the recipients to provide technical assistance or other kinds of dissemination-consultation to other nursing schools. While it can be anticipated that they may occur pro forma over the course of time, there appears to be no specifically designed role for this kind of assistance. Collaboration with existing programs such as the current Health Research Services Administration (HRSA) funded Geriatric Education Centers (GECs) which have a mandate to provide this kind of help might be exercised. Unfortunately, none of the RWJ programs are located in the same geographic regions as the existing GECs (Michigan, upstate New York, New England and federal Region IX).

Beverly Enterprises (BE) TNH Program

Of the three programs under discussion, this program has been least visible because program announcements have not been broadcast as widely as the other two and it has been focused in the nursing homes owned by Beverly Enterprises (BE), the for-profit corporation which is also parent to a sponsoring foundation. Beverly Enterprises consists of 850 nursing homes and retirement centers, some with home health and pharmacy components. Much of the information about this TNH program was provided by the Beverly Foundation and by Dr. Pipes, director of program development for the corporation, supplemented by proceedings of a Beverly Foundation-sponsored TNH conference in 1984.[56]

The purpose of this TNH program is to draw nursing homes into the mainstream of medical care,[57] as well as to permit BE to exercise it leadership in the long-term care indsutry,[34] especially among proprietary facilities. While there is a major focus on the involvement of schools of medicine and nursing, the enhancement of the interdisciplinary team approach to patient management is an important program thrust. A special prorgam emphasis is on nursing home administration and management and on the problems of organizing services so as to take better care of the nursing home patient.[34] Through university-affiliated programs of research and education and community college training programs, BE anticipates that not only will patient care in it own facilities be improved, but replicable and successful industry-wide models of patient care will result. It is anticipated that research will focus on alternatives in community and acute care, an issue of importance because of the influx of sicker patients into nursing home beds.[34] Another program objective is that physicians and nurses will, through exposure to positive long-term care experiences, consider it as a career potion. Finally, another desired program outcome is that the image of nursing homes will be improved, with less reliance on the media as the source of information about long-term care.[34]

BE has funded 25 TNH programs that have involved schools of medicine, nursing, pharmacy, and long-term administration.[57] Several of the programs are targeted specifically to training future practitioners, while others have focused on methods of improving care, such as the assessment and management of urinary incontinence and the creation of a short-stay training program for family members. In those cases where an individual program involves more than one discipline, medicine and nursing are characteristically involved.

In addition to the funding of student training rotations and studies of particular intervention programs in the nursing home setting, BE makes funds available to insure that the academic institution and the nursing home are involved in a series of joint activities: appointments, operational planning, and the development and implementation of research on patient care. This collaboration, however, is not to be based on the teaching hospital model of control by the educational institution; rather, the model to be created is an evolving partnership. This is an arrangement for which few guidelines exist but is necessitated by the concerns of stockholders of the for-profit nursing home.[34] The evolution of this new model is crucial because it can serve as a blueprint for university affiliations with proprietary homes, which constitute the vast majority of nursing homes in this country. Most university affiliated programs, including the NIA and RWJ TNH programs, are with not-for-profit facilities.[9]

In developing this partnership, the basic BE strategy has been to get faculty to spend more time in the nursing home by providing incentives. At the same time it is expected that participating universities will also provide resources. House rounds two or three times a week, and greater faculty involvement in patient care and in the conduct of inservice training are yielding positive results in terms of improved patient care.[34]

Dissemination of the results of the studies and of the other activities do not seem to occur systematically. Presumably dissemination of patient care improvements is provided within the BE network. BE sponsored a TNH conference held a year ago with proceedings due out shortly.[56] However, detailed information about the BE TNH program was not provided. Journal articles do not appear to be a dissemination mechanism used by this TNH and given BEs for-profit status, it is unlikely that programs of technical assistance to non-BE nursing homes will be forthcoming. Thus, the model-building capacity of this program will not be particularly widespread, outside the BE system. Similarly, as is true of all the TNH programs, small proprietary homes are less likely to be able to build upon the experience of BE's large proprietary network.

Besides this highly parochial character of the BE TNH program, other criticisms can be levied, some similar to those raised in connection with the other two programs. The BE TNH program is targeted to four disciplines, rather than on one or two; however, the main target disciplines are medicine and nursing. Other professions and the multidisciplinary team care concept are little in evidence.

The extent of student (and faculty) involvement is hard to track and while research, education and service improvements all appear to be about equally important, very little is known about the quantity or quality of education and training, and whether it is being conducted as a direct result of the TNH program. Similarly, it is difficult to ascertain if model educational programs are being created. Unlike the NIA and RWJ programs, there is little basis for comparison among the 25 BE programs, because of their different foci. Unlike the RWJ program, there appears to be no built-in evaluation component that will measure whether the sites are exemplary and conducive to the training of students. Presumably a preliminary evaluation might be conducted jointly by the participating facility and university to determine if educational program objectives have been achieved.

As can be seen from the above discussion, the three existing TNH programs have some decided strengths and weaknesses. These programs have been successful in bridging the gap between the university and the nursing home and in getting faculty involved to a greater extent in patient care activities of the affiliated nursing home facilities. How facility personnel are involved in the educational activities of the universities, whether as providers or recipients, remains obscure. It is even less clear as to what roles facility staff may play in research design and research training and whether the presumed involvement will continue once the funding has terminated.

It is also difficult to determine if funding for research in nursing homes alone will lead to education of practitioners for care of the elderly in that setting. It seems unlikely unless the university recipient has previously been using that setting for instructional purposes. Similarly, while it is highly probable that a focus on the training of a single discipline will yield improved training for that group, it is hard to guage the extent of the spillover effects for students ouside that discipline. A focus on two disciplines, i.e., medicine and nursing, may impact training for physicians and nurses, but the needed education of other health professionals in these existing TNH programs seems to be getting short shrift.

It is clear from the descriptions of the three programs that, taken as a group, their primary focus is not on education for a wide range of current and future practitioners. The RWJ TNH program avoids some of these "trickle down" phenomena and clearly, education for both current and future practitioners is being implemented now. The RWJ program, while highly focused on education, is designed primarily for nurses. The BE program has some emphasis on education, mostly physicians and nurses, but it is clear that the primary focus is on developing methods of patient management that can be applied in the near term. The NIA program, by contrast, emphasizes research, mainly on diseases and chronic deficits that have relevance for nursing home populations, with educational activities specifically not supported. Thus, in the opinion of this writer, the current TNH programs have some deficits when it comes to providing models for education of practitioners for care of the elderly, especially in the realm of multidisciplinary team care. If a model is to be found, one must search for programs that consistently use the nursing home for instructional purposes and/or for other settings that are equally relevant for teaching geriatric care.

CONCLUSION

Over the next decade and well into the next century, concerns about the education of practitioners for care of the elderly will continue unabated as the number and proportion of the elderly in the total population increase. Where and how this education is conducted will also be shaped by other factors, especially long term care policy. While the nursing home is not going to go out of business and therefore, will remain an important site for the training of practitioners, alternative sites for elder care and for training of practitioners are, and will continue to be, developed and refined. The newly-created, federally-funded S/HMO (social/health maintenance organization) experiment and California's Multipurpose Senior Services Program of comprehensive assessment and the care management services, are but two examples of financing care delivery that may, in turn, shape educational programs for both current and future practitioners. These and other long-term care reforms, the adding of occupational therapy to the list of Medicare reimbursed skilled services, and the provision of grants to schools of nursing for the training of nurses aides, for example, will probably have direct impact, not only on the training of those specific groups of practitioners, but on all those health-related disciplines involved in care of the elderly.

There are other forces that may also affect care delivery and therefore, training. Certainly one of the most intriguing is the projected physician glut which some see as being a powerful marketplace incentive for greater involvement of doctors in nursing home care.[34] If this were to occur, then TNH and TNH-like programs might be sought but by physicians in the same way TH programs are now. It is likely, however, that unless special training incentives are provided, such as geriatric fellowships for physician training as medical directors of nursing homes, that this greater involvement will be slow in coming. It is clear that this increased physician role in nursing home care will have impacts on other health-professionals and practitioners, most notably nurses who currently dominate the nursing home. As we have seen, the RWJ TNH program is designed to enhance that dominance; an increased physician involvement would challenge that supremacy.

Another marketplace phenomenon that will also have major effects on training is the increased competition by hospitals and skilled nursing facilities to get into all aspects of long term care. There are movements by large hospital chains to buy up existing nursing homes. Similarly, there is an increase of nursing homes developing home-health and other community-based programs. This vertical integration may do more to promote the rapid mainstreaming of the nursing home into the health care system than the small handful of TNH programs can ever be expected to achieve. Additionally, the greater number of these integrated programs may be in a far better position to provide the necessary education of large numbers of practitioners than the TNH programs which are clustered in a limited number of geographical areas. Whether a research foundation for that training will be incorporated into those integrated programs is far more uncertain. This may be the greatest contribution that the TNHs have to offer, and yet, the continuation of that research in the post-funding period is also open to uncertainty.

There is no question that the current TNH programs provide an opportunity to integrate research, education and care in the nursing home setting in a way that more classical educational nursing home programs have not and are not likely to be by the vertically integrated, market-driven programs described above. But there are a number of problems with the TNHs. The multiple agendas and objectives go well beyond those of education and training. Improving the quality of care, opening career options, mainstreaming the nursing home into the health care system, reducing costs, improving nursing home management, and increasing knowledge about chronic illness are the major outcomes defined by the TNH programs. There are some dangers in expecting this much from programs with relatively short periods of funding.

More importantly for the topic at hand, it is clear that education of a wide range of practitioners is not a major objective of the TNHs, despite the obvious need for such multidisciplinary training. The education of doctors and nurses is dominant, with nursing home employees receiving some training as well. This focus is not likely to encourage broad multidisciplinary collaboration, although it may certainly promote better collaboration between physicians and nurses in the nursing home setting. Coupled with the impacts of the DRGs resulting in the discharge of sicker patients to nursing homes, a possible outcome of this focus is the greater medicalizing of the nursing home and its taking on the role of a subacute care hospital.

Given the educational needs of a broad group of health practitioners, the limited number of TNHs and their multiple objectives, it would seem inappropriate to rely on the TNHs to provide a great deal of training. While the TNHs might become regional training resource centers, that development is not likely to occur, unless some funding is provided for that level of activity. The TNHs, rather, should be regarded as an exemplary mechanism for the training of a small group of health professionals and paraprofessionals. As a set of organizations they will have their educational impacts over the long run, especially on medicine and nursing. They will probably not play a major role in training a wide range of practitioners—that task may be better accomplished by some other kind of institution or program. But the TNHs have the capacity to demonstrate to practitioners and the public a number of approaches to the improvement of nursing home care through a combination of quality research, care and education. It is in this capacity that the TNHs have much to teach us all.

REFERENCES

1. Bok, D.C. Needed: a new way to train doctors. *Harvard Magazine*, May June, 32–43, 70–71, 1984.

2. Panel on the General Professional Education of the Physician and College Preparation of the Association of American Medical Colleges: Conclusion and recommendations. *Chronicle of Higher Education*, September 26, 1984, pp. 15–20.

3. National Institute on Aging. *Report on Education and Training in Geriatrics and Gerontology*. (Administrative document). Washington, D.C.: Department of Health and Human Services, National Institute on Aging, 1984.

4. McPherson, C., Liss, L., and McLeod, D. Basic concepts for geriatrics/ gerontological education. *Gerontology and Geriatrics Education,* 4(2): 11–21, 1983.

5. National Institute of Mental Health. Grant Announcement: Research on mental illness in nursing homes. Washington, D.C.: Department of Health and Human Services, September 1984.

6. California AB2614 establishing five University of California schools of medicine-based academic geriatric resource centers. Eligibility criteria.

7. Wren, G.R. Internship for nursing home administrators. *Nursing Homes* 21(9): 15, 1972.

8. Hart, M.E. Dietetic traineeships, I, planning and philosophy of new programs. *Journal of the American Dietetic Association,* 64(5): 511–2, 1974.

9. Libow, L.S. The teaching nursing home: Past, present and future. *Journal of the American Geriatrics Society* 32(8): 598–603, 1984.

10. Williams, T.F. Introduction. In Steel, K. (editor): *Geriatric Education.* Lexington, Massachusetts. Collamore Press, 1983, pp. 15–16.

11. Institute of Medicine, *Aging and Medical Education.* Washington, D.C.:IOM National Academy of Sciences, 1978.

12. Aronheim, J.C. Sounding board: Pitfalls of the teaching nursing home: A case for balanced geriatric education. *New England Journal of Medicine,* 308(6): 335–6, 1983.

13. Kane, R.L., Solomon, D.H., Beck, J.C., Keeler, E.B. and Kane, R.A. *Geriatrics in the United States.* Lexington, Massachusetts: DC Health, 1981.

14. Kerzner, L.C. Medical education opportunities offered by long-term-care institutions. In: Steel, K. (editor): *Geriatric Education.* Lexington, Massachusetts: Collamore Press, 1983, pp. 41–44.

15. Shannon, R.P. Medical education at the Monroe Community Hospital: A long-term setting—one student's experience. In: Steel, K. (editor): *Geriatric Education.* Lexington, Massachusetts: Collamore Press, 1983, pp. 45–48.

16. Kane, R.L. The potential of the nursing home in medical education. In: Clark, D.W., Williams, T.F. (editors): *Teaching of Chronic Illness and Aging.* Bethesda, Maryland: NIH, 1976, pp. 13–18.

17. Williams, T.F., Izzo, A.J., and Steel, R.K. Innovations in teaching about chronic illness and aging in a chronic disease hospital. In: Clark, D.W., Williams, T.F. (editors): *Teaching of Chronic Illness and Aging.* Bethesda, Maryland: NIH, 1976, pp. 21–30.

18. Schneider, E.L. Sounding board: Teaching nursing homes. *New England Journal of Medicine,* 308(6): 336–7, 1981.

19. Steel, K. Geriatrics for the educator and the educated. In: Steel, K. (editor): *Geriatric Education.* Lexington, Massachusetts: Collamore Press, 1983, pp. 3–11.

20. Jelly, E.C., and Hawkinson, W.P. Geriatric education in a family practice residency program—an interdisciplinary health-care team approach. *The Gerontologist,* 20(2): 168–72, 1980.

21. Garrell, M. The organization of a teaching nursing home: an eight-year experience. *Journal of Medical Education,* 58(6): 482–3, 1983.

22. Sherman, F. and Sonneborn, M. Medical student education in teaching nursing homes (mimeo), 1984.

23. Pawlson, L.G. Clinical education in the nursing home: Opportunities and limits. *Journal of Medical Education,* 57(10, pt 1): 787–91, 1982.

24. Kirkpatrick, R.D. The teaching nursing home (letter). *New England Journal of Medicine,* 308(26): 1604–6, 1983.

25. Kapp, M.B. Nursing homes as teaching institutions: Legal issues. *The Gerontologist,* 24(1): 55–60, 1984.

26. Somers, A. Long-term care for the elderly: Policy and economic issues. In: Schneider, E.L., et al. (editors): *The Teaching Nursing Home—A New Approach to Geriatric Research, Education and Clinical Care.* New York: Raven Press, 1985, pp. 71–78.

27. Kane, R.L. and Kane, R.A. A guide through the maze of long-term care. *Western Journal of Medicine*, 136(6): 503–510, 1981.

28. Last, J.M. Teaching about chronic illness and aging. In: Clark, D.W. and Williams, T.F. (editors): *Teaching of Chronic Illness and Aging*. Bethesda, Maryland: NIH, 1976.

29. Wright, I.S. A look into the future of geriatric medicine. *Journal of the American Geriatrics Society*, 21(1): 55–57, 1973.

30. Beck, J., Ettinger, R., Glenn, R., Paule, C. and Holtsman, J. Oral health status impact on dental students' attitudes towards the aged. *The Gerontologist*, 19(6): 580–585, 1979.

31. Liu, F. and Palesch, Y. The nursing home population: Different perspectives and implications for policy. *Health Care Financing Review*, 3(1): 15–22, 1981.

32. Manton, K.G., Liu, K. and Cornelius, E.S. An analysis of the heterogeneity of U.S. nursing home patients. *Journal of Gerontology*, 40(1): 34–46, 1985.

33. Brody, E.M. The social aspects of nursing home care. In: Schneider, et al. (eds.): *The Teaching Nursing Home—A New Approach to Geriatric Research, Education and Clinical Care*. New York: Raven Press, 1985.

34. Pipes, L.J. Interview conducted January, 1985.

35. Calkins, E. Role of veterans administration hospitals as bases for academic units in geriatric medicine—a historical perspective. In: Steel, K. (editor): *Geriatric Education*. Lexington, Massachusetts: Collamore Press, 1983, pp. 53–58.

36. Posner, J. et al. The teaching nursing home (letter). *New England Journal of Medicine*, 308(26): 1604–1606, 1983.

37. Liebig, P.S. Mental health care of the elderly in a time of scarcity. *Administration in Mental Health*, Winter: 124–132, 1984.

38. Mezey, M.D., Lynaugh, J.E. and Aiken, L.H. The Robert Wood Johnson Foundation teaching nursing home. In: Schneider, E.L., et al. (editor): *The Teaching Nursing Home—A New Approach to Geriatric Research, Education and Clinical Care*. New York: Raven Press, 1985, pp. 79–87.

39. Gillick, M.R. Is the care of the chronically ill a medical perogative? *New England Journal of Medicine*, 309(3): 190–193, 1984.

40. Katz, S., Papsidero, J. and Halstead, L. Team care and chronic illness: A framework for teaching comprehensive care. In: Clark, D.W. and Williams, T.F. (editors): *Teaching of Chronic Illness and Aging*. Bethesda, Maryland: NIH, 1976.

41. Winograd, C.H. Implementing geriatric curricula. *Journal of the American Geriatrics Society*, 30: 415–16, 1982.

42. Evaluation of the federally funded geriatric curriculum development program (mimeo). Vienna, Virginia: Mandex, Inc. 1984.

43. Hagan, D. Nursing homes as training sites for licensed practical nurses/licensed vocational nurses. *Journal of Long Term Care Administration*, 8: 1–12, 1980.

44. Pawlson, L.G. Education in the nursing home: Practical considerations. *Journal of the American Geriatrics Society*, 30(9): 600–602, 1982.

45. Butler, R.N. Teaching nursing home models. In: Schneider, E.L. et al. (editors): *The Teaching Nursing Home—A New Approach to Geriatric Research, Education and Clinical Care*. New York: Raven Press, 1985, pp. 99–104.

46. Libow, L.S. Teaching models. In: *Perspectives on Geriatric Medicine*. DHHS, PHS, NIH#81-1924, 1980.

47. Margolis, E.J. and Bishnu, S.K. Nursing home: place for teaching geriatrics. *New York State Journal of Medicine*, 81(11): 1683–6, 1981.

48. Butler, R.N.: The teaching nursing home. *Journal of the American Medical Association*, 245(14): 1435–7, 1981.

49. Aronson, M.K. Implementing a teaching nursing home: Lessons for research and practice. *The Gerontologist*, 24(5): 451–4, 1984.

50. National Institute on Aging. Announcement: teaching nursing home award, October 1981.

51. National Institute on Aging. Guidelines for prospective applicants: NIA teaching nursing home (TNH) awards for geriatric research, November 1982.

52. Response to questionnaire by Johns Hopkins TNH program, January 1985.

53. The Robert Wood Johnson Foundation, *News Release*, February 26, 1982.

54. The Robert Wood Johnson Foundation, Teaching Nursing Home Program, June 1981.

55. Mezey, M.D., Lynaugh, J.E. and Cherry, J.E. The teaching nursing home program. *Nursing Outlook*, 32(3): 146–150, 1984.

56. Schneider, E.L., Wendland, C.J., Zimmer, A.W., List, N. and Ory, M. (editors), *The Teaching Nursing Home—A New Approach to Geriatric Research, Education and Clinical Care*. New York: Raven Press, 1985.

57. Pipes, L.J.: The Beverly Enterprises teaching nursing home program. In: Schneider, E.L. et al. (editors): *The Teaching Nursing Home—A New Approach to Geriatric Research, Education and Clinical Care*. New York: Raven Press, 1985, pp. 71–78.

Educating Practitioners
for the Care of the Elderly:
The Teaching Nursing Home?
A General Policy Perspective

Mathey Mezey, RN, EdD, FAAN

In her paper Dr. Liebig reflected on standard format for "a teaching nursing home" and how currently funded teaching nursing home programs measure up to it. I will examine selected issues which Dr. Liebig raises, and provide a somewhat different perspective and alternate conclusions from those in her paper.

Dr. Liebig assumes that the major purpose of the teaching nursing home (TNH) is educating students. In relation to the funded TNHs, this is an incorrect assumption. The currently funded homes have perhaps misled the academic and lay public as to what "trainees" they propose to educate. The NIH and RWJ (Robert Wood Johnson) Teaching Nursing Homes mandate activities which, by definition, involve primarily faculty or potential faculty, for example, advanced practitioners, fellows and young researchers. This is quite obvious when one looks at the outcomes for which these programs are held accountable. The NIH Teaching Nursing Homes focus on research productivity. While initially conceived as projects to increase the education and preparation of nurses in nursing home care, the Robert Wood Johnson Foundation TNHs will be evaluated on clinical outcomes rather than on curriculum revisions or educational programming. The Beverly Enterprise Teaching Nursing Homes concentrate primarily on new systems of care. All of these outcomes require faculty rather than student involvement. Therefore, at this stage of the funded teaching nursing homes, student training is not the priority task.

The decision to focus on faculty rather than student preparation is best understood by reflecting on the historical antecedents of these decisions. The National Institute on Aging (NIA) primarily funds medical research. Despite the presence of a large captive research population, the relative ease of access, and opportunities for longitudinal studies, medical research in nursing homes prior to the NIA TNH awards was minimal. Moreover, very few highly respected, published researchers were interested in the aged. The NIA chose to entice established researchers and, probably to a greater extent, bright, young but as yet uncommitted investigators to research in aging. The Robert Wood Johnson Foundation TNH was conceived in 1979.[1] At that time very few nurses, less than 8 percent of the registered nurse work force, worked in nursing homes, and the number of faculty knowledgeable about nursing homes was almost non-existant. Therefore, there was good reason to concentrate on faculty preparation as a first step in the development of the nursing home as a clinical laboratory.

A second criticism made in Dr. Liebig's paper relates to the relative parochialism of the teaching nursing homes. While I do not disagree with Dr. Liebig's general conclusions, again some background helps to put these decisions in perspective. Let me use the Robert Wood Johnson Teaching Nursing Program as an illustration.

According to Vladeck[2] in 1979 there were 1 million employees taking care of nursing home residents. Of these, less than 7 percent were registered nurses. In 1983, in one TNH site, a 250 bed hospital-based facility, the percentage of the total nursing department, i.e., registered nurses, licensed practical nurses and aides who were nurses, was 8.9, a ratio of 23.1 beds for each registered nurse. Currently there are 18,000+ nursing homes, each of which has a Director of Nursing, who comprises half of the facility's management team and is frequently the only health professional in the facility. As of 1980, only 420 nurses held a masters degree with a primary focus in geriatrics, and very few masters programs offered courses focused on long term care. In 1977 there were only 8 masters programs in gerontological nursing.[3,4,5]

In light of these facts, it becomes quite apparent why the Robert Wood Johnson Teaching Nursing Homes have chosen to first "put their own house in order" before actively pursuing the involvement of other professional schools. These projects have in fact specifically chosen to somewhat restrict their scope of influence to nursing, and I would suggest rightly so, in that their mandated goals are sufficiently demanding as to warrant their undivided attention.

Despite their purposefully limited scope, there are some generalizable accomplishments of the funded teaching nursing home programs.

First, they have attempted to establish long range relationships between academic disciplines and nursing homes that are more than brief, circumscribed encounters for specific but brief student experiences. Even in the case of research, the patient registries established through the NIA Teaching Nursing Home Programs are mechanisms for fostering long range involvement.

Secondly, the teaching nursing homes have infused a professional presence into the nursing homes. They have contributed to a critical mass of professional people who spend some of their time in the nursing home facility, thus augmenting efforts of already capable nursing home staff, and providing a vehicle for exchange of ideas and discussions. Moreover, the teaching nursing homes encourage a more reflective environment which may or may not result in more or less aggressive approaches to patient care.

Thirdly, for better or worse, the teaching nursing homes have transported nursing home "stories" to the academic setting. Whether this has resulted in increased respectability is unclear, but there is an increased awareness and presence of nursing home issues. In a somewhat analogous situation that came about as a result of women's liberation when women who worked at home felt compelled to explain why they did not have a paying job, professional schools now feel obliged to explain why they have no relationship with a nursing home. Similarly the nursing home is seen as a respectable academic and/or community resource. The nursing home is now a viable player, maybe not the first draft choice but nevertheless in the game. However, nursing homes remain only one small piece of the geriatric curriculum in professional schools, and in fact, the nursing home remains the "stepsister" in the curriculum, with geriatric faculty continuously needing to "persuade" other faculty to include a nursing home experience.

Whether teaching nursing homes will or should approach a more congruent standard, as Dr. Liebig suggests, remains to be seen. While it is easy to agree on very general goals, there is, I would suggest, lack of consensus as to specific TNH goals. At this stage in development, we need to be clear as to what aspects of nursing home care can in fact be influenced by academic affiliations and what changes will occur irrespective of, or are outside the influence of, academic forces.

Take for example the "medicalization" of nursing homes. I

would suggest that the picture of the nursing home as an institution concerned with patient comfort, noninvasive procedures, peaceful death, etc., as suggested by Liebig is a myth. Rather, nursing homes are and have been, extremely heterogeneous institutions and "medicalization," where it is occurring, is an *inevitable* result of the convergence of demography and financing. Long term patients are now older and sicker. They have complicated chronic conditions and increasing episodes of acute illness. One of four is hospitalized each year. Yet availability of acceptable medical care continues to be a major problem in many nursing homes. While the extreme frailty of these patients is outside our control, TNHs can choose whether to exclude or include within their program bounds. Earlier in these proceedings, we heard of the risks of "over-medicalizing" the care of long term residents. There is, however, also a risk in non-involvement. If academic health centers concern themselves only with short-stayers, long term patients will be moved even one step further away from mainstream health services and, therefore, become at even greater risk of abandonment and warehousing than they have in the past.

Similarly, outside of the TNH control is the reimbursement for nursing home care. The total dollars expended, the lack of articulation between Medicare Part A and B and between Medicare and Medicaid, regulations which require at best only one RN in a facility in 24 hours, irrespective of the total number or case mix of patients; all these factors markedly influence the relative degree of interest in nursing homes as teaching institutions.

The future of TNHs is somewhat dependent on the future agendas of medicine and nursing.[6] In reviewing the geriatric education literature, Dr. Liebig concludes that, to physicians, nursing home residents constitute "treatment failures." One wonders if this is true, and if so, whether such an attitude will persist for medical schools and individual physicians in the face of an anticipated physician surplus. We have some evidence that physicians do not enter geriatrics even in the face of high economic incentives, but the question remains open.

Unfortunately, Dr. Liebig's ability to draw an accurate picture of nursing's commitment to long term care is hindered by a reliance on the medical literature. The nursing literature, both representing the stance of official organizations and leaders in geriatric nursing, documents an ongoing commitment to care of older people in nursing homes for reasons not only restricted to education, but rather reflecting an acknowledgement of the congruence of the mission of nursing and the care of nursing home patients.[1,7-11]

There is good evidence that nurses, especially those with advanced clinical practice skill, do in fact find that nursing homes are satisfying, acceptable, and in some instances preferable work environments. Such nurses cite the emphasis on "care versus cure" and the ability to practice congruent with educational preparation as positive aspects of nursing home employment.[12-23]

Nursing homes need to come to grips with how to deliver rational care to nursing home patients. The issue of collaboration between nursing and medicine will best be accomplished if both groups can focus on the care needs of patients and how that care can most rationally and realistically be delivered.

REFERENCES

1. Aiken, L. Nursing priorities for the 1980s: Hospitals and nursing homes. *American Journal of Nursing*, 81(2):324–30, 1981.

2. Vladeck, B. *Unloving Care*. Basic Books: New York, New York, 1980.

3. Gerder, J. Graduate Medical Education National Advisory Committee (GMENAC) Report, Volume VI, Nonphysician Health Care Provider Panel, HHR, 1981.

4. Mezey, M., Lynaugh, J. and Cherry, J. Teaching Nursing Home: A report of joint ventures between schools of nursing and nursing homes. *Nursing Outlook*, 32(3), 1984.

5. Mezey, M., Lynaugh, J. and Aiken, L. The Robert Wood Johnson Teaching Nursing Home Program. In: Schneider, E. (Senior Editor), *The Teaching Nursing Home: A New Approach to Geriatric Research, Education and Clinical Care*. Washington, D.C.: National Institute on Aging, NIH, 1984 publication date.

6. Mechanic, D. and Aiken, L. A Cooperative Agenda for Medicine and Nursing. *New England Journal of Medicine*, 307(12):747–750, 1982.

7. Clinton, G., Bigas, C. and Linares, E. Nurse practitioner role in chronic congestive heart failure clinic in hospital time, costs, patient satisfaction. *Heart Lung*, 12(2):237–40, 1983.

8. Kane, R.L., Hammer, D. and Byrnes, N. Getting care to nursing-home patients: A problem and a proposal. *Medical Care*, 15(1):74–180, 1977.

9. Rogers, T., Metzger, L. and Bauman, R. Geriatric nurse practitioners: How are they doing. *Geriatric Nursing*, 5(1):51–54, 1984.

10. Rosenaur, J. et al. Prescribing behavior of primary care nurse practitioners. *American Journal of Public Health*, 74(1):12, 1984.

11. Runyan, J.W. The Memphis Chronic Disease Program, Comparisons in outcome, the nurse's expanded role. *Journal of the American Medical Association*, 264–267, 1975.

12. Brody, S.J., Cole, L., Storey, P.B., and Wink, N.J. The Geriatric Nurse Practitioner: A new medical resource in the skilled nursing home. *Journal of Chronic Disease*, 29(53):7–543, 1976.

13. Ebersole, P., Smith, A., Dickey, E.W. and Gamroth, L. Roles and functions of Geriatric Nurse Practitioners in long term care as viewed by physician, GNP, and administrators. *American Health Care Association Journal*, March:2–7, 1982.

14. Gabrielle, et al. Geriatric Nurse Practitioner in the nursing home. Unpublished report, 1980.

15. Gerdes, J. Report of the Rural Mountain States Gerontological Nurse Practitioner Program. Mountain States Health Corp. Boise, Idaho.

16. Groth-Junker, A. Home Health Care Team: Randomized Trial of a new team approach to home care. Paper presented at the Annual Meeting of the Gerontological Society, 1983.

17. Henderson, M. A GNP in a retirement community. *Geriatric Nursing*, 5(2):109–112, 1984.

18. Leroy, L. and Solkowitz, S. The implications of cost effectiveness of medical technology: Case study #160. *The Costs and Effectiveness of Nurse Practitioners*, Office of Technology Assessment, July, 1981.

19. Lynaugh, J., Gerrity, P., and Hagopain, G. Patterns of practice: Masters prepared Nurse Practitioners. Unpublished document.

20. Sultz, H. et al. A decade of changes for Nurse Practitioners, Part I. *Nursing Outlook*, 31(3):137–142, 1983.

21. Sultz, H. et al. Nurse Practitioners: A decade of change, Part II. *Nursing Outlook*, 31(5):216–219, 1983.

22. Sultz, H. et al. Nurse Practitioners: A decade of change, Part III. *Nursing Outlook*, 31(5)266–269, 1983.

23. Sultz, H. et al. Nurse Practitioners: A decade of change, Part IV. *Nursing Outlook*, 32(3):158–163, 1984.

Educating Practitioners
for the Care of the Elderly:
The Teaching Nursing Home?
A National Policy Perspective

Knight Steel, MD

The paper of Phoebe Liebig is like a marvelous *boeuf bourgignon*. Her presentation of a confusing array of quite disparate chunks of meats and vegetables were all mixed together in exactly the proper proportions and bound together with an easy to read stylistic sauce so as to deliver a most satisfying and illuminating main course.

Such a meal is complimented by the heady wine of Dr. Mezey and will no doubt be topped off by a serving of crepes suzette or cherries jubilee prepared by Dr. Gaitz. It is left to me to make the salad! I therefore see my job as a sous-chef who is asked to prepare a complimentary item to the main course, modest in size and limited in ingredients, yet with enough vinegar to make the jaded gourmet take notice. Because of time constraints, my presentation on the national perspective of the teaching nursing home will deal almost exclusively with physician education and have three quite distinctive components.

Let me begin with a statement of fact. Dictum #1, as I call it: Talk money for money talks. There is absolutely no way there can be a significant national effort in the development of an academic base for any professional, paraprofessional, allied professional, or non-professional group in the setting of a nursing home without money. Yet many features of the present era and the foreseeable future mitigate against finding new sources of revenue. Even if we were to be numbed by the constant crying and carrying on about diminishing NIH support, which is an everyday occurrence at least at my institution, we can appreciate the degree to which research grants from the federal government are becoming restricted when we read about it in the *Wall Street Journal*. States are making major efforts to control costs just as surely as the federal government. Indeed state funding and their primal relationship to Medicaid is certainly of far greater significance to nursing homes than federal funding. In Massachusetts, which I know best, there are grave concerns about the rising cost of Medicaid. I doubt I could convince anyone in state government in Massachusetts to fund education within our Medicaid budget!

Perhaps we can learn from the experience of teaching hospitals. How have teaching hospitals funded their training programs for physicians? A major part of faculty support comes from patient care. Additionally, state funds are available to state institutions; the Veterans Administration supports its own; and then there are research grants. Very little, it seems, comes to the institution explicitly to underwrite the costs of teaching. The educational efforts are seen to be subsidized by clinical care, line item funds, and research. The "students" are also "subsidized" while undergoing housestaff training, at least up until the present time, in that *accredited* residency programs are supported by third-party payers. Medicare is especially pertinent in this regard. Note the importance of accreditation—I'll return to that point again.

Contrast this situation with that found in nursing homes. Where will the faculty be funded from? Federal research grants in total are at best level funded accounting for inflation and teaching, and nursing homes are unlikely to be able to compete with teaching hospitals. (Parenthetically one must ask if they should?) Patient care in nursing homes is funded predominately by Medicaid and since they usually only pay about $10 or so per patient *per month*, no significant amount of faculty support can be found here. This leaves either the state or the VA or another unidentified angel for support. I only hope this brief discussion is of some value to our host, the President of The University of Texas Health Science Center at Houston, when he goes to the Legislature of the State of Texas for monies to underwrite a teaching nursing home here.

With respect to the "students," I see no likelihood that third-party payers will find the money for them the way they did for housestaff at accredited hospitals. Housestaff and fellows will therefore need subsidy from elsewhere.

Let me return now to the subject of accreditation and credentialing. I cannot emphasize too much the need for geriatric medicine to be intimately involved with two processes: the credentialing of persons and the accrediting of programs. There is not time now to elaborate, but I am delighted to note that the appropriate accrediting and credentialing boards and committees either have or are about to address some of the needs of geriatric medicine and the teaching nursing home.[2,3] Under any circumstances, if the boards for physicians, or for that matter other professionals, have questions about geriatric medicine included in their examinations and, if the accrediting agencies, such as the Accreditation Council for Graduate Medical Education, require rotations in nursing homes for residents in internal medicine, family medicine, neurology, psychiatry, and rehabilitation medicine, then funds for teachers and students alike will *have to be found*.

Let me stop talking about money and change subjects abruptly. I would remind you that the components of a salad, lettuce, which we have addressed (pun intended!), and tomatoes, for example, are quite disparate. I expect I'll be considered a heretic among the faithful, but I have some difficulty with the concept of multidisciplinary teams. What is the team supposed to do? I mean exactly what is the product of the convening process? Is it to maximize each individual patient's function in the most cost-effective way? If this is true, then different skills may well be needed in different circumstances for different persons. Furthermore, our present professionals may not be the best ones to do the job required. Thus, I am struck by the fact that the separation of nursing knowledge and social work knowledge, insofar as it is relevant to the frail elderly, is often more semantic than real. Legal issues are raised in these discussions, but a social worker and physicians, or perhaps, a nurse along with periodic physician consultation, are often able to handle most patients as well as a team, I suspect, and at less cost to the third-party payer. Parenthetically, I would stress that physicians in the next decade will need to understand the social system much better than they do at the present time (including reimbursement mechanisms), if they are to be able to provide the best care. Reliance on social workers will not be a viable option in many clinical situations where judgments as to the course of treatment will depend increasingly on payment for and availability of services.

My last subject for this potpourri of thought, perhaps, should have been the first, I've addressed payment mechanisms and who should be on the team. (Indeed, should there be a team?) What is needed is also a consideration of what will be taught. Ethics and humanitarian concerns are considered of primary importance by some. I, for one, doubt we can do much in this area. God knows I doubt the government will fund it! In my opinion, there's no substitute for example. When our chiefs walk into nursing homes, when they go to the bedside of demented souls with contractures, and when they ask about family concerns, then and only then, I believe, will students appreciate the importance of the humanistic elements of medicine. Should we be teaching about methods of rehabilitation? I would respectfully point out the dearth of knowledge in these and related areas and the difficulty of teaching when the knowledge base is as inadequate as it presently is. I would also respectfully suggest that considerable health services research could be carried out quite appropriately in nursing homes. This would raise important "local" issues for discussion on rounds, especially general medicine sections, and be a nidus of interest to attract faculty and students. It might just pay for both as well!

These then are the components of my salad—funding issues, personnel issues, and substantive issues of pedagogy. I've added a little vinegar for spice and I hope a little oil to ease the way for a new and better program in those components of geriatric medicine which take place in nursing homes.

REFERENCES

1. Koenig, R. Lab letdown: Medical researchers face serious problems getting federal grants. *The Wall Street Journal*.CCV(67):1,8, 1985.

2. Steel, K. Geriatric medicine is coming of age. *The Gerontologist*, 24(4):367-372, 1984.

3. Steel, K. Geriatric medicine from neonate to toddler: Adapted from the Presidential Address to 41st Annual Scientific Meeting of the American Geriatrics Society, May 18, 1984, Denver, Colorado (in press as an Editorial in the *Archives of Internal Medicine*).

Educating Practitioners
for the Care of the Elderly:
The Teaching Nursing Home?
A Regional Policy Perspective

Charles M. Gaitz, MD

Dr. Liebig gave us an excellent review of the current status of teaching nursing homes: that is, nursing homes in which practitioners receive some of their formal training. The usefulness of such institutions, and their shortcomings, led me to certain conclusions. Among these are:

1. Teaching nursing homes are not necessarily the ideal *core* institution for a training program in any discipline.
2. Teaching nursing homes are an ideal setting for certain kinds of training, e.g., the long term care of multiply impaired elderly.
3. Teaching nursing homes have not been used by medical schools in this area, nor have the medical schools been obliged to explain why such institutions have not been incorporated into their teaching programs. I shall give some examples later, however, of ways in which such institutions have been used by medical schools in this region.
4. The association of nursing homes with medical schools has mixed blessings for both partners. Presumably, the quality of care will improve, but the nursing home administration loses some control. Furthermore, the residents of the nusing homes may not accept medical school staff members as their physicians, or they will accept them only until they experience emergencies and want to return to the physician who treated them earlier in life. This creates problems, among which are the threat to the medical school faculty's image, the disruption in the continuity of care, and the tendency of some personal

physicians to disrupt care by becoming involved in the care of patients.

5. Though the merger has some positive aspects, it seems desirable to leave to nursing home administrators such aspects as negotiations with licensing agencies. This gives the school some protection if, for example, deficiencies in housekeeping and dietary setting become publicized.

6. It is essential to clarify what constitutes a teaching nursing home, constrasted with a nursing home in which teaching occurs.

Inasmuch as my remarks represent a regional perspective, I will share with you a few examples of the involvement of medical schools in this region and the Texas Research Institute of Mental Sciences with nursing homes.

Baylor College of Medicine, Houston

While students are on a six-week rotation in community medicine, they serve about 40-hours at one of two nursing homes, supervised by Baylor College of Medicine faculty members. This is primarily an experience in which students observe long-term care, with minimal exposure to ancillary services. Although these limitations are recognized, no more faculty time is available currently to expand this teaching effort. In addition, residents in family medicine assume primary medical responsibility at two nursing homes for a one-month rotation. Here again, the breadth of activity is limited by the faculty time available to provide a broader teaching experience.

The University of Texas Health Science Center, Dallas

The Center houses a long-term care gerontology center on its campus, but it provides little clinical experience at the present time. The Department of Neurology is planning an Alzheimer's disease unit at a local nursing home, and medical students probably will serve rotations there when the service is established.

The University of Texas Medical Branch, Galveston

During an introductory course on patient evaluation, medical students examine patients in a nursing home two half-days per week under the supervision of medical school faculty. The school's family practice training program is not involved. The medical school already has a geriatric psychiatric service and is contemplating establishment of a 24-bed geriatric medicine service in the teaching hospital, but there are no immediate plans for more involvement with nursing homes.

University of Oklahoma College of Medicine, Oklahoma City

Family practice residents in the Departments of Family Practice and Psychiatry assume primary medical care for many of the patients in a nursing home, and a part-time psychiatric social worker does consultations and meets with residents and nursing staff.

North Texas State University College of Osteopathy, Fort Worth

I have just learned that this institution is beginning to build a close affiliation with a nursing home, but no details are available to me.

Texas Research Institute of Mental Science, Houston (TRIMS)

To expand on what I noted above, the Baylor College of Medicine Department of Community Medicine and Seven Acres-Jewish Home for the Aged established an affiliation several years ago. Long before that, almost 30 years ago, I became the psychiatric consultant at Seven Acres and have continued to serve in this role, and I also direct the gerontology fellowship training program for psychiatrists and psychologists since 1979. The fellows rotate to Seven Acres for a half-day a week for six months. I provide supervision, sometimes individually, but usually in a group meeting with social workers, nurses, and occasionally administrative staff members. The fellows learn much about staff interaction, and they gain experience in treating nursing home residents over a relatively long period. They do consultations, evaluate recently admitted residents, and treat both acutely and chronically ill elderly persons. The home also has a day care program in which the fellows participate.

The TRIMS geriatric fellowship program has incorporated a nursing home as a training site since its inception. Fourteen psychologists and six psychiatrists have completed at least one year of training, and two psychologists and two psychiatrists are currently in the program. Support for stipends comes from a grant from the National Institute of Mental Health, but about one-third of the stipends are supplemented by TRIMS funds. This was necessary because the federal stipends were too low to allow us to compete with other alternatives available to eligible students. We have found the nursing home experience to be very valuable to our trainees, but of course, they are strongly committed to working with the elderly, in contrast to other students who are more or less required to do the rotation. In addition to their rotation at Seven Acres, our fellows have for several years provided in-service training at a nursing home in a Houston suburb. This has been a useful experience, too, because the fellows have become familiar with the operation of a home that is not as adequately staffed and academically oriented as Seven Acres.

We believe the nursing homes setting is one of several in which geriatric fellows should be trained. Our fellows also work in the TRIMS outpatient clinic, the local Veterans Administration Medical Center. In a general hospital psychiatric services, and in consultation-liaison services; they make home visits and sometimes become involved with day care centers, housing projects, and senior citizen centers. We sometimes arrange tutorials for specific training; some of the fellows, for example, have worked with a neuro-psychologist who is in private practice.

Obviously, our emphasis is on the *curriculum* and what needs to be taught rather than on the *site* of teaching. It is more important to find ways of interesting practitioners caring for the elderly than to provide a single ideal setting for training.

I suspect an emphasis on semantics has confused our discussion. How does a teaching nursing home differ from other specialized services like a neurosensory or a cardiology center? We can become so concerned about training sites that we will avoid issues more relevant to the delivery of appropriate services. Students can learn about geriatric care in a variety of places. Each school faculty should make connections with institutions and agencies that are available and cooperative. Medical students in Galveston, for example, will benefit from the establishment of geriatric medicine service regardless of whether they have an opportunity to work in a nursing home environment. Teachers must design a good curriculum; where the teaching occurs is less important.

I have no doubt that a well funded, widely publicized national program to establish teaching nursing homes would persuade many medical schools that they need a teaching nursing home. But to be more pragmatic, the pattern of working with existing and potentially useful agencies offers more hope than does a policy of demanding specifically that a teaching nursing home be associated with every medical or nursing school.

My experience and that of others has led to a strong conviction that the provision of comprehensive care to elderly persons requires a continuum of services and settings. A multidisciplinary approach is very effective but sometimes is not available. This does not alter the needs and condition of our patients. It simply requires that practitioners of each discipline recognize the complexity of needs and provide services to the extent possible in each setting.

We probably have been too preoccupied with debating whether a social or a health model is better for delivering services. Such arguments may be used as a rationalization for not getting on with the treatment of needy elderly people. Fixing responsibility is an important early step in treatment plan, but all professionals in all settings responsible for caring for elderly persons are responsible for providing comprehensive care.

In most communities at the present time elderly people gain access to service by different paths. The concept of a teaching nursing home as providing single access is a pleasant thought, but it is not reality. Not all of the elderly would be served if such a plan were to be put in operation. Elderly people today are being treated in nursing homes, hospitals, senior citizen centers, outpatient clinics, day care health centers, sometimes access to care is through religious institutions, social agencies, nutrition centers, and government agencies. This is likely to continue. Access to service may be through various professionals, including physicians, social workers, nurses, ministers, and psychologists. All professionals and institutions to which people turn for help have opportunities to be useful and, at least in our region, this approach is likely to prevail. No single discipline or institutional approach can fill all needs.

If teaching nursing homes are established as a primary site for research, service, and training, there must be clear communication about priorities; basic versus applied research issues, for example, need to be discussed early and policy decisions made. This may require communication between the funding bodies of the nursing home and the academic staff of the medical school. If the funding body values service or profit more than research or training, such issues need to be resolved early in the development of a teaching nursing home.

To summarize:

1. Training programs should use facilities that are available and whose managers will be cooperative.
2. Students, regardless of discipline, deserve an opportunity to observe and treat elderly persons in a variety of settings.
3. Among the potential settings, a teaching nursing home offers special opportunities. Students who observe long-term care will discover that multiply handicapped people in nursing homes deserve close attention and can be treated effectively; that their suffering can be alleviated and their quality of life improved.
4. Institutions are sometimes motivated by a desire to survive and, therefore, act in somewhat mysterious ways. To fill empty beds, acute-care hospitals may develop rehabilitation or nursing home units. Nursing homes develop day care centers and homecare programs, and housing projects provide infirmaries and even nursing home care. For the time being, it seems more reasonable to support such efforts and assure a high quality of care than to set up rigid territorial limits of interest and responsibility.
5. The time has come to stop identifying long term care with a *place* where people are treated for a long time, and to stop debating whether institutions are designed to offer only acute or chronic care, short- or long-term service, medically or socially oriented treatment. Instead, we should get on with the job of applying what we know to wherever people in need happen to be. And we should continue the research that will permit us to treat elderly people even more effectively than we are able to do today.

Educating Practitioners
for the Care of the Elderly:
The Teaching Nursing Home?
Panel Discussion

Ms. Elaine Brody: Dr. Gaitz is correct, we have to get on with the job and stop the debate. At the Philadelphia Geriatric Center, we have probably admitted and cared for between 15,000 and 20,000 people over the years. Not one of those individuals has ever been admitted to our nursing facility because of a diagnosis, unlike a hospital. Instead, they are admitted because they cannot function on their own and don't have the social support to do so. Our task is not to make them full-time professional patients, to remake nursing homes in the image of the acute hospital with the medicalization or the nursing routine dominant; this results in the tail wagging the dog. You don't go into a person's home and make it into a full-time hospital because they have chronic ailments. The whole rhythm of life, and the whole atmosphere have to be different.

There are few of us in this room who do not have at least one chronic ailment. We have diagnoses. We are functioning pretty well, fortunately. The diagnoses of the people in the institutions may be remarkably similar: arthritis, cardiovascular disease, etc., but they function very differently and that's what makes the difference. Their lives in those institutions should resemble the normal rhythm of life as much as possible.

Dr. Robert Kane: We need to step back and decide, first of all, what it is that we want to educate practitioners about in caring for the elderly. Indeed, many of the principles that we enunciated yesterday bear close scrutiny. If we are looking at policies that are related to educating various types of practitioners for the care of elderly, much of the advice that Dr. Steel gave us about sources of funding, indirect effects on curriculums such as accreditation, and certain kinds of knowledge bases built into requirements for certification, is probably going to be much more effective in setting directions for

243

policies than trying to develop some innovation like the teaching nursing home.

In discussing education of practitioners to care for the elderly, we have left out a major player, the organization which has probably contributed the most to that effort, the Veterans' Administration (VA). They have actually put real dollars into the task, as opposed to putting money into research or other kinds of indirect subsidies to build the academic substrates that we confuse with education. The next group that has done the most, for good or bad, is the Health Care Financing Administration (HCFA), because it turns out that if you want to educate practitioners, what you really need to do is structure an environment. The environment in which people function probably has much more to do with how they behave than what their teachers told them in school. Indeed, HCFA has done a very good job of creating a very bad environment through the kinds of policies that it has been able to develop.

I would like to raise a couple of issues that were hinted at before, but perhaps deserve some re-affirmation in regard to the educational aspects that they represent. One is the whole question about Medicare payment systems. While it is certainly true that Medicare pays a miniscule amount of nursing home care, it pays for a rather substantial amount of service care under Part B. The policies that evolved under Part B adversely affect the care delivered to nursing home patients. They have done this in several ways: they do not encourage physicians to spend any time with nursing home patients at all; they mandate that you make one visit per month whether the patient needs it or not. It is a fixed payment approach. You can just go down the list of how the payment system is structured and discover, not only are there no fiscal incentives, but there are strong disadvantages to delivering any kind of meaningful care. The tradeoff between technology and cognition, which we alluded to before is nowhere more intensely felt than in that area.

Now if that weren't bad enough, Medicare took another step, which I think is even more serious; it deliberately excluded the group who really wanted to give good care to nursing home patients, geriatric nurse practitioners, by passing a regulation that required on-site supervision by a physician. First, you can't get physicians on-site anyway, and second, Medicare eliminated an important source of people who were keen to give that kind of care. So, it is hardly surprising that there are very few nurse practitioner students who want to go into geriatric nurse practitioner training programs; there are no jobs for them when they get out. There are very few things that they can do under the current Part B regulation system.

We face very serious questions about how we educate people, because there is not very much out there to attract them. The career path for a physician who wants to enter geriatrics is probably good for those who have very strong altruistic tendencies. This has not been a major selection criterion in most medical schools, however. They tend to look for other kinds of characteristics. Geriatrics is not a high-paying profession, it requires spending a great deal of time with patients, but the basic reimbursement system for medical services in this country today does not reward that kind of behavior.

Finally, we have to look very carefully at the teaching nursing home. There really are two classes of teaching homes, neither of which fit the general model of nursing homes. The predominant models, the Johnson and NIA models, deal with a group of nursing homes that are the exceptions to the rule. They are very carefully selected institutions, generally, not for-profit. The Beverly and the Hill Haven models are rather unexplored territory because nobody really knows what those are. One has a certain suspicion, however, that what those corporations are buying is some sort of socially redeeming importance for themselves; it isn't totally clear just what they're purchasing in the name of a teaching nursing home. If we look at the teaching nursing homes in the public eye, we have to be very careful to note that these are not typical nursing homes. For example, the HRCA model that Harvard uses as a teaching nursing home isn't even licensed as a nursing home; it is licensed as a chronic disease hospital. You have to be very careful about how the terminology is used.

Dr. Stanley Reiser: Bob Kane's remarks set an important agenda for us. The issue is, what should be the views that we teach in the various health professions to deal with the problems of the elderly? If you look at the consistent model of curricula in these schools, you find that it is directed at a population that the elderly does not represent. For example, the theory of disease that is taught as a theory of biology has very little to do with social interaction. Having learned this theory very well, how can students cope with the multiple problems of an elderly population?

There is a great debate in medicine about where and how one should train people interested in the elderly. Should it be in a family practice setting? A department of internal medicine? Is geriatrics a specialty or is it simply a branch of internal medicine? I have heard this question debated endlessly, with no satisfactory conclusion to it. That's a very elementary kind of question that you would think we could answer before we get into the details of what sort of care they should have.

There is also the issue about the design of nursing homes. Every nursing home that I have visited looked like a hospital. They are set up like hospitals, they have nursing stations, hospital beds; the whole thing says "hospital." Of course, the way we are talking about it, is that it is not a hospital, so the issue of design should concern us.

I agree that the agenda is not the nursing home per se, but the basic issue of what geriatrics is and how we learn it.

Dr. Eli Ginzberg: I want to reinforce what Dr. Steel said, in part, that the discussion must be linked very closely to dollar flows. The first thing that is obvious to me is that we haven't flowed very many dollars into the care of the typical nursing homes in this country. At best they are passable, at worst, a third of them should be closed down.

Second, in a period of physician surplus, which is surely coming, if it is not already here, it is unlikely that the existing subspecialties in medicine and major specialties, including internal medicine, are going to give up anything to a newly-defined group called Gerontologists. It just does not work that way in the real world. Why should anybody give up a part of their scope of practice at a time when it is very hard for them to fill their appointment books.

Third, there is a significant lack of minimum medical attention to people who are "locked up" in nursing homes. The first challenge to a medical profession that is concerned about access to care should be that these elderly people, some of whom need medical attention, should get it. They are not getting it. That is a very simple place to begin. Unless you can answer the simple questions, you better not get very fancy. That is the minimum responsibility of the medical profession and academic health centers, to see that we don't neglect the large numbers of elderly that we have dumped in nursing homes.

The final point follows from what Ms. Brody said. Many of the problems of dealing with elderly have much less to do with physicians than they have to do with people who have some skills in moving someone from limited functions back to fuller functionality, so we can get them out of a nursing home. This raises the whole question of how one puts together equipment and social supports and income flows. Physicians are at the tail end of being knowledgable about such matters. I don't know who is going to do that very well, but it does not look to me, from what I know about modern medicine, that physicians are the people who are able and interested, and there isn't any financing for them to really become concerned about that.

Dr. T. Franklin Williams: As with other segments of the population, we start with the patient and then build our teaching and research into the environment of care. That is what has stimulated turning to the nursing home environment, as well as to home care services, and similar settings where older people predominate, for teaching purposes. There are some 70 medical schools that are teaching in nursing homes. This brings out Dr. Gaitz's point that one might try to make a distinction, but I'm not sure it's a wise one, between teaching in nursing homes and teaching nursing homes. I would rather aim more towards the role of the nursing home as the essential setting for the training of practitioners.

In a report the Public Health Service made to Congress a year ago on training for geriatrics and gerontology, the first principle, agreed upon by all branches of the PHS, was that *all* students preparing for careers in health and other human service professions should receive training in the aging process and the strengths and problems of older people. That is the basic place we start when we talk about teaching. In the coming years, students have got to understand aging and the problems of older people, and that includes experience with those who are in nursing homes, as well as those who are at home. We face the problems of money, but I think the principles are clear.

Dr. James Haughton: Fifteen years ago, I went to Chicago and one of the things I inherited was a county nursing home. In the past, it had been the county poor house. I had learned a few things in New York about older people and their health care needs. One was that many nursing home patients are ill, perhaps not ill enough to be in hospitals, but they are ill and somebody has to provide medical care for them. You can call it medicalization if you wish, but that is the reality. Another thing I learned was that long term care facilities, at that time, were isolated from sources of medical care. Thirdly, I had learned that no one was teaching doctors continuing medical responsibility for people of this type. You can't teach a resident in an acute tertiary hospital how to take care of a patient for 12 months. And, fourthly, I had learned that the status of these patients changes from day to day. They go back and forth across boundaries.

Those were the problems that I thought needed to be solved. Over the next six years, we converted that institution into a long term facility with five levels of care. We had an acute hospital on the premises, a skilled nursing facility, an intermediate facility, an acute rehabilitation facility and, in time, we created a home care program. We could not find doctors trained to take care of these people across that spectrum, so we started a training program. That was a financial burden. Since it was not an accredited program, we could not include the cost of those trainees in the per diem rate that the state paid. We went to the AMA and tried to convince them that there was such a thing as geriatric medicine and that perhaps the Liaison Committee on Graduate Medical Education (LCGME) should start considering the possibility of accrediting such a program. We were unsuccessful. Fortunately, we had a state health director who was wise enough to recognize the need. He found a way to accredit our program within the state so that we could get Medicaid reimbursement for the salary of our residents. These residents had at least two years of internal medicine or we would not accept them; some had already finished their training in internal medicine.

We had several departments in the institution, but those departments were not geographic areas, they reflected the needs of the patients who were in the institution. We had a department of cardiology, urology, oncology, and so on, because those were the areas of care that people needed. Residents did not rotate through those departments, they were assigned patients as they were admitted and took care of those patients no matter where the patient was in the institution and no matter what the patient's problem was. We found that in a given month, a single patient might have spent five days in the acute hospital, four or five days in the skilled nursing division, and the remainder of that month in the intermediate facility. Many patients, because of that program were able to go back home to their families. What I had observed in New York was that many such patients were abandoned to nursing homes without medical care and were bouncing back and forth between the hospital and nursing home, many times staying in the hospital too many days because nobody kept the nursing home bed available for them.

It is possible to put together resources that work and create the mechanism that makes them work. We were able to get paid for a single patient on two or three different levels of care during the same month because the state of Illinois realized that was the reality of the aged population, they do move back and forth across those boundaries. Since we are doing things to allow people to live to be 90, we have got to create the kinds of mechanisms that make it possible for those people to have a decent life when they reach that age and to get the kinds of services they need. In many instances that is going to include medical care no matter what the facility is. I don't know if we are doing them a service by calling that the medicalization of their environment.

Dr. Donald Young: Bob Kane's remarks about payment policy cry out to be challenged. I will restrain myself at this point. It is easy to point to flaws in payment policy, I have done it many times. I sense a tone that one hopes the federal government payment policy will solve problems that the academic community and the health services delivery community are not capable of solving. The discussion to this point has left me no clear idea what the problem or the question really is.

If I were to return to Washington today with my magic wand to fix those payments policies, I don't know how I would do it. The government does very well with policies when things are black or white. It has an immense amount of trouble with gray. I am very much in the middle of gray at the moment.

On the other hand, if you look at what is happening to medical education in the Medicare program, there are multiple funding mechanisms: billing for patient care, research, indirect costs, and direct costs of medical education. Those have all been hidden until the emergence of prospective payment. They are now highly visible and they are also very vulnerable. The academic community that has received those payments on the physician side is currently scurrying to attempt to justify why those payments have been given, in order to maintain them.

Those of you interested in the elderly, nursing homes, teaching, faculty development, patient care, and research, have to come together to understand what it is that you want, how it might logically be sold to the Congress and how payment and funding policies might allow you to accomplish the goal you want.

Dr. T. Franklin Williams: I want to add what seems to me a matter of principle, a very simple black and white principle at that. Whatever applies in paying for training for health professionals in acute teaching hospitals should apply in nursing homes, or home care places, or any place else where federal money is used as a part of the support for training. It should apply across the board.

Dr. Donald Young: Occasionally I find myself acting like, thinking like and behaving like a bureaucrat, and I feel that urge coming over me at the moment. It is black and white to you. It is not black and white to the structure of the Medicare statute, Medicare regulations, and implementation policies, because of the complexity of the program. The current structure and policies of the Medicare program have not kept pace with the world as it exists today.

Mr. Robert Ball: Let's put aside the issue of paying for education for a moment. Dr. Kane's comments reminded me that perhaps what we need, as far as Part B of Medicare is concerned, is a fundamental reexamination of the policy toward payment of physicians' services in nursing homes. The basic statute was designed to pay for all necessary physicians' services in nursing homes or anywhere else. A regulation was then designed to prevent a particular abuse that arose at the beginning of Medicare, gang visits by physicians going from bed to bed very fast, to build up fees. Evidently, this regulation has, in reality, prevented needed medical care. That seems to me disgraceful! The bureaucracy should get on that or we better go in court and sue them.

Dr. Young: I agree that fundamental restructuring is necessary. The payment level has to be determined by the usual customary and reasonable methodology, that's the large part of the $10 per visit. The one visit per month issue is a separate issue and the gang visit issue relates only to the code that is chosen for billing purposes. The problem from the Medicare perspective is relatively minimal. The problem is much more on the Medicaid side.

Dr. Robert Kane: The other reformation that you have got to look at, one which has come up before Congress three times, is broadening the coverage for Part B payments to include people like geriatric nurse practitioners.

Mr. Robert Ball: A change in statute may be highly desirable. I just wanted to give Dr. Young what he is asking for, and that is an assignment when he goes back to re-examine the Part B regulations on physician services.

Dr. Lawrence Green: A lot of these comments assume that if we could pay for physician services in nursing homes, we could get physicians to teach more about the elderly in medical schools; if we could pay for the teaching in medical schools, we could get them to teach more. One lesson I learned as a faculty member and relearned as a bureaucrat is that medical school faculty don't necessarily teach in medical schools what we think we have structured the incentives for them to teach about. Whether it is perversity or self respect, physicians who teach in medical schools seem to teach about that which they are interested in. They are interested in that about which they are doing research. There is much to be gained by looking critically at building the support for research on some of these problems that will provide the incentive for medical school faculties to get more involved in this area. That will achieve more directly and more effectively teaching in medical schools about geriatrics than most of the curriculum reforms and regulatory reforms.

Dr. Knight Steel: Dr. Young, I appreciate your position and I'm impressed with some of your thoughts. Perhaps you would like to speculate on what you think should be done, in answer to your own question. You understand the congressional and Washington scene so well, what would you advise us to do?

Dr. Donald Young: That is very difficult to answer shortly. Medicare pays doctors in hospitals as teaching physicians under a variety of mechanisms. There was what was called the teaching physician regulations; it was extraordinarily controversial and went back and forth with statutory change. That would pay the teaching physician, but it has never been implemented. It was modified in the Reconciliation Act of 1980. The department has never issued the regulations from that. It relates to what is called the hospital-based physician regulations. That is mechanism number one.

The mechanism that was being talked about for physicians is the usual Part B office visit, nursing home visit type of thing, where the doctor is paid specifically for the services provided. There is a problem there with the level of payment, it relates to the usual/ customary/reasonable methodology and historical patterns of payment. Those have changed today and that is no longer useful. That's why certain surgeons get $5,000 an hour and certain internists get $10.00 an hour. That is the historical pattern and cannot be changed by bureaucratic control. The issue of using geriatric nurse practitioners or other non-M.D. types also relates back to the enabling legislation in Title XVIII. There is minor room for interpretation by the bureaucracy. They have chosen not to use that.

The gang visit is a real problem and was an issue of abuse. The irony is that the Inspector General is now saying "you have a gang billing rule for nursing homes that should apply to hospitals too. Doctors should not get the same amount if they have five patients in the hospital. Let's reduce their per hospital visit." So what is being suggested is not fixing the old problem, but taking it to another phase. The question is what is a reasonable amount of payment and how often should the patient be seen? It was pointed out that many of the patients in nursing homes are not patients, they are residents. We got to the one-a-month for a series of social reasons because there are large numbers of people in nursing homes whom doctors never treated. So the bureaucracy limited visits to once a month after consultation. They had to come up with a number because they were under immense pressure. However, that once a month, which was a minimum, has now also become a maximum. That's the usual characteristic of the floor banging into the ceiling when you come up with arbitrary numbers.

So we have problems with payment amounts under Part B, problems with the payment which is under Part B but on a salary basis to teaching physicians, called compensation related charges, problems with gang visits. Then there is the whole issue of indirect versus direct payments which add on to other payments now being attached to the academic center. There is no easy solution, but I can give you some advice on how to proceed. One would be to maximize your billing when you are a physician taking care of patients. You can get several visits a month if there is good medical reason for it.

Dr. Mathy Mezey: In the state of Oregon, geriatric nurse practitioners are certified and can bill under Medicaid. In the Teaching

Nursing Home Program, we have several geriatric nurse practitioners who work in Oregon nursing homes. Unfortunately, they are rendered ineffective in these settings because almost all of the situations where their expertise would be called upon in terms of managing changes in patients status, working up onset of acute conditions, etc., are billed directly to Medicare Part B. As a result, while these geriatric nurse practitioners are reimbursed for care to patients who qualify for Medicaid in clinics, they are unable to receive reimbursement for exactly the same activities rendered to the same patients under Medicare in certified nursing homes. This kind of example is seen in many different instances all over the country.

Dr. Donald Young: You are absolutely right and I can give you many reasons why that came about, not to justify that they were good, but it does have something to do with physician supervision requirements. Whenever we have moved to do something about physician supervision, the storm of protest, particularly from organized medicine, has been overwhelming. The best example, one that has been well studied, is the nurse midwife issue.

Rebuttal

Phoebe S. Liebig, PhD

I agree that there are problems, as I certainly know in my own geriatric education center, of trying to get faculty involved in teaching about the elderly. I agree that the National Institute on Aging's purpose was to entice researchers. On the other hand, you have to look at who got funding and ask whether those people were uncommited to geriatric research. Academics are indeed very clever, and one of the things we all do is try to snowball as much funding for the same kinds of programs so that we're not going at it from spotted efforts and can build up a program of a critical mass.

As I pointed out in my paper, we have teaching nursing home programs at present. But what happens to them once that funding is gone? I am going to assume that all of these programs have a finite life as well as finite resources. I don't see more programs coming out of the National Institute on Aging very rapidly, and the Robert Wood Johnson does not seem inclined to do another round. I assume that one of the things that the teaching nursing home is trying to do, is to get people to see the career options in the field. We had abundant evidence in the discussion towards the end of this period that the career options may be there but the payment mechanisms for them may not be.

I am interested in Knight Steel's concept of the credentialing of persons and accrediting of programs. I don't know if that's something that all the health professions want to move into, but perhaps we are now at that point in terms of the education of health professionals, at least in some professions. Certainly, I know in Psychiatry there are now questions on the National Board that relate to geriatric patient care.

On the issue of health services research in terms of the nursing home base, I don't see a lot of that. And most of what I read in the research coming out of teaching nursing homes is not health services research. I think Bob Kane is quite unusual in that regard.

One of the things that Bob Kane brought up was the role of the

VA in educating people who are going to be taking care of the elderly tomorrow or next week. If we did not have the VA program in this country, we would have to hide our heads in shame in terms of educating practitioners. The numbers may not be huge, but it has been a consistent, focused approach, which has benefited the universities affiliated with VAs. We have to raise our hat to the VA and the people who had the foresight, like Paul Haber, to say that this is something that the VA should be taking on. For those of us who are women, I worry about the model there; but here is a program that is working. Bob Ball asked where we could look for programs that have worked: the VA education program, in terms of geriatrics, has been successful. That's where many of our geriatric fellows who are going into academic medicine have come from.

Another thing I would like to discuss is the problem of attracting students to geriatric medicine, the conflict between altruism and general characteristics of physicians. Perhaps one way, instead of relying on altruism, is to do what Harvard is going now in restructuring its whole geriatric medicine curriculum in a program call the Pathway. Ten percent of that curriculum is specifically dedicated to geriatrics. It may require that kind of self-kicking for medical schools to say we are going to try this sort of experimental approach. I think this is going to be a really interesting thing to see, whether or not it works, because it is a curriculum within a curriculum. Not all students at Harvard Medical School will be receiving this.

On the issue of who is going to pay for geriatric education, we are beginning to see some movement in the states to resolve this. State-funded programs, mandated—"thou shall teach geriatrics or thou shall not be accredited"—is one approach, but we are also seeing some "carrot" approaches. California, for example, now has some academic geriatric resource programs which are funded by the state. Not many, but they certainly are providing the same kind of levels as the Robert Wood Johnson program. The teaching nursing home is a part of their requirements.

On the question of who is going to pay for geriatric education, I would like to take a page from Robert Ball's book and say, how about an earmarked tax? Massachusetts, for a number of years, had an earmarked tax. I can remember as a kid, you went to a restaurant and part of the tax on that bill was for older persons' care. Maybe this is something which we should go back to at the state level. How about a tax that says this is for geriatric education of practitioners in our state? Of course, there is the problem that those practitioners may go to other states and practice. One of the things that we have to be looking at is other ways to get better-educated professionals to take care of older people.

The other thing that has not been discussed here is the considerable loss of training money from federal sources over the last few years for people who will go on to either be faculty and train the next generation, or who are practitioners themselves. We have seen a considerable compression, if not of morbidity, of vitality in funding for training. If we think that educating current or future practitioners is an important activity, then we need to seek out some ways that will make that happen. There are other ways of looking at this, and there is no question that a number of schools have been doing this for years without much outside help. Franklin Williams' tabulation of 70 medical schools that have affiliations with nursing homes for both research and teaching is simply another implication that this has been going on. It will continue to go on.

CHAPTER 6

Health Promotion and the Elderly:
Why Do It and Where Does It Lead?
Position Paper

T. Franklin Williams, MD

It is necessary to consider health promotion in the context of one's overall concept and understanding of aging, of what being "elderly" means. The implications of biological aging were discussed earlier, but as background for this session I need to give my own changing perspective as well as what I judge to be changing perspectives in society, and then address the question, why health promotion for older people?

Contrary to earlier (and even recent) views of aging, the aging process *per se* is being found to be relatively benign, with preservation of functions on into very late years, *if* a person is spared chronic diseases. The most recent evidence on cardiac function, for example, indicates that in healthy people in their 70s and 80s, without even subtle evidence of coronary artery disease, maximum cardiac output on a standard stress test, falls in the same range as in a healthy, young person; there is no evidence of any decline with age. Similar findings now exist for most persons, absent disease, with regard to maintaining mental function, and I expect that we will see similar trends in other organ and functional areas.

Thus, age *per se* will, I believe, be seen as a less significant variable in affecting older people's degree of independence or choices; rather we will be dealing with the specific collection of a combination of chronic diseases which each individual person may have acquired. Diseases are by definition conditions which are not a part of the "normal" process, but are at least theoretically mutable, preventable, modifiable, and treatable. Thus, for older people just as for younger, the goals of health care are the same, i.e., maintenance of health, treatment of acute and chronic conditions with the best available knowledge, and restoration of function and independence whenever possible. Such a rehabilitative philosophy is at the heart of geriatric medicine[1] and is properly included in a broad concept of health promotion.

It may be stated also that such a goal is clearly what older people seek for themselves: most older people want to continue to live in the lifestyle they have already chosen and developed, with continuation of their own independence and options. Personality as well as physical and mental functioning continues remarkably stable into later years.[2] However, the long-standing ambivalence about aging that has characterized most societies and cultures[3] continues to persist: people tend to venerate, but also to fear and deplore old age, and to say, "It's just old age" as a resigned explanation of symptoms and changes,[4] in Western as well as Eastern cultures (although with some differences). Such ambivalence, such a negative view, in my judgment, underlies the intense concerns about "doing too much" for or to frail older people, a concern for which there is little direct supporting evidence. At least one study indicates that even in terminal situations the wishes of patients, families and health professionals can be in agreement about supportive care rather than presumably fruitless efforts to cure.[5]

A powerful factor in shifting such conflicting views of aging toward more positive perceptions is, I believe, the common experience in most families, now, for the first time in history, of having generally healthy and vigorous very old relatives or friends. Furthermore, health promotion is a natural part of the increasing interest in taking responsibility for one's own health, i.e., self-care. Carrying out health-promoting activities for oneself, such as dental care, tends to replace with hope what may otherwise be helpless feelings about one's own health. All in all, my expectation is that we will see more and more commitment to health promotion and health maintenance for older persons, as naturally as we see its importance in people of all other ages, because that is the way most older people want it, and younger people will want it for their older relatives (and themselves in the future). In addition, that is the way health professionals see their goals, possibilities and responsibilities.

WHAT ARE THE POSSIBILITIES
FOR HEALTH PROMOTION FOR OLDER PEOPLE?

Despite widespread expressed interest in such goals and efforts, we as yet have only limited information based on research, about what can be accomplished. The Office of Technology Assessment, the Public Health Service, the U.S. Preventive Services Task Force, and other groups have attempted to draw up lists and guidelines for prevention and health promotion in the elderly. The Institute of Medicine, National Academy of Sciences, has just begun an initiative on "Health Promotion/Disease Prevention for the Second Fifty." In this paper it is possible only to point to some of the unanswered questions or issues which come up for almost all of the proposed health promotion activities. The following examples are illustrative.

Avoidance of injury—this would appear to be one of the safest and most desirable health promotion activities for frail older people. Efforts can fruitfully be diverted to removal or correction of an modifying individual risk factors in the older person, such as decreased vision or hearing or unsteadiness of gait. This last common problem may be approached through investigation of causes, appropriate specific treatment where possible, physical therapy to improve function of muscles and joints, and use of cane or walker if needed. The National Institute on Aging encourages more research of factors involved in falls in the elderly. But when carried to extremes, such as restraining frail older people in chairs for fear of falls and fractured limbs, such activities have severe physical and psychological costs. Thus, in the area of avoidance of injury, the costs as well as benefits, must be weighed.

Vaccination, e.g., for influenza and pneumococcus—these procedures carry only limited risks and appear to benefit the majority of older people, but the relative effectiveness of pneumococcus vaccines is still debated.

Ceasing smoking and reducing misuse of alcohol and drugs—accomplishing these goals is, at any age, beneficial financially as well as in terms of health. We all know the difficulties involved in accomplishing them, however.

Control of hypertension—the benefits of effective treatment of diastolic hypertension in terms of prevention of strokes and their sequellae at all ages, are well established. Clinical trials are currently under way, supported by the National Heart, Lung and Blood Institute and the National Institute on Aging, to determine the benefits as well as risks of treating systolic hypertension in the elderly.

Maintenance of good nutrition—here the problem is that we have very little information about what is, in fact, good nutrition for older and very old people. In the Recommended Dietary Allowances (RDA) of the National Research Council, everyone aged 51 and older was classified in one category, and the recommendations were based on studies done in younger subjects. In only a few areas, e.g., the need for calcium and vitamin D to minimize osteoporosis, do we have some careful studies on older people themselves. These studies indicate a need for a larger daily intake of calcium, and probably vitamin D as well, in older women in particular, than the RDA has called for. Basic studies are needed, and some are under way, to establish what is required of various nutrients to maintain balance in healthy older people. Studies will also be needed to determine nutritional needs in the presence of the various diseases and related medications that are commonly present in older people. Findings must be weighed against the question of what ill effects may occur, in what time period, if older people for reasons of personal preference deviate from what appears to be optimal nutrition. The role and possible risks of high-fiber intake needs further evaluation. Overall, it must be emphasized that good nutritional practices need to begin early in life and continue throughout the life span.

Exercise and fitness—again we have only minimal data on what amounts of what types of exercise may contribute what benefits to older people. The common view has been that muscular mass declines inexorably with age, and that declining physical activity should perhaps be accepted as the norm. But recent studies are beginning to challenge such views. In one recent series of papers, it is reported that previously sedentary older people who voluntarily undertook endurance training, had the same order of increases in their aerobic capacity as did young previous sedentary subjects, as well as improved glucose tolerance.[6,7,8] We need to know much more about the possible benefits of various degrees of exercise, in terms of daily vigor, modification of disease course, and survival. We need to learn how to deal with the common occurrence of not continuing exercise programs, once begun.

Modification of stress—it seems reasonable, and is supported by animal research, that avoiding or decreasing the impact of stress may have a favorable effect on the immune system and on susceptibility to disease, but it would be most helpful to have a better understanding of these relationships in older persons. All stress is not necessarily bad.

Response to rehabilitative efforts—if one applies this term broadly to include protheses for hearing and vision, physical and occupational therapy modalities, rehabilitative surgery like joint replacements, and other supportive and restorative efforts including strengthening social supports, it seems clear that these can be called health-promoting when they restore or maintain function and independence. For healthy people, health promotion may mean working for marginal, but nevertheless important, benefits, whereas for high-risk groups, health promotion must be approached in terms of the risk factors and chronic diseases already present.

Primary care health maintenance—prompt, effective primary care for acute illnesses and for chronic conditions would appear to qualify as health promotion.

The role of social opportunities—with the increasing numbers of relatively health, long-lived retirees, there is the need for increased and varied social opportunities, including opportunities for satisfying contributions to society, as a part of promoting health.[9]

HEALTH PROMOTION: WHERE DOES IT LEAD?

As illustrated above, health promotion for older people, when viewed with the breadth which I think is appropriate, calls for a comprehensive range of activities, on the part of the individual older person and as well as health professionals, and independence. To the degree that health promotion is successful, I anticipate functionally healthier, happier, more satisfied older people, and, derivatively, their families.

For the health professions, I see the response to such a challenge as requiring more knowledge about aging and the diseases of old age, and further development of comprehensive, multidisciplinary approaches to care for older people. I see the need for the Health Maintenance Organization approach, conceived broadly to include the full range of health professions, or its equivalent (e.g., well-organized groups or independent practice associations).

For payment sources, I see the need to have prepayment arrangements which provide incentives for health promotion and health maintenance. In such arrangements, the costs of health-promoting activities, including effective, well-chosen rehabilitative measures, should prove cost-saving for everyone.

REFERENCES

1. Williams, T.F., (editor). *Rehabilitation in the Aging.* New York: Raven Press, 1984.
2. McRae, R.R. and Costa, P.T., Jr. *Emerging Lives, Enduring Dispositions.* Boston: Little Brown, 1984.
3. de Beauvior, S. *The Coming of Aging.* New York: Warner, 1970.
4. Sankar, A. It's just old age: Old age as a diagnosis in American and Chinese medicine. In: Kertzer, D. and Keith, J. (editors). *Age and Anthropological Theory.* Ithaca, New York: Cornell University Press, p. 250, 1984.
5. Loomis, M. and Williams, T.F. Evaluation of care provided to terminally ill patients. *The Gerontologist,*23:493-99, 1983.
6. Seals, D., Hagberg, J., Hurley, B., Ehsani, A., and Holloszy, J. Endurance training in older men and women: I. Cardiovascular responses to exercise. *Journal of Applied Physiology,* 57(4):1024-29, 1984.
7. Seals, D., Hurley, B., Schulta, J., and Hagverg, J. Endurance training in older men and women: II. Blood lactate response to submaximal exercise. *Journal of Applied Physiology,* 57(4):1030-33, 1984.

Health Promotion and the Elderly:
Why Do It and Where Does It Lead?
A General Policy Perspective

Jonathan E. Fielding, MD, MPH

Dr. Williams has provided an excellent synopsis of some priorities for health promotion in old persons. He points out that the development of many chronic diseases, frequently associated with the "aging process" are far from inevitable. To most fruitfully analyze opportunities, four general observations may be helpful:

1. Health promotion and disease prevention are related but not synonymous. Some activities may achieve both objectives. For example, exercise may both reduce heart disease risk and help maintain or improve personal mobility, an important component of health status. Some actions, such as seat belt use, primarily have disease prevention as a target. Others, such as seeing friends often, may be primarily health promoting, although also possibly contributing to lower incidence of some diseases. In recommending policies we should be clear with respect to how each of these objectives can be achieved.

2. Health promotion directed *primarily* at the elderly can never be more than partially effective. Our understanding of risk indicators and the natural history of many chronic diseases strongly suggest that health promotion should begin earlier in life. Some studies suggest that the most effective target population is young children. At that age, important health habits, such as eating practices, are usually established. Three-quarters of all smokers begin before age 20. Alcohol consumption habits also tend to become established during the teenage years.

3. Different health behaviors exhibit different patterns of change with age. Some disease-preventing behaviors such as

aerobic exercise tend to decrease with age. By contrast, some risktaking behaviors such as speeding and performance of risky sports appear to decrease with age. We need to learn how to prevent declines in the former group and try to establish better risk reduction approaches by examining and learning from the latter group of behaviors.

4. While health promotion and disease prevention rely primarily on individual behavior, the behavior is, in large part, conditioned and, in some instances, clearly determined by the physical and social environment. The mandatory seat belt law in New York could lead to an increase in usage rates from under 20 percent to 60–80 percent. A social norm that holds smoking as uncultured and impolite to others can create a fertile environment for personal smoking cessation.

Armed with these general observations, what is a potentially effective strategy for providing health promotion to older Americans? I will review each of Dr. Williams well-considered opportunities for health promotion and disease prevention. My comments will be limited to the "well" population, i.e., those without a chronic disease.

Avoidance of Injury

Older Americans are much more likely than younger ones to die in a motor vehicle accident. Their increased risk derived primarily from their increased vulnerability to the effects of the accident, with a smaller contribution to risk from an increase number of accidents per mile driven. Suggested strategies to prevent all types of injury among the elderly include:

• Encouragement of safety belt use, generally associated with a 40–60 percent decrease in risk of a serious injury or death;
• Laws making safety belt use mandatory;
• Encouragement to drive a crashworthy motor vehicle (larger and heavier vehicles confer a reduced risk of injury; within weight classes crashworthiness still varies considerably);
• Installation of non-skid surfaces in bath, tubs, bathroom floor, stairs, etc.; and

- Adequate lighting of potentially hazardous areas, e.g., stairs, entry to home, path from home to garage and/or street, etc.

Vaccination

Yearly influenza shots seem reasonable based upon the sharp increase in influenza mortality at about age 65. However, most older Americans are not immunized. Judicious use of amantadine hydrochloride, which has roughly equal effectiveness against the more virulent influenza A as the strain-specific vaccines, is also appropriate, especially in the face of epidemics and individual exposures.

The efficacy of *Pneumovax* is still questionable, with several trials having not demonstrated a clear benefit. The frequency of pneumococcal pneumonia is low and the strains included in the vaccine account for perhaps as little as 20 percent of pneumonias in the elderly. The ability of the vaccine to affect the course in the majority of those innoculated is unclear. However, the low cost of a single injection and the potential benefit make it difficult to argue against those who recommend it based on prudence.

Smoking Cessation

Smoking cessation makes sense at any age, but the risk of most smoke-related cancers in ex-smokers takes 15 or more years to decrease to that of non-smokers. Serious pulmonary diseases may be forestalled with smoking cessation, but are not reversible. Smoking-related cardiac risk on the other hand, declines quickly post cessation. Most careful studies using the best available behavioral techniques achieve cessation rates of 20–35 percent. However, the creation of social and physical environments which discourage smoking can be more helpful in reducing smoking prevalence than the availability of free cessation classes. Stressing both the health and financial benefits of cessation even after many years of smoking, may also prove motivational to older people. Helping people believe they can quit and the use of nicotine gum also appear to improve results. However, removing the pleasure of smoking may also be traumatic and can lead to depression and anxiety, especially for individuals with limited other pleasures. Cessation activities need to provide substitutes, such as exercise and stress relaxation.

Alcohol/Drug Use

Alcohol abuse is a continuing and serious problem in older adults and an important contributor in serious injuries and malnutrition, as well as cirrhosis, gastritis and other well known conditions.

Adverse effects of prescription drugs, either purposefully prescribed or taken in doses and for time periods beyond those prescribed, are a problem whose risk potential increases with age. Physician and family vigilance and computerized personal drug registries now maintained by many pharmacies can help reduce the risk of side effects due to interactions and to overdose.

Good Nutrition

Once again, good nutritional habits early in life increase the likelihood of good health and adequate nutrition at older ages. High fat intake not only increases heart disease risk, although to a lesser extent with advancing age, but also some cancers, including breast, and probably colon and prostrate. While the protective effect of high fiber intake on colon cancer incidence remains controversial, nobody denies its beneficial effect on the most common gastrointestinal condition—constipation—often accompanied by hemorrhoids, one of the most dreaded diseases based on a cursory review of television ads. While osteoporosis may be slowed or stopped by some combination of calcium, vitamin D, estrogens and exercise, reversing bone loss, which often starts in women in their 30s and 40s, appears extremely difficult to achieve. Adequate calcium supplement should start well before achieving "elderly" status. Calcium deficiency has been increasingly implicated as a cause of hypertension, one of the most frequent chronic conditions in older people.

Post-menopausal low dose estrogen may be a health promotion replacement both as a preventive agent for osteoporosis and to reduce atrophy of female reproductive tract.

While low salt intake may assist some in preventing blood pressure increases with age, sodium appears to make a significant contribution to hypertension in only a minority of the elderly who have high blood pressure. The benefits and risks of vitamin therapy, with the exception of megadoses, deserves much greater exploration, particularly with respect to the elderly. Intake of Vitamin A, possibly others, may reduce risk for some cancers, especially lung and colon.

Dr. William's call for enlarged efforts to develop age-specific RDAs deserves strong reinforcement. Although reduced calorie needs with aging has been well-documented, the degree of decrease or increase in requirements for different nutrients remains largely unexplored.

A final nutrition-related issue that deserves health promotion emphasis is obesity, which tends to increase with age in many socioeconomic groups. Serious risks for ill health directly related to excess weight and body fat include some reproductive cancers, hypertension, elevated total serum cholesterol, Type II diabetes mellitus and some forms of osteoarthritis, specially of the weight bearing joints. We have limited information on the best and safest ways to assist older people to reduce their weight or what ideal weight is in older people. Rapid weight loss may render older people particularly vulnerable to dehydration, infections or other serious health problems.

A health promotion issue related to both nutrition and self-image is the state of both teeth and gums. Early initiation of flossing and other preventive measures can reduce tooth loss due to gum disease. Starting at age 60, 65, or 70 is usually too late. However, initiation of these procedures at any age can reduce or stop peridontal disease. Poor dentition interferes with adequate nutrition and can affect self-concept and socialization.

Exercise and Fitness

Dr. Williams has sufficiently summarized the evidence for continued capacity for aerobic fitness with advancing age. But a major problem of exercise with older as with younger people is recidivism. Most of us have difficulty maintaining an exercise habit. In younger age groups not exercising may not affect usual functioning due to significant reserves. With increasing age reserve declines, comes greater vulnerability to reduced fitness if the habit is not maintained. In older people, aerobic fitness should be complemented by strength-building exercises. The ability to carry the groceries or the vacuum cleaner may be enhanced through such activities. In addition, stretching exercises and exercises designed to maintain coordination may have the potential to reduce the frequency of falls and other musculo-skeletal injuries.

One clear benefit of exercise relevant to all age groups is its anti-depressant effect. Group exercise also provides a natural opportunity for socialization for all ages.

Modification of Stress

We might broaden this topic to include the promotion of psychosocial functioning. Both the perception of stress, objective measures of usually stressful events, and the way people cope with stress, affect health along several dimensions. Inappropriate reactions can reduce opportunities for socialization. High degrees of perceived stress may not only affect the immune system but the gastrointestinal system, vascular system, many metabolic processes, and cognitive function.

However, stress is not necessarily bad. A certain amount is stimulating and supports continued function as a mature and contributing member of family and other socially defined groups. Lack of sufficient stressors may be a particular problem for some older people.

Social support, i.e., the number of close family members and friends as well as the frequency with which they are seen, has been established as an important contributor to disease prevention as well as personal satisfaction. In the Alameda County study, those with few social supports were found to be a greatly increased risk of dying of all causes in all age groups studied.

Rehabilitative Effects

Whether prostheses, physical and occupational therapy comfortably fit under the name of either health promotion or disease prevention is less important than their clear contribution to improved physical and mental health status.

A FEW CONCLUDING POINTS

1. Specific exclusion of preventive services under Medicare is expensive and indefensible based on the weight of current scientific evidence.
2. A number of medical procedures are very important and effective in screening of older persons, including frequent

hearing and vision checks, assessment of fecal occult blood and periodic sigmoidoscopy, blood counts for those at nutritional risk, blood pressure determinations and, for women, pap smears, clinical breast examination and mammography.

3. Much health promotion and disease prevention can occur in a clinical context. Comprehensive primary care systems, especially those with incentives for health maintenance, can support age-, sex- and risk-related periodic health examinations which include both procedures and counseling.

4. An important part of health promotion is education. Older people tend to be quite interested in health maintenance. Providing them with information to help themselves should be a high priority.

5. We need to change expectations of many practitioners. We want practitioners who do not consider rapidly declining function as inevitable. We want them to be aware of benefits of health promotion and disease prevention activities and understand that they play a critical role as trusted figures to encourage continued personal growth and health in all dimensions in their patients.

In summary, both health promotion and disease prevention, beginning early in life, but continued throughout life, provide a majority opportunity, at generally low cost, to improve the physical and mental health of older Americans.

Health Promotion and the Elderly: Why Do It and Where Does It Lead? A National Policy Perspective

Lawrence W. Green, DrPH

National policy for health promotion has been articulated in the Surgeon General's Report, *Healthy People,*[1] and in *Promoting Health, Preventing Disease: Objectives for the Nation.*[2] In the former, a chapter was devoted to the elderly as one of five age groups in a life-span analysis of what we ought to be able to achieve by 1990 if we began applying in 1980 what we knew then. It assumed no scientific breakthroughs during the decade, but a more focused and concerted effort in disease prevention and health promotion through the 1980s. The broad goal for the elderly was "to improve the health and quality of life for older adults and, by 1990, to reduce the average annual number of days of restricted activity due to acute and chronic conditions by 20 percent, to fewer than 30 days per year for people aged 65 and older."

That broad goal, The Surgeon General's Report asserted, should be supported by the accomplishments of two subgoals: "Increasing the number of older adults who can function independently," and "reducing premature death from influenza and pneumonia." "Reducing Functional Dependency" was the subtitle of the background paper on health promotion for the elderly, co-authored by Dr. T. Franklin Williams, and produced for the Surgeon General by the co-sponsor of this conference, the Institute of Medicine.[3] Dr. Williams makes no reference to this national policy background in his paper for this conference, possibly out of modesty. In his current position as Director of the National Institute on Aging, he would not have assumed, as many have, that these documents no longer carried the force of policy, having been produced in the Carter Administration.

Miraculously, the Reagan Administration adopted these documents as policy. Dr. Edward Brandt, when be became Assistant

Secretary for Health, went a big step farther. He instructed the agencies of the Public Health Service to prepare their next fiscal year's budgets using the *Objectives for the Nation* as their justification for requests. This caused many of the agencies to turn the corner in their adoption of disease prevention and health promotion initiatives. Some, including many of the National Institutes of Health, accomplished the rebudgeting with creative bookkeeping, simply redefining much of what they did as prevention. For example, virtually all the research of NIH on children or childhood diseases, growth and development, was reclassified as prevention research on the grounds that it might lead to earlier intervention to promote health or to prevent diseases or their sequelae. Comforting as this might have been to those in Congress and elsewhere who sought assurances that NIH was devoting more of its resources to disease prevention and health promotion, it did not represent as much change in the allocation of resources or research priorities as we need to advance the objectives for the nation, especially for the old.

THE RELATIVE NEEDS AND POTENTIAL OF THE ELDERLY

Dr. Williams' first point is that the elderly have as much to gain as younger people from health promotion, *if* they have been spared the experience of chronic disease. "Age, per se, will . . . be seen as a less and less significant variable affecting older people's degree of independence of choices . . ." This seems, on the surface, a manifesto for health promotion, a policy goal worthy of priority in the agenda of the Department of Health and Human Services, a hypothesis worthy of sponsored research from the NIA. Older people should reasonably expect to obtain as much marginal benefit from health promotion, but they necessarily start from a lower average baseline of deteriorated capacity. The reality today is that a minority of the elderly reach advanced years without some chronic diseases in the process, so it would be hazardous to overgeneralize the expectations of functional capacity on the basis of the experience of those free of any chronic disease.

The point is that the objectives of health promotion for the elderly must be set at a more modest level of outcomes, even though their gains may be as great in relative terms. To expect otherwise is to set policy destined for disappointment.

THE PLACE OF REHABILITATION

Dr. Williams' second point is that a "rehabilitative" philosophy is at the heart of geriatric medicine and should be included in health promotion for the elderly. This presents no problem for geriatric medicine, but strikes a discordant note with health promotion. Isn't rehabilitation at the opposite end of some continuum from health promotion? Is there not some danger, as Dr. Stallones pointed out to me, of counting rehabilitation as health promotion when budget allocations move money intended for primary prevention into tertiary medical care?

We find some clue to the paradox of rehabilitation as a part of health promotion in Dr. Williams' next point. What older people themselves seek, he says, is to continue to live in the lifestyle they have already chosen and developed, with independence and options. This, he implies, is health maintenance for the elderly, in general, and health promotion for those with some remediable impairments. Later, he gives a further clue as to how these disparate elements tie together. Rehabilitation he defines broadly to include prostheses for hearing and vision, physical and occupational therapy, all of which are health promoting when they restore or maintain function and independence.

For most of us, healthy and relatively unthreatened, health promotion means tinkering at a narrow margin of benefit from nutritional, exercise and stress management practices, in return for some real or imagined improvements in quality of life. Happily, even the imagined improvements are notable because they do not compete for attention with severe deficits, losses or deteriorating sensory and motor capacities, aches and pains, or grief and bereavement. Attention to these latter concerns in the elderly and other high-risk groups may be necessary before much can be expected to be palpable from the efforts of health promotion in the narrower sense. Without palpable feedback and reinforcement, the personal effort that must go into health promoting practices will not endure for lack of perceived reward.

If we define health promotion restrictively as primary prevention in the purest sense of interventions only in the absence of any symptoms, then health promotion has little to offer those who are at highest risk of lifestyle-related diseases and conditions and, perhaps, nothing to offer most of the elderly. If we adopt a broader view of health promotion for the elderly, as Dr. Williams has, to include rehabilitative interventions to restore such fundamental lifestyle capacities as vision and hearing, then it has more immediate pertinence to the elderly. While I was in the federal Office of Health Information and Health Promotion, we defined health promotion as any combination of health education and related organizational, economic and environmental supports for behavior conducive to health. For the sake of consistency, I would find the intersection of health promotion and rehabilitation at the behavioral level rather than the medical.

Much needs doing to get older people to overcome their own vanity and stereotypes about aging so that they will avail themselves of the medical and prosthetic devices that would help offset their declining sensory capacities. Eyeglasses and hearing aids represent rehabilitation devices; getting people to accept them and use them requires health promotion as defined in federal policy. Similarly, physical therapy is usually considered a rehabilitative maneuver; getting people to adopt the exercises designed to control their symptoms of back pain is a behavioral dimension of rehabilitation consistent with health promotion as defined above.

THE POLITICAL FUTURE OF HEALTH PROMOTION

Dr. Williams' next two points relate to the political future of health promotion for the elderly. He notes that society's ambivalence toward aging underlies the concerns of professionals about "doing too much" for or to the frail elderly, not wanting to usurp their independence or fruitlessly pursue cures to their degenerative conditions. These concerns, by implication, should lead to more intensive efforts to prolong or maintain health in old age, compressing morbidity (to borrow Dr. Fries' term) into a narrower and narrower range of the final months, weeks or days of life.

The other factor Dr. Williams cites as evidence of a future for health promotion is essentially numerical. Our commitment to health promotion and health maintenance for the elderly will increase, he says, because more people reaching old age in generally good health will want it. Furthermore, their adult children want it for them. These growing numbers represent a political force for health promotion.

If Dr. Williams' thesis is true, then it follows that priorities for *types* of health promotion ought to be based on *what* they want most. Even if you don't buy that, this is the way priorities should be set, in a democratic society and free-market economy, it is how they do get set. The projection of priorities by this "demand" equation is predictive, not necessarily prescriptive. Do we know what they want? How do the elderly themselves view the issues we have debated here?

Facing criticisms that the *Objectives for the Nation*[2] did not adequately reflect the special needs of minority groups, we surveyed some 600 members of five minority groups to nominate people they would want to represent their views in refining the *Objectives for the Nation*. The representatives chosen met with officials of the appropriate federal agencies. The following is a summary of views expressed by participants during the meeting on strategies for promoting health for elderly Americans.[4] (See Table 1.)

The *Objectives for the Nation* did not adequately address some of these specific needs of the elderly. Local control of decision making and resources, and more participation by older persons, will facilitate adaptation of the objectives to address the needs of elderly people.[5]

Table 1
Health Promotion and Preventive Care Priorities, as
Ranked by Elected Representatives of Elderly Americans

Health Care Area	Ranking*
Health Promotion	
Smoking cessation	5
Reducing misuse of alcohol and drugs	4
Exercise and fitness	2
Improved nutrition	1
Stress Control	3
Preventive Health Services	
Immunizations	3
Hypertension control	2
Sensory deprivation control **	1
Periodic retirement, life-style, and health assessment	4

* 1 is high; 5 is low
** Category added as especially applicable to the elderly

BALANCING MOTIVATIONAL, EPIDEMIOLOGICAL, AND ECONOMIC ANALYSES

Another reason to give credence to these rankings or preferences, even if you deny the political force they may represent, is that they might reflect the motivational level several speakers here have said is missing. Much has been said of resistance to behavior or lifestyle changes conducive to health, and of financial incentives and penalties to induce such changes in behavior. The foregoing analysis of priorities for health promotion reflect what representatives of the elderly themselves say they want. By starting with needs that people themselves feel, the motivational barriers should be less and the commitment to changes made should be more firmly internalized than behavioral changes made in response to financial incentives and threats of penalties.

If we start with some combination of epidemiological and medical diagnoses of what the elderly need, economic analyses of what they can afford, and social or educational diagnoses of what they want, I believe we can shape policies for health promotion that will have greater benefits and greater durability.

REFERENCES

1. *Healthy People: The Surgeon General's Report on Health Promotion and Disease Prevention.* DHEW publication No. (PHS) 79-55071. Washington, D.C.: Government Printing Office, 1979.

2. Office of Health Information and Health Promotion. *Promoting Health, Preventing Disease: Objectives for the Nation.* U.S. Department of Health and Human Services, Public Health Service. Washington, D.C.: Government Printing Office, 1980.

3. Filner, B. and Williams, T.F. Health promotion for the elderly: reducing functional dependency. In: *Healthy People: The Surgeon General's Report on Health Promotion and Disease Prevention. Background Papers.* U.S. Department of Health, Education, and Welfare, Public Health Service, Office of the Assistant Secretary for Health and Surgeon General. DHEW (PHS) Publication No. 79-55071A. Washington D.C.: Government Printing Office, 1979.

4. *Strategies for Promoting Health for Specific Populations.* DHHS Publication No. (PHS) 81-50169. Washington, D.C.: Government Printing Office, 1981.

5. Green, L.W. Some challenges to health services research on children and the elderly. *Health Services Research,* 19(6): 793–815, Part II, 1985.

Health Promotion and the Elderly: Why Do It and Where Does It Lead? A Regional Policy Perspective

Robert Bernstein, MD, FACP

I thought Dr. William's paper was excellent. I can't add very much and I can argue with even less. It was important for him to start out discussing the definition and dynamics of aging; maybe it is even more important to discuss the perceptions of aging. Not just perceptions of the aging individual, but also the perceptions of those folks surrounding that individual we are talking about.

On the matter of health promotion, the relationship of the "normal" versus "abnormal" processes of aging is important, abnormal being that influenced by disease. We usually only think of chronic diseases in that connection, but certainly acute diseases must be included. It is well known that health promotion can be most profitable in avoiding chronic diseases. Cancer screening/cancer prevention is becoming a prominent field on its own. There are certainly some very exciting prevention activities, some we had known earlier, and some of the new information on diet that has already been alluded to. Avoidance of some known hazards of today's living certainly are matters for health promotion. Traditional public health involves health promotion/disease prevention and virtually all the programs that public health deals with in the traditional program areas involve entire populations, including the aged.

I disagree with my good friend Dr. Green in his discussion of rehabilitation versus health promotion, if I understand him correctly. Health promotion is not all black and white, an all or none situation. In my view, we need to go into this health promotion business with the idea that everybody can get some good out of it. A step in the right direction brings us closer to that final objective. He made reference to National Public Health Objectives, the *1990 Objectives* set by the Department of Health and Human Services.

We in Texas, including many people and agencies outside of our Health Department, had a meeting here in Houston and several follow-up meetings in which we have set health objectives. A great deal of deliberations involved the aging. Health promotion, or wellness, as people sometimes call it, is a formal and major program of ours. There is much too much talk and too many meetings about it, not enough research, as mentioned in Dr. Williams' paper, and certainly not enough action!

Aside from all of the aspects that have been mentioned about promotion, we must reinforce a very important concept. It is that a person's health is his or her responsibility, not their mother's, father's or doctor's or whatever. Formal health promotion lays that responsibility and burden right on the individual. Thus, education is involved, and as mentioned earlier, this is mainly self-education and self-help. Dr. Fielding alluded to that.

The most lucrative target, without question, is children in school, grammar school and up. They are the ones who are developing their lifestyles and they don't yet need that "toddy" in the evening like some of us do. The youngsters are more amendable to such "good health" education. Give them the facts without scaring them. Let them work their own way out of it and we will be better off. While that does not help today's aged population, it will certainly have a great bearing on the Aging Conference that will convene fifty years from now.

There is another point about this self-education that has been discussed. That is, the hopeless and helpless feeling that we all know exists in some of the aged and certainly some who live in nursing homes. Some feel like they have been put "out to pasture" to die. A very important aspect of this program is the hope that it can give them. They hope that somebody is interested in their future, not just for the moment. I attempted to get some state money for a dental progam within nursing homes. It was not just to make them look better or to pull those teeth that needed it. We believed the residents might realize that if someone is "worried about my teeth, they must be thinking I am going to live awhile." For those of you have not been in nursing homes, check their hairdressers, usually you will see long waiting lines. These "niceties" really are vital to those who have an interest in the future.

Incidentially, we co-lead a Texas program originating from the federal government, entitled "Health Promotion for the Aging." We work with the Department of Aging here in Texas on that. We have a plan, we have had statewide public hearings. Obviously, we want the promotional information to get out and want to target population to follow some of the advide that we believe is important. So we hope for success; it is too early to know. We have a great theme for the program, "Wellness is Ageless," and it is not copyrighted.

Most of our earlier discussions about using nursing homes for education of the professionals, I agree with. I wonder where we will find the money for such programs. I am worried about pay for the nurse aides. We are all interested in supporting a better life for those in nursing homes. Most states are similar to Texas in this regard. We pay the nurses aide, that is, the hands-on person in nursing homes, minimum wage; so they bounce back and forth between jobs. We have tried to do something about it, but to no avail; namely, to get the state to augment that pay a little. Now they are talking about education for aides and certifying them. They can go down the street to Safeway without all that hassle and make the same money—it is a terrible problem.

We have some 254 counties in Texas. We have counties with nursing homes that have a few hundred people in them. We cannot get a physician to go to some of them. If there is one in the area, he or she is too busy. I do know that the Texas Medical Association has tried very diligently; they have a permanent nursing home committee to look into these problems. They have also been able to get pertinent information into the curriculum of most of the medical schools. In the long run, that will certainly improve the lot of the aging, including those in nursing homes.

Health Promotion and the Elderly:
Why Do It and Where Does It Lead?
Panel Discussion

Dr. Queta Bond: We need to reshape our thinking about the need for health promotion and disease prevention for older people. Although youth is most often the target of health promotion, as a recent paper about smoking cessation in older persons has shown, you can document very clear advances to health at older ages. We need to think about offering these kinds of programs for the elderly. To do this, physician and health professional training in this area is essential.

We also need new ideas for reimbursing these kinds of services. It is true Medicare is paying for pneumococcal vaccine and so forth, and the social HMO is supporting greater incorporation of prevention into services, but we need more incentives for doing health promotion and disease prevention. It is also critical to expand our research efforts to develop the necessary knowledge base to support effective programs and services. As Dr. Williams pointed out, there is very little research on health promotion targeted for this older population.

I want to make a comment about rehabilitation, Dr. Green. We at the Institute of Medicine think of prevention as primary, secondary and tertiary. Primary is more health promotion, secondary is disease identification in its early stages and prevention of further symptoms, and tertiary is rehabilitation.

Dr. Charles Sprague: There has been a gross deficiency in our discussions on the importance of research. The single allusion to basic research thus far, was a comment Dr. Fries made that maybe 25 years hence, recombinant DNA research may have something to offer in terms of clarifying mortality/morbidity data. Virtually, everything with respect to health promotion and prevention had to do with modification of lifestyle.

We have information today that has far-reaching implications for the elderly population. In the case of arteriosclerosis, the work of Drs.

281

Goldstein and Brown is noteworthy. They are studying what is thought to be the commonest genetic disorder in humans, familial hypercholesterolemia. One in every 500 people have this disorder, but one out of every 20 patients admitted to coronary care units have it. What is involved is a defect in the number of receptors on cell surfaces that allow cholesterol to enter the cell from the blood. As a result, children are born with enormously elevated levels of cholesterol and die from coronary heart disease within the first few years of life. Drs. Goldstein and Brown, in collaboration with others, have found drugs that will influence the genes responsible for receptive production. Even in patients who ingest large amounts of cholesterol, these receptors, even though normal in numbers, are sluggish and can be activated with drug therapy. This knowledge will have a tremendous impact on the frequency of arteriosclerosis and its complications.

In the case of diabetes, within the last year we have been able to detect genetic markers that will allow us to determine the population at risk for Type I diabetes, which may result in blindness, kidney failure, amputations and so forth; a real killer. With these genetic markers and the ability to define the population at risk for diabetes, and knowing the natural history of diabetes, I would not be at all surprised that we will find within the next decade a way to prevent diabetes from occurring. Not treating it with islet cell transplants and so forth, but actually preventing it by identifying the population at risk and seeing what triggers diabetes in that susceptible individual. The likelihood is that it will turn out to be a virus.

Twenty-five years from now there will be tissue typing at birth for a number of the chronic debilitating diseases, neuromuscular diseases, some metabolic disorders, some mental disorders where there is a genetic predisposition. You could determine what individuals are predisposed to and perhaps immunize them, much as we do for various infections, against chronic disabling disorders.

Let's not minimize the importance of basic biologic research in dealing with the elderly population.

Dr. Eugene Stead: I would like to take an exception to Dr. Williams' notion about organ function. There are two kinds of approaches to finding out about the elderly. One is the scientific approach which is liable to error. The other is just go talk to a few old folks. Tinsley Harrison said many years ago, ''I am just as smart as I ever was, but I am not as smart as many hours a day." That has applicability to all testing of old people. I myself have 20/20 vision when I go to the ophthalmologist. When I sit and read a book, I rapidly lose that 20/20 vision. I cannot hold it during the course of a 12 hour day like I used to. I have, for the last seven years, climbed to the tenth floor of the VA hospital every day. In year one, I went up in one minute and 40 seconds; today, it takes me three minutes and 20 seconds. The general notion that organ function does not decline is absolutely foreign to every elderly person's experience. I hope that Frank will live long enough to appreciate it.

Dr. Steve Schroeder: The issue of paying for preventive services comes up a lot. We hear much criticism of the low level of payments for preventive services. We have to think that one through very carefully, however. In the world of internal medicine, one could theoretically justify following the American Cancer Society guidelines: bring someone in every year, do a mammogram on a woman, a flexible sigmoidoscopy on individuals of both sexes, and, in the process, run up staggering bills that would have questionable benefit. Let's take a little more flexible look at payment for preventive services.

The five priorities that Larry Green mentioned are not things that doctors are going to do, even if you make payments for health promotion or disease prevention more liberal. In fact, I am not sure that these are things that doctors are capable of doing better than other people. Before we fall into the usual trap of asking for more money for preventive services, in a time when money is tight, we should know the best way to spend that money.

Dr. Karl Shaner: In my work with older people, I find that the people who pay attention to all the health promotion literature that we produce are middle class, upper middle class, educated people. That is not the great majority of the sick elderly. Unfortunately, the people who need information on nutrition, need to have their living environments controlled and improved, or need to stop spending money on alcohol and cigarettes, are not the ones who are going to respond to the kinds of health promotion talk that we are hearing here. Everything that we are talking about makes a lot of sense and has a lot of virtue, but the message is not getting through to many of those who need this kind of help.

Dr. James Haughton: Twenty years ago I did something in New

York that I thought was great for old people. Some of them wrote back to me and said, "Doctor, I have been doing it this way for 40 years and I don't care what you doctors say, I am now 80 years old and I am going to continue to do it my way." There was nothing I could do about it. Furthermore, if they had done what I was thinking was great for them, they may not have lived as long as they had. Sometimes our older people think that they have earned the right to live their own lives and all of our notions about health promotion are not going to change their minds.

Dr. Robert Kane: You can find anecdotal data to support almost any position with regard to the elderly and their health habits. I am very concerned about a number of issues that I think we need to recognize up front about the elderly. One is that the elderly, particularly the poor elderly, are spending an inordinate amount of money on worthless medicaments of various types. If one could, in some way, redistribute the effort that goes into reading the *National Enquirer*, onto other kinds of informational resources, one would mobilize a very strong motivation for behavior change. The elderly are not necessarily any different from the rest of the population in seeking the miracle cure. That is why Herbalife just opened a 20 story building in Los Angeles. There is a market out there for that kind of stuff and I think we are foolish to ignore it. It is always amazing to me that we wind up in meetings like this saying that we cannot change the people's behavior; people are getting rich changing behavior. We should not become nihilistic and write these people off.

On the other hand, there is another movement within the gerontology circles, which is potentially disturbing, the self care movement. There are major meetings trying to organize the elderly to try and take better care of themselves, as though this was somehow an anathema to medical care. We wind up creating barriers between the self care people and the health care people, when probably one of the most important self care things you can do, is learn how to deal with the health care system.

One of the most important preventive issues which has not been raised, is the most prevalent disease of the elderly, iatrogenesis. One of the things we need to teach the elderly how to do is how to deal effectively with the health care system. We talked earlier about making the health care system more responsive to the needs of the elderly. We could look at it the other way around, and say another strategy that may be equally important is to try and mobilize the elderly to make intelligent, purposeful demands on the medical care system. There are things they can do to get better information to and from their physicians. Indeed, there is growing evidence that physicians, particularly in a competitive market situation, will respond to consumer pressures. We should get the consumers to exert more of those pressures.

I am concerned about some of the things which appear to be potential benefits, but are also open to tremendous exploitation. I think Steve Schroeder is right to question the value of simply paying for prevention. If I may quote some anecdotal data, my mother, who is geriatric by the international definition, but a very functional lady, occasionally goes to a podiatrist. She called me up one day very upset because she found out that this podiatrist was asking her to sign a blank Medicare form to make it easier for her. She then found out what he was putting on this form. It turned out not only was he charging for a routine podiatric visit, but also charging for a whole series of preventive foot services, which were apparently reimbursable under Medicare. It turned out that this man's average bill was over a $100 per visit for essentially cutting toe nails. That is what happens in a fee-for-service system when we start covering individual kinds of services. If we were to begin to cover the preventive services on a fee-for-service basis, we would find ourselves paying for a lot of questionable, marginal therapies, even though it may be in the best intentions of people advocating preventive medicine.

The other option is to look toward something like capitation. Frank Williams has been optimistic about what capitation offers. I share some of his optimism, but I also need to express a little bit of caution of what is likely to happen with capitation. We have, as a population, been known as the land of the slogans. Perhaps, one of the most misleading slogans that we have ever encountered is the "Health Maintenance Organization," which is not designed to maintain anything but its own financial health. Anybody with any appreciation of prevention recognizes that the fundamental social contract of prevention is a contract which talks about investments. Most of the payoff from prevention does not occur today or tomorrow, it occurs years from now. If you want to sell health insurance, you want to sell it to the healthiest population. You offer benefits that will attract the healthy. The elderly are even more vulnerable to that kind of selective marketing. There is some evidence that selective marketing is going on within Medicare HMOs. While I think the capitation concept makes a lot of sense and may be the way to get around some of these concerns about the fee-for-service billing for preventive services, it will only work when it is tied into geopolitical responsibility and not left to the free market system.

Dr. Charles Gaitz: If we paid more attention to the aged as individuals, and Dr. Stead certainly emphasized this, we would get away from the notion that health maintenance can be separate from mental health. We have played this down. It would be meaningful if we only promoted programs that dealt with the stresses of old age. There is good evidence of interactions between social and physiological and physical factors, to the point that we should be paying much more attention to stresses that come on in old age. For example, we should help plan for retirement and help people who are grief-stricken. There is an infinite number of things that can be done that don't require a tremendous amount of effort. We should be more cognizant of the fact that these are important issues in the list of things that relate to health maintenance. We must be concerned with the factors affecting mental health.

Dr. Eli Ginzberg: On that last point, there is story about a lady in Israel who used to come to the clinic every morning, and then she did not come for five days. She came on the sixth day and the physician asked what the matter was. She said, "Oh Doc, I was sick, so I had to stay home." So the question of the mental state and the socialization about health is obviously critical. Given the estimate that five million people are involved in some kind of self help organization, which must contain many who are elderly, it is clear that a lot of people who have disabilities, chronic illnesses, and so on, are not finding the medical profession responsive or not finding their pocketbooks in a condition that they can use the medical profession. We should not be insensitive to that kind of social response to something that is going on out there, if these figures are anywhere near right.

Some of you must have read Dewitt Stetten's piece in the *New England Journal* some years ago, which indicated that somebody like him, at the top of the profession, with money to pay for medical care, couldn't get the most simple help out of his colleagues about his loss of sight. His story is just unbelievable, which means that putting everything back on the medical profession does not seem sensible. With Steve Schroeder's comment about the payment for preventive services reminded me that Dr. Spock's book saved us about 50,000 pediatricians because he wrote a simple book to teach high school-educated mothers to take care of their children. I have never understood why we don't have two or three books on the major chronic diseases of old age to provide the same kind of reassurance, insight and suggestions to elderly people, most of whom read.

I could not agree more with Robert Kane, that the interest of an HMO is in their financial survivability, and it is supposed to be. This notion we are having now of putting Medicare patients into HMOs is not sound. The healthy ones will go into HMOs, the HMOs will reject the unhealthy ones, and the total cost to the federal government will go up. That is another way of trying to remind you all that we play games between need, services, financing, and intermediaries who want to make a buck. That is a circle that we don't square.

Mr. Robert Ball: For better or worse, I spent a considerable part of the last thirty to thirty-five years designing, modifying, thinking up different kinds of reimbursement schemes for a variety of benefit packages. This health promotion, disease prevention area has always been very troublesome. The question is really, is there anything that you would propose reimbursing under Medicare that it does not now pay for in this area, other than to establish an advisory group of outstanding experts who would recommend to the Secretary what to cover? And that seems to me to say that we really don't know what works for older people. I wish we did.

Rebuttal

T. Franklin Williams, MD

Ann Somers, who was unable to be here and regretted it very much, sent me some "random thoughts," as she called them and the headings fit in very well with the comments here. She emphasized the risk of undernutrition; that is, getting too thin as well as getting too fat. She discussed polypharmacy and pointed out the issues there about health maintenance. In the British system, it is important to note that the consultant physician can only prescribe drugs for a few days and the general practitioner has to renew the prescription if it is going to be continued. There is, therefore, at least a physician who knows what everybody is taking. There are ways to manage this issue of polypharmacy. Ms. Somer's third topic was inadequate family support in relation to health maintenance.

Concerning the necessity for considering health promotion in older people in the presence of multiple chronic diseases, I certainly agree, and I did not stress this in my paper as much as I should have. I am grateful for Dr. Sprague's comments about the research side. We unequivocally are making and will be making marvelous advances that will help us modify or prevent the course of the major chronic diseases that are the major contributors to loss of health and functioning in older people.

On the matter of self care, I am very glad to see that both Dr. Fielding and Dr. Bernstein brought this out. I would not agree that it has been exaggerated, however. It is a very fundamental issue and I would refer people to the summary of the World Health Organization on Self Help and Care for Older People. The final version of this summary is a very useful document in pointing out the multiple ways it is being approached around the world, including the types of organizations that Dr. Ginzberg referred to. This is all to the good and it is up to us to try to relate this to our professional activities.

In relation to Mr. Ball's question, the best thing would be to do exactly what he and Ann Somers have suggested before, and that is to have some type of board that would make such recommendations. We have the experience of the Canadian Commission approach to this, which did a very sound job. This is the kind of thing that can only be done by a commission or advisory committee, which would periodically review a set of practices that could be paid for as routine preventive services. Then, other elements could be recommended to be incorporated into general services that, perhaps, would not be billed for separately, but accepted as part of good practice.

CHAPTER 7

Medical Care for the Elderly in Other Western Countries: Lessons for the United States Position Paper

Steven A. Schroeder, MD

Health care for the elderly in the United States today stands at the crossroads. Compared with most other Western countries, the United States provides virtually unrestricted medical care for its elderly citizens, particularly hospital-based technological services. It does this through a system that seems maximally designed to feature these types of care, but one that seems much less responsive to the provision of other services needed by the elderly—such as home care, long-term care within institutions, and hospice care.

Perhaps as a logical outcome of this country's focus on acute-care services, it now finds itself under attack for being too expensive on the one hand and not providing acceptable chronic care services on the other hand. When the structure and performance of the United States' medical care system is compared with that of other Western countries, the reasons for this attack become more apparent. This paper starts by comparing the structures of Western medical care systems, moves next to a description of their performance, analyzes reasons for the differences in structure and performance and closes with a discussion of the policy implications of these differences for the care of the elderly.

COMPARISON OF THE MEDICAL CARE SYSTEMS

General Characteristics

Table 7-1 summarizes selected general aspects of the medical care system in the United States compared with other Western countries. Perhaps the most striking difference is the absence of universal health insurance coverage in the United States. It is estimated that about 13 percent of the United States population, or about 30 million people, have no health insurance coverage. For the most part, these people have too many assets to qualify for Medicaid, are not eligible for other health insurance programs, or are disqualified from governmental programs because they are not United States citizens. By contrast, virtually the entire population of

TABLE 7-1

GENERAL CHARACTERISTICS OF THE MEDICAL CARE SYSTEMS
OF THE UNITED STATES AND OTHER WESTERN COUNTRIES

Characteristics	United States	Other Western Countries
Population coverage medical care	About 87% of population covered through government or private health insurance	Essentially universal for coverage for all countries except Africa
Assignment to primary physician countries)	No	Occurs in some countries (United Kingdom, the Netherlands, New Zealand, the Scandinavian
Referral to specialists	Either by self-referral or physician referral	From the general practitioners in most countries although self-referral occurs in some (e.g., West Germany, Belgium)
Payment of physicians	Dominantly fee-for-service for generalists and specialists. Capitation and its variants in health maintenance organizations	Variable patterns including fee-for-service (fee schedule), West Germany, the Netherlands; capitation (United Kingdom, general practitioners in the Netherlands); and salary for specialists in United Kingdom, West Germany

every other Western country, except for the Union of South Africa, has basic health coverage, both for hospital and out-patient care.

For the other categories shown in Table 7-1, the differences between the United States and other Western countries are not as dramatic. Although many nations, such as the United Kingdom, the Netherlands, New Zealand, and the Scandanavian countries, designate an assigned primary care physical for each individual, many others, including the United States, do not. Similarly, although access to specialist physicians is controlled by generalists in many countries (e.g., Norway, the United Kingdom, the Netherlands, and New Zealand), in others, including the United States, the patient may self-refer directly to a specialist physician. Finally, although few countries feature fee-for-service payment of physicians as prominently as the United States, fee-for-service, along with capitation on salary, is how physicians are paid in several other countries.

Differences in the Supply of Medical Resources

The three most important supply factors that determine the use of medical resources are institutions, personnel, and equipment. Representative categories from each of these are listed in Table 7-2. One measure of institutional capacity is the supply of acute-care hospital beds. Here, the United States is actually on the low side compared with other countries, having about five beds per 1000 persons, a similar number to that found in the United Kingdom, Canada, and Belgium, but substantially fewer than the 11 per 1000 in West Germany. However, there is room to believe that United States' hospitals are more intensively staffed and supplied. For example, a recent comparison of a prestigious university hospital in the United States with one in each of four European countries showed that the United States hospital (University of California at San Francisco) had from 1.5 to 2.5 times as many total employees, 2 to 8 times as many staff physicians, and 2 to 3 times as many houseofficers per adjusted occupied bed as its European counterparts.[5] It also had a much higher proportion of intensive care beds (even though it had fewer such beds than the average United States teaching hospital) and more CT scanners.

Perhaps the most visible component of medical-service personnel is the physician. As shown in Table 7-2, the current and projected United States' concentration of physicians is unremarkable com-

TABLE 7-2

THE SUPPLY OF MEDICAL RESOURCES (1-4)

Resource	United States	Other Western Countries
Acute care hospital (per 1000 persons) 1980	5	5 (United Kingdom) beds to 11 (W. Germany)
Physicians (per 100,000 persons),		
1980	191	159 (New Zealand) to 249 (Belgium)
1990	243	171 (United Kingdom) to 340 (Belgium)
Selected Technologies		
CT scanners (per 1,000,000 persons), 1979	5.7	0.6 (United Kingdom) to 4.6 (Japan)
Magnetic Resonance Imaging Facilities	64 percent of world supply was in United States as of August 1984	

pared with other Western countries. Although in 1980, it had somewhat more physicians than New Zealand (159/100,000 persons) or the United Kingdom (162/100,000), it lagged behind Belgium (240/100,000), West Germany (229/100,000) and France (220/100,000), as well as Italy, Israel and the Scandanavian countries. Estimates for the year 1990 project the United States to remain substantially below many European countries, although it will continue to have slightly more physicians than the United Kingdom, Canada and Australia.[1]

Although the United States does not stand out as having an unusually high concentration of physicians, it is unique in its large concentration of specialists. In 1980, 84 percent of all active physicians in the United States who had completed residency and/or fellowship training were specialists, including internal medicine and pediatrics, but excluding family practice. Comparable figures for other countries were 27 percent (United Kingdom), 46 percent (West Germany), and 62 percent (the Netherlands). These figures may be somewhat inflated, since the United States, in contradistinction to other countries, features internists, pediatricians, and gynecologists as primary care physicians. However, the United States' concentration of such non-primary care specialties as cardiology, gastroenterology, general surgery, ophthalmology, orthopedic surgery, psychiatry and neurology appear to be among the highest in the world.[1]

One specialty that is found in very low concentrations in all Western countries is geriatric medicine. In no country that I know of do geriatricians constitute more than one percent of the total physician population. However, in several, most notably, the United Kingdom and New Zealand, there is an explicit governmental commitment to the growth and development of geriatric medicine as an important feature of medical care for the elderly. Within these countries, the roles of geriatricians vary, including functions as consultant and as primary physician for the elderly.

The last row in Table 7-2 lists the concentration of two selected diagnostic medical technologies, the computerized tomographic scanner (CT) and magnetic resonance imaging, to illustrate the diffusion of medical technologies in general. In the category of medical technology use, the United States clearly stands out as the most lavishly endowed, with only Japan having even half as many CT scanners per population,[3] and with the United States having twice as many magnetic resonance imagers as the rest of the world combined.[4]

In summary, the United States' concentration of acute-hospital beds and physicians seems about average compared with other Western countries, although its hospitals may be more intensively staffed and equipped. However, it far exceeds other countries in its relative proportion and absolute concentration of specialist physicians and in its supply of technologies, such as CT scanners and magnetic resonance imagers.

DIFFERENCES IN DEMAND FOR MEDICAL SERVICES

Unlike the supply of medical resources, it is more difficult to measure demand directly. However, there appear to be at least two indirect measures that attest to a higher demand for medical services in the United States than in other Western countries. The first measure is the rate of medical malpractice litigation. Although precise figures on the number of such suits and the size of successful claims are not known, it is common knowledge that malpractice litigation is much more frequent, and awards much higher in the United States. Evidence for this is the contrast between the $1.7 million annual malpractice premium paid by the 550-bed University of California, compared with premiums ranging from nothing to $45,000 per year for four comparable (but larger) hospitals in Belgium, West Germany, the Netherlands and the United Kingdom.[5] Reasons given for this huge difference in litigation include the American jury system, our high concentration of lawyers, the incentive provided by U.S. lawyers' contigency fees, and higher expectations by U.S. patients. The last reason, higher patient expectations, is the second indirect measure of consumer demand. During my recent visits to numerous Western European countries, I had the opportunity to talk with many patients and physicians. It was the strong conviction of most experts, many of whom had first-hand experience with the medical care system in the United States, that the levels of sophistication, expectation, and willingness to question physician authority were substantially greater among U.S. patients than in any other country.

OUTCOMES OF THE MEDICAL CARE SYSTEMS

The Costs of Medical Care

The costs of medical care, as a proportion of Gross National Product in 1980, are displayed in Table 7-3 for seven Western countries. More recent data from the United States show that medical care had increased to about 10.8 percent of the GNP by 1983, and it should be at about 11 percent in 1984. It is estimated by many that the United States has probably passed West Germany, and may now only trail Sweden as the country that spends the most of its resources on medical care.

Utilization

As shown in Table 7-4, the United States has a relatively high rate of admissions to acute-care hospitals. However, because of its short length of stay in the United States, its overall number of patient days per population is low compared to most other Western countries.

One reason for the high rate of hospital admission in the United

TABLE 7-3

COST OF MEDICAL CARE AS A PERCENT
OF GROSS NATIONAL PRODUCT, 1980 (1,2)

Country	Percent of Gross National Product
United States	9.4 (10.8 in 1983)
West Germany	10.2
The Netherlands	8.9
Belgium	7.5
Australia	7.3
Canada	7.3
United Kingdom	6.2

TABLE 7-4
USE OF ACUTE-CARE HOSPITALS, 1980 (1)

Measure	United States	Belgium	West Germany	The Netherlands	United Kingdom
No. of admissions per 1000 persons per year	173	139	157	110	93
Mean length of hospital stay (days)	7	12	15	13	13
Patient days per 1000 persons per year	1,212	1,666	2,357	1,433	1,207

States is shown in Table 7-5, which compares rates of coronary
artery bypass graft surgery among eight different countries. Although the United States does not differ appreciably from other
countries in the prevalence of coronary artery disease and in
mortality resulting from the condition, it clearly has a pro-surgical
style of treatment. Similar, although less dramatic, differences can
be seen in the frequency of other elective surgical procedures such
as cataract excision, hysterectomy, hip replacement, and so on.
There is some reason to believe that much of the higher rates of
performance of such procedures occurs in elderly persons.

TABLE 7-5

FREQUENCY OF CORONARY ARTERY BYPASS SURGERY PER
MILLION POPULATION, 1978 (3)

Country	Frequency
United States	483 (estimated at about 800 for 1983) (5)
Ireland	233
Australia	150
The Netherlands	78
United Kingdom	74
Sweden	37
West Germany	25
France	19

Less is known about the intensity of treatment of chronic medical conditions. However, if the experience with one such condition, end-stage renal disease, is representative (and there is no reason to think that it is not) then the United States also treats such conditions more intensively than occurs in other countries (Table 7-6). Although some differences across countries do exist in the incidence of chronic renal disease, the differences shown in Table 7-6 are felt to represent differing willingness to commit resources for dialysis and renal transplantation rather than responses to differing levels of kidney disease.[6]

Health Status

All Western countries have achieved impressive improvements in mortality during the past two decades. Whether measured in terms of infant mortality, in life expectancy from birth, from age 65, or from age 75, people are living longer. Although other measures of health status, such as morbidity and functional status, are less easy to define, there is a general impression that they have also improved. Among Western countries, one of the most dramatic improvements in mortality statistics has occurred in the United States. Formerly having one of the highest infant mortality rates, it has now caught up with many Western countries (see Table 7-7) although it still lags behind the Scandinavian countries, the Netherlands, Japan, France, and Canada. In 1983, infant mortality in the United States had fallen to 10.8 deaths in the first year of life per 1000 live births, probably moving it ahead of such countries as the United Kingdom and Belgium, whose recent rates of improvement have been slower than the United States.

What may be less well known is that the United States does even better in life expectancy from birth, and stands at the top of all countries in life expectancy from age 65. How much of the improved longevity for seniors is attributable to good medical care, healthier life styles, genetics, prosperity, or "other" factors is unclear. Nevertheless, it is tempting, given the high consumption of medical services by the elderly in the United States to posit at least a partial cause-and-effect relationship.

DIFFERENCES IN NATIONAL STYLES OF MEDICAL PRACTICE

Many of the differences in national systems of medical care and their resultant outcomes can be explained by differing "styles" of medical practice. Whether these differing styles result from or cause the differing levels of investment in medical resources is, of course, impossible to determine. Nevertheless, at the multiple possible steps in the sequence of medical care for a symptomatic patient (or even

TABLE 7-6

ACCEPTANCE RATES OF NEW PATIENTS FOR TREATMENT
FOR CHRONIC RENAL DISEASE (PER MILLION POPULATION) 1981 (6)

Country	Rate (per million)
United States	about 61
Sweden	51.3
West Germany	49.7
France	42.3
The Netherlands	34.8
England	25.4
East Germany	23.0

TABLE 7-7

HEALTH STATUS INDICATORS (7)

Country	Infant Mortality Rate (1980)	Life expectancy at birth (1978-80) male/female		Life expectancy at age 65 (1978-80) male/female	
United States	12.5%	70.3	77.9	79.5	84.0
Australia	10.7	71.2	78.2	78.6	82.8
Belgium	12.3	69.5	76.2	77.7	81.4
Canada	10.0	71.4	78.9	79.4	83.7
Denmark	7.9	71.7	77.6	78.7	82.9
France	9.7	70.8	79.1	79.3	83.9
Japan	7.5	74.1	79.6	80.1	83.4
Italy	14.1	70.7	77.4	78.8	82.3
The Netherlands	8.6	72.5	79.5	79.1	83.8
Spain	10.3	71.8	78.0	79.4	82.5
Sweden	7.0	77.8	79.1	79.4	83.2
United Kingdom	12.0	70.7	76.8	77.6	79.3
West Germany	12.6	69.9	76.8	78.1	81.9

an asymptomatic patient with a potential surgical condition, such as cataracts) different Western countries are likely to follow different paths. As shown in Figure 7-1, using a 78-year old woman with a breast lump as an illustrative case, in the United States she would be much more likely to follow the sequence in the upper part of the flow diagram, while in the United Kingdom choices would be more likely to follow the earlier and lower pathways. The process whereby medical care is thus limited have been described in the most detail for the United Kingdom.

Aaron and Schwartz, in their book, *The Painful Prescription: Rationing Hospital Care*,[7] document the degree to which the British limit the use of X-rays, treatment of chronic renal failure, total parenteral nutrition, CT scanning, intensive care treatment in hospitals, and coronary artery bypass surgery compared to the United States. They describe several mechanisms that serve to make the British limit-setting possible. Most important are the physicians,

SEQUENTIAL STEPS IN MEDICAL CARE OF THE ELDERLY

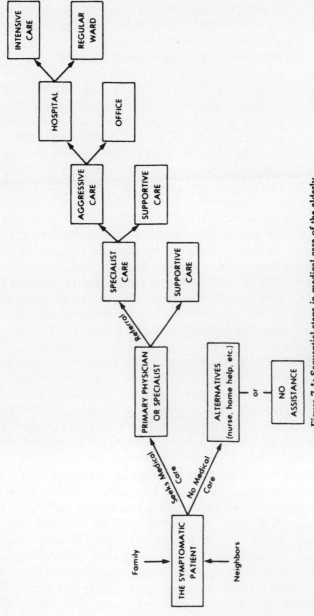

Figure 7-1: Sequential steps in medical care of the elderly.

who, in the belief that medical resources are finite, make explicit and implicit rationing decisions. Physicians may limit services directly, by not offering them in the first place, or refusing to provide them if requested. In addition, the lengthy queues for most elective procedures can serve to delay, sometimes forever, the performance of some procedures that the physician does order. However, this limit-setting by physicians would not be possible without a permissive political climate, a relatively dormant medical-legal process, and a comparatively undemanding public.

A closer look at a single condition, end-stage renal disease, illustrates in more detail how much rationing occurs in the United Kingdom. In order to understand the low rate of therapy for renal failure for the entire population, but especially for the population age 65 and over, over 700 doctors including general practitioners, consultants, and nephrologists were asked to rate whether 16 sample case histories should be eligible for end-stage renal disease treatment in their district. Consultant physicians had the highest rejection rate (7.4 cases), followed by general practitioners (6.9 cases), and nephrologists (4.7 cases). The six cases least likely to be recommended for treatment were (starting with the most frequently rejected): a 29-year old man who was positive for hepatitis B virus; a 52-year old male alcoholic; a 30-year old male with schizophrenia; a 50-year old male with ischemic heart disease; a 51-year old female with breast cancer; and a 67-year old Asian who speaks no English. Patients most often recommended for treatment were a 55-year old woman with asthma, a 72-year old retired male veterinarian; a 36-year old man with paraplegia; and three diabetics, two in their 50s and one age 25 and blind. By contrast, 19 responses from general medical colleagues of North American nephrologists rejected on the average only 0.3 patients, compared with 3.6 in Western Europe.

Although no comparable data on limiting care exist for Western countries other than the United Kingdom, my impression is that the situation in most lies about mid-way between the United States and the United Kingdom. This opinion is based on crude utilization data for such services as CT scanning and coronary artery bypass surgery, as well as impressions gained from visiting medical facilities in five Western European countries (Belgium, Denmark, France, West Germany and the Netherlands) and talking with physicians and other medical care experts from many other countries. As in the United Kingdom, it is hard to determine how these national styles of practice get established. They seem to reflect differing levels of demands by physicians and patients and differing determinations of the adequacy of supply by government.

Since the elderly in every Western country are the largest consumers of medical care, and since the United States has both the largest utilization of expensive health care by the elderly and the longest life expectancy for those who reach age 65, it is tempting to say that the increased U.S. life span results from the elderly receiving more medical care. However, at least two observations suggest caution in arriving at such a conclusion. First, Canada, a country that spends much less than the United States on medical care (Table 7-3) enjoys a comparably long life expectancy from age 65, and has a better infant mortality rate and life expectancy from birth. Second, there are alternate hypothesis, e.g., such as healthier lifestyles and more prosperity, for the increased life span of elderly Americans. In fact, the past two decades have seen dramatic improvements in the health habits within the United States, including decreased consumption of cigarettes and animal fats, and increased exercise. Each of these changes may have made important contributions to increased life expectancy, independent of medical care.

ACUTE CARE VERSUS LONG TERM CARE IN AN ERA OF CONSTRAINED RESOURCES

The combination of the United States' costly system of medical care and the aging of its population create a major policy dilemma that, although not unique to this country, is perhaps more troublesome here than elsewhere. As Blendon and Altman have summarized, recent public opinion polls in the United states seem to show a profound reluctance by the American public to endorse any reductions, or even changes, in the current systems of medical care, except perhaps to favor decreases in expenditures for the poor.[8] Yet, if current patterns of medical care utilization continue, and the proportion of the elderly keeps rising (as will certainly occur), then equally certainly, the amount of money spent on medical care will also increase.

One is tempted to ask, "So what? What is the big problem here? Medical care is expensive, people want it, and as a nation we can afford it. If it takes 11 percent, 12 percent, 14 percent of our gross national product, that is money well spent.'' There are two problems with that response. First, the current political and economic situation consisting of declining tax revenues, increasing national debt, and increasing claims by the military on a relatively static federal budget means that there will be severe pressures to limit federal expenditures on medical care. Although the rate of increase in medical care expenditures has declined, it is still rising almost twice as fast as the overall economy. Thus, given the recent increased support for medical cost containment from the business community and from labor, it is likely that politicians will be reluctant to let expenditures for medical care continue to climb at their current rate.

The second problem posed by a laissez-faire approach to escalating medical expenditures is that of opportunity costs, and here is where the needs of the elderly are most involved. In a sense, medical care can be seen to operate under a sort of Gresham's Law, with acute care driving out chronic care. It is significant that Blendon and Altman did not dwell on findings of public opinion polls regarding the wishes of elderly persons about long-term care and chronic illness. For it is in this area that the conflict with acute care emerges. Most Americans do not wish to end their lives in nursing homes, preferring instead to be cared for in their own homes. However, such care can be very expensive as pointed out in this conference. In my opinion, it is unlikely that the resources for needed new services for home health care and for nursing home reform can simply be added to an already swollen national medical care budget.

In this respect, the United States may have less flexibility to respond to the service needs of its aging population than do other Western countries that spend less on medical care and, therefore, seem to have more to give to social services and long-term care. Countries that spend 8 or 10 percent of the GNP on medical care may find it easier to add new social services, or even, paradoxically, to cut back on medical services in exchange for more and better long-term care in the community and in institutions.

It would seem that three broad strategies are available to the United States regarding its future investment in acute and long-term care.

1. *Let medical care costs continue to increase in the expectation that a booming economy can sustain them.* In this ''rosy'' scenario, continued economic growth postpones or

prevents the necessity of further rationing and permits gradual (albeit reluctant) increases in long-term care. This scenario is the least politically contentious of the three, but is dependent on a shaky premise, that of continued sustained economic growth. It also assumes that no major increase in resources for long term care would occur.

2. *Keep medical care costs at about current levels and let politics and the marketplace decide the share between acute and long-term care.* This scenario, which in various forms summarizes many current medical cost containment proposals, would entail continued pressures of the sort recently represented by the Prospective Payment System for Medicare hospital payment, increasing incentives to join Health Maintenance Organizations, freezes on physicians' fees, etc. The underlying assumption of this strategy is that the current mixture of medical services, which by international standards is relatively heavy on the acute side, is appropriate, and that the major policy goal is the prevention of major expansion of acute-care services. Given what we have learned about the existing supply and demand for their services, it is unlikely that this strategy would result in many new resources accruing to long-term or community care.

3. *Assume that total medical costs will increase slightly, if at all, but shift resources from the acute to the chronic sector.* This scenario, currently the least likely of the three, assumes that the welfare and desires of older people dictate a reordering of priorities and resources within the medical care system. It hypothesizes that people would accept slightly less aggressive/intensive care if they could be assured of better access to home health services that would keep them out of nursing homes, and better quality of care should they have to be institutionalized. Compared with other Western countries, the third strategy seems the most difficult to follow in the United States, for it would require major reorientations of the expectations of both providers and patients.

Comparing these three strategies, it is apparent that only the third would involve any substantial increase in resources for long-term care services, and that it would also be the most difficult to implement at this time. In order for the third strategy to be successful, a new lobbying group would have to coalesce. Such a group would likely consist of the elderly themselves, the long-term care industry, relevant medical personnel such as social workers and community health professionals, and possibly the geriatricians.

What seems most apparent from comparing the United States' health experience with other Western countries is that its high costs and intense use of costly acute-care services will make it more difficult to provide those community and long-term care services that will be needed by an increasingly elderly population. Whether other countries will follow the United States' pattern or whether we will find ourselves increasingly isolated is not yet clear, but, in my opinion, despite its relative prosperity, the United States would appear to have less flexibility to respond to long-term care needs of its elderly than almost any other Western country.

REFERENCES

1. Schroeder, S.A. Western European responses to physician oversupply. *Journal of the American Medical Association,* 252:373–84, 1984.

2. World Health Organization. *Statistics Annual, 1983.* Geneva World Health Organization, 1983.

3. Banta, H.D. and Kemp, K.B. *Background Paper No. 4: The Management of Health Care Technology in Ten Countries.* Washington, D.C.: Office of Technology Assessment, 1980.

4. Steinberg, P.E. and Cohen, A.B. *Health Technology Case Study No. 27: Nuclear Magnetic Resonance Imaging Technology: A Clinical, Industrial and Policy Analysis.* Washington, D.C.: U.S. Congress, Office of Technology Assessment OTA-HcS-27, 1984.

5. Schroeder, S.A. A Comparison of Western European and U.S. University Hospitals. *Journal of the American Medical Association,* 252:240–246, 1984.

6. Challah, S., Wing, A. J., Bauer, R., Morris, R.W., and Schroeder, S.A. Negative selection of patients for dialysis and transplantation in the United Kingdom. *British Medical Journal,* 288:1119–22, 1984.

7. Aaron, J.H. and Schwartz, W.B. *The Painful Prescription: Rationing Hospital Care.* Washington, D.C.: The Brookings Institute, 1984.

8. Blendon, R.J. and Altman, D.E. Public attitudes about health care costs: A lesson in national schizophrenia. *New England Journal of Medicine,* 311:613–16, 1984.

Medical Care for the Elderly in Other Western Countries: Lessons for the United States A General Policy Perspective

Robert L. Kane, MD

Dr. Schroeder concludes with a very important observation about the constraints on flexibility in the United States to respond to long-term care needs of the elderly. His conclusion is reminiscent of observations made by several Europeans about the United States. They note that our efforts to ensure freedom by explicit statements tend to limit our exercise of these freedoms rather than expand them. Much of the health policy in this country has reflected this tendency to make explicit policies that are left more implicit in other countries. This is certainly one of the points noted by Aaron and Schwartz.[1]

Dr. Schroeder has focused his observation primarily to medical care of the elderly. I prefer to broaden the discussion to look at health care in general, including elements of long-term care.

The differences then between the United States and Europe may be more impressive in the qualitative areas than in the quantitative. Part of the difficulty in interpreting cross-national data is the difference in definitions. Project HOPE recently attempted to develop cross-national data on long-term care, relying heavily on reports prepared for the 1982 World Assembly on Aging.[2] Because the United States has only very limited forms of national health insurance, its rate of public health care expenditures as a percent of the Gross National Product was the lowest of the countries studied in Western Europe and Canada. However, in Table 7-8, which expresses this as a percent of public health expenditures devoted to the elderly, the U.S. rate exceeds Canada, the Netherlands, and Switzerland. If one looks at total public expenditures on the elderly as a percentage of GNP, a similar trend emerges. The United States

TABLE 7-8
PUBLIC HEALTH CARE EXPENDITURES FOR THE ELDERLY

COUNTRY	Public Health care expenditures in 1980 as a percent of GNP	Percent of Public health expenditures devoted to the elderly
United States	3.9	29
Canada	5.8	21
Denmark	6.4	43
France	6.1	35 to 40
Germany	6.2	NA
Netherlands	6.5	25
Norway	5.8	50
Sweden	8.9	NA
Switzerland	4.5	25
United Kingdom	5.2	33

Source: US Senate, 1984

is not generous toward the elderly, but its rates of expenditure exceeds that of Canada and Norway (Table 7-9).

As an additional point of comparison, we can look at the proportion of persons aged 65 and above who are housed in institutions or in group living quarters. The latter category refers to the substantial use of sheltered housing as a substitute for the traditional nursing home in this country. Although caution must be exercised in looking at such gross cross-national data because of the differences in age structure, the figures in Table 7-10 argue that the rate of institutionalization of the elderly in the United States is lower than that for all of the countries noted except Germany.

Heterogeneity of care patterns in various countries are matched by the heterogeneity of the elderly themselves. Discussions about "the elderly" and about "geriatrics" tend to use these terms as though they represented a homogeneous population. Even the most basic demographic data suggests this is not the case. Like any group, the elderly are made up of numerous sub-groups. Most of the elderly are very functional, but some need substantial amounts of assistance. According to 1979 National Health Interview Survey, the number of adults per 1000 who needed assistance from another person in one or more basic physical activity or home management tasks ranged from 70 in the 65 to 74 year old age group to 436 in the 85 and over group.[3]

This variation is also seen in health expenditures. Data from the National Medical Care Utilization Expenditure Study indicate that in 1980 over 60 percent of the elderly spent less than $500 per year on health expenditures. (Interestingly, this proportion did not change with age.) However, 10 percent of the elderly spent over $3500 per year during that same year.[4]

This point is not simply one of semantics. The Achilles heel of

TABLE 7-9

TOTAL PUBLIC EXPENDITURES ON THE ELDERLY
AS A PERCENT OF GNP FOR SELECTED COUNTRIES

COUNTRY	YEAR	PERCENT GNP
United States	1981	5.9
Canada	1982	5.4
Denmark	1980	10.1
France	1980	9.8
Germany	NA	NA
Netherlands	1982	8.2
Norway	1981	5.7
Sweden	1982	14.5
Switzerland	1980	13.4
United Kingdom	1980	7.7

Source: US Senate, 1984

7-10

POPULATON AGE 65 AND OLDER IN INSTITUTIONS
AND GROUP LIVING QUARTERS AS PERCENT
OF TOTAL POPULATION 65 AND OLDER
FOR SELECTED COUNTRIES

| COUNTRY | YEAR | Percent of Elderly in Institutions | | |
		Insti-tutions	Group Qtrs	Inst. Grp Qtrs
United States	1980	5.3	0.5	5.8
Canada	1978	7.1	1.6	8.7
Denmark	1980	5.3	0.9	6.2
France	1980	5.2	1.4	6.6
Germany	1980	3.6	0.9	4.5
Netherlands	1980	4.0	7.1	11.1
Norway	1981	5.1	5.7	10.8
Sweden	1981	3.1	6.1	9.2
Switzerland	1976	5.7	NA	NA
United Kingdom	1980	3.9	5.4	9.3

Source: US Senate, 1984.

health and social interventions for the elderly seems to be targeting. Study after study have failed to show impressive effects when the experimental group is compared to the control group. Closer examination of the data suggests that the control group had a low incidence of the catastrophic event, whether it be nursing home admission, death, or decline in functional status. The effective projects appear to be those which have been most focused on the appropriate target group where there was a clear potential for benefit from the intervention.

Similarly, the discussions about the appropriate role of technology for the elderly must also recognize this distinction. The United Kingdom's approach to rationing, described by Dr. Schroeder, can be readily interpreted as a reflection of ageism. It is epidemiologically incorrect to assume that technologies devoted to chronic disease are inappropriately directed toward many of the elderly. New techniques to examine the value of interventions such as the management of end-stage renal disease[5] and long-term care[6] are addressing quality of life measures rather than simple survival.

In some cases, it is difficult to convincingly relate the data between improvements observed and modes of care. As Dr. Schroeder notes, the life-expectancy at age 65 in the United States has shown a rather dramatic improvement, particularly in recent years. However, there are some interesting observations with regard to that data that illustrate the difficulty in making clear causative statements. As shown in Figure 7-2, the rate of improvement continues to be greater for women than for men. There is certainly no reason to assume that older women are getting better medical care than older men. The same figure indicates that the differences between the races have essentially disappeared. However, it is not clear which changes over the last several decades have been responsible for improved status of the non-white elderly population.

For many of the elderly, their fate is tied to the general shape of the health care system. The only difference between the functional elderly and other members of the population is that the former rely heavily on coverage under a federally administered health program of health insurance. To the extent that this program treats its beneficiaries differently than other insurance programs, they may be discriminated against. For the elderly with significant burdens of chronic illness, the situation is quite different. These individuals are more likely to become dependent on a long-term care system, which in the United States is funded under a welfare authority. The pernicious effects of this type of care sponsorship represents a commitment to two-class care, where the criterion for eligibility is poverty and the benefits must be kept sufficiently low to encourage private persons to first use their own resources. The possibilities for rehabilitation, consumer choice and quality of life are clearly constrained by such an approach.

Although the development of long-term care services is more often the responsibility of the social service system than the medical care system in many of these Western countries, the availability of interested and knowledgeable geriatric medicine expertise can be a very critical factor in developing effective programs. Examples of

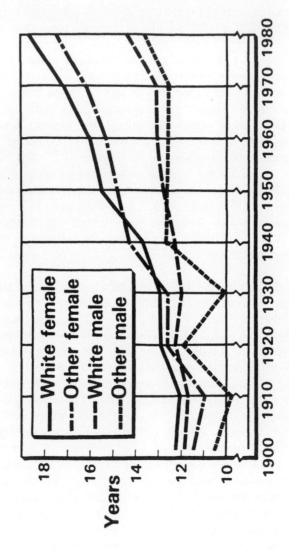

Figure 7-2: Life expectancy at age 65, 1900 to 1980.
Source: Kane, Ouslander, Abrass, 1984.

such creativity can be found in several of these Western countries. Within the United Kingdom, geriatric leadership has been an important element in the growth of innovative health services for the elderly.[7,8] Although geriatricians are not numerous in these Western European nations, their presence has led to at least an increased recognition of the need for specially targeted services for the dependent elderly. Projections of similar requirements for this country suggest that we are far from the even bare minimum numbers needed to begin to meet the demand.[9]

Although the availability of universal, unduplicated coverage by primary care physicians is not a constant feature of all health care programs in the western world, where it does exist it has clear advantages over the more entrepreneurial, less coordinated system found in the United States. Physicians remain the professionals most likely to be in contact with an older person. Where the responsibility for care can be appropriately fixed, the potential for closer linkages between medical and social services is enhanced.

Several countries offer good models of how long-term care services, operated under a social mandate, can respond to the specific needs and preferences of the client. Perhaps some of the best models are found in several Canadian provinces where well-developed models of case management and a mixed menu of community-based and institutional services are available.[10] Although the linkages between the acute medical sector and the long-term care sector are not necessarily well-forged, there is nonetheless the opportunity to make policy decisions about allocation of resources at a higher ministerial level. In fact, in several Canadian provinces, the expenditures on hospital care are declining as the expenditures on long-term care are increased.

Although most Western countries have programs specifically targeted to the elderly, these programs build on a base of health insurance and social care provision that is virtually universal. The fiscal isolation of the elderly in the United States has created a number of problems. On the one hand, there is a growing sentiment that the elderly are benefiting disproportionately from public programs.[11] Part of this mythology has resulted from the tendency to keep two sets of books in the United States, one for private dollars and the other for public dollars. In a sense, this separation has severely limited our degrees of freedom in seeking new solutions. Public funds in the United States come from all sorts of constraints on eligibility and utilization. Creativity must be directed toward utilizing the resources in such cases rather than trying to evolve more appropriate programs.

One of the lessons available from the experiences of the Western countries is the importance of basing programs at the local level.[12] Although most Western countries are physically smaller, less populous, and more homogeneous than the United States, social programs are generally run at the local level, usually at a level corresponding to a municipality or country. Extrapolating to a country as large, complex, and heterogeneous as the United States, one can readily appreciate the need for locally organized, fiscally responsible units of administration. Such a philosophy is compatible with that of the current administration which is seeking to deemphasize the role of the federal government and to place residual responsibility on other units. The growing enthusiasm for capitation, manifested by the new TEFRA regulations for Medicare coverage of HMOs reflect this approach, as does the increased use of 2176 waivers under Medicaid. What has not yet evolved is a clear demarcation of responsibility along geopolitical lines. At the present time we continue to try and merge the entrepreneurial ethic with these new developments.

Capitation and capitalism can mix but they may produce some untoward consequences. One of the great concerns is selective marketing in which such programs are offered preferentially to those who represent the least risk to the providers. In this sense, the concept of a geopolitical entity as the general organizing unit for capitation may have more appeal. The rise of the proprietary forces in medicine and long-term care in the United States distinguishes it from other western countries, although it may be exporting some of this culture.

The paradigm of proprietary provision of services funded by public funds leads inevitably to regulation. Our efforts to develop useful, enforceable and meaningful regulations in the area of health care delivery, especially in long-term care have not been very encouraging. The fascination with codification of professional orthodoxy appears to be a very American trait. We have responded with the same behaviors that gave rise to the Bill of Rights. It remains to be seen whether the same propensities to restricting freedom by trying to enunciate it will ensue.

REFERENCES

1. Aaron, J.H. and Schwartz, W.B. *The Painful Prescription: Rationing Hospital Care.* Washington, D.C.: The Brookings Institute, 1984.

2. U.S. Senate Special Committee on aging. *Long-term care in Western Europe and Canada: Implications for the United States.* Washington, D.C.: U.S. Government Printing Office, 1984.

3. Feller, B. Americans needing help to function at home. *Advanced Data, Vital and Health Statistics, #92.* National Center for Health Statistics, DHHS publication #83–1250, Hyattsville, Maryland: Public Health Service, 1983.

4. Kovar, M.G. Expenditures for the medical care of elderly people living in the community throughout 1980. *National Medical Care Utilization and Expenditure Survey: Data Report #4.* DHHS publication #84-2000, National Center for Health Statistics, Hyattsville, Maryland: Public Health Service, 1983.

5. Evans, R.W., Manninen, D.L., Garrison, L.P., Hart, L.G., Blagg, C.R., Gutman, R.A., Hull, A.R., and Lowrie, E.G. The quality of life of patients with end-stage renal disease. *New England Journal of Medicine,* 312:553–79, 1985.

6. Katz, S., Branch, L.G., Branson, M.H., Papsidero, J.A., Beck, J.C., and Greer, D.S. Active life expectancy. *New England Journal of Medicine,* 309:1218–24, 1983.

7. Isaacs, B. and Evers, H. (editors). *Innovations in the Care of the Elderly.* Dover, New Hampshire: Croom Helm, 1984.

8. Coakley, D. (editor). *Establishing a Geriatric Service.* London: Croom Helm, 1982.

9. Kane, R.L., Solomon, D.H., Beck, J.C., Keller, E., and Kane, R.A. *Geriatrics in the United States: Manpower Projections and Training Considerations.* Lexington, Massachusetts: D.C. Heath, 1981.

10. Kane, R.L. and Kane, R.A. *A Will and a Way: What Americans can Learn about Long-term Care from Canada.* New York: Columbia University Press, 1985.

11. Preston, S.H. Children and the elderly in the U.S. *Scientific American,* 251(6):44–9, 1984.

12. Kane, R.L. and Kane, R.A. *Long Term Care in Six Countries: Implications for the United States.* DHEW publication #(NIH) 76-1207, Washington, D.C.: U.S. Government Printing Office, 1976.

Medical Care for the Elderly in Other Western Countries: Lessons for the United States A National Policy Perspective

Ethel Shanas, PhD

Dr. Schroeder outlines some of the similarities and differences of health care systems in the United States and in other western countries and then indicates how these differences in national styles of health care affect the health of the elderly. As he points out, the United States, in contrast to most western countries, lacks a system of universal health insurance. In most western countries, access to specialist physicians is through general physicians and a system of referrals. The patient in the United States, however, has direct access to any specialist he or she chooses, unless his or her chosen specialist limits his or her practice only to referrals from other physicians. In all western countries, including the United States, geriatric medicine is a specialty with low concentrations of physicians. Again, in actual practice, many internists in the United States are primarily geriatricians without being so identified since their practice is heavily weighted with older people. United States hospitals have a relatively high rate of admissions to acute care, intensive care of patients within the hospital, and extensive use of advanced medical technologies.

In my comments, I will discuss public expenditures for health care of the elderly in the United States and other western countries, the role of the family in the provision of health care, and health of the elderly as a sociomedical problem.

EXPENDITURES FOR HEALTH CARE OF THE ELDERLY

Expenditures for health care in the United States have risen rapidly within the last two decades. Dr. Schroeder reports that health care expenditures in 1983 were estimated at 10.8 percent of the

Gross National Product. An information paper of the Senate Special Committee on Aging, using statistics compiled by Organization for Economic Cooperation and Development (OECD), estimated that public expenditures for health, as distinct from total health expenditures, were 4 percent of the total GNP in 1980, compared to 1.3 percent in 1960.

While strict comparability of data from country to country cannot be assumed, in every country such expenditures appear to be strongly related to the proportion of the elderly in the population. The proportion of Gross National Product expended on public expenditures for health for the American elderly does not seem to be excessive compared to the expenditures made by other western countries. Persons 65 years of age and over are now about 11.1 percent of the American population. Public health expenditures in their behalf are about 29 percent of all such expenditures or 1.1 percent of the GNP.

The Netherlands has almost the same proportion of elderly in its population as the United States, 11.5 percent. Twenty five percent of all public expenditures for health, or 1.6 percent of its GNP, is spent for the elderly. The Scandinavian countries and France, all of whom have greater proportions of elderly than the U.S., spend more of their GNP on public health expenditures in behalf of old people.

The major difference between the United States and the Netherlands, as well as other western countries, is not so much in the proportion of GNP spent on health care for the elderly, but in how these expenditures are distributed between acute care and other care services. An aging population requires not only medical care, but also maintenance care. Western European countries place greater emphasis on community care compared to the United States. Day hospitals, rehabilitation programs, homemakers, home health aides, and sheltered housing are all developments which serve to maintain old people in the community. While each of these modalities of care can be found in the United States, nowhere do we find an emphasis on these services comparable to that reported from Western Europe. The Senate document referred to earlier notes that all western countries, including the United States, report problems with the coordination of services, the integration of medical and social services, and the design of programs to target those most in need.

THE ROLE OF THE FAMILY

In both the United States and western European countries, the family is the chief provider of care for the frail elderly. An analysis of factors affecting the service utilization patterns of dependent elderly in the community emphasizes the role of family support:

> Outside services are likely to be introduced into the household of a frail older person living alone or with nonrelatives at fairly low and simple levels of need. In contrast, the likely use of such services is postponed until higher levels of need for dependent elderly who live with either a spouse or other relative.[3]

Findings from mid-1970s national surveys of the elderly in Denmark and the United States are relevant here. Among persons over 80 living at home in both countries, four of every five have living adult children. In Denmark, about seven of every 10 men and five of every 10 women with children either live with an adult child or within 10 minutes of a child. Comparable figures for the United States are seven of every 10 men, and eight of every 10 women. For the majority of individuals over age 80, a middle-aged child in the 50s, 60s or even 70s had assumed responsibility either for care in a joint household or for the provision of the necessary services to nearby elderly parents that make life in the community possible for the latter. Such care can mean doing the shopping or help with transportation, or it can mean the tasks associated with care of the bedfast, the provision of personal care, meals, medication, et cetera. In both Denmark and the United States, as well as in other western countries, the grandparent generation is taking care of the great grandparent generation.

In all western countries the traditional caretaker for the frail elderly has been a woman family member, either a daughter or daughter-in-law. With the steady increase of women in the paid labor force, these family caretakers may no longer be available to the elderly. Some European countries have recognized the services of family caregivers by paying them for the caretaking activities. Policymakers and the social services in the United States need to recognize the contribution of family caregivers to the elderly. Payments to caretakers may be unnecessary. Community services, however, should be available as needed to elderly persons both with and without families, and to their family caretakers.

SOCIOMEDICAL ISSUES

In an analysis of the implications of his findings for the United States, Dr. Schroeder sets out three strategies which the United States may follow in steering a course between the provision of health services to the elderly and controlling expenditures for health. The first, which Dr. Schroeder rejects as unrealistic, is simply to let medical care costs rise; the second, is to let politics and the marketplace decide the shares between acute and long-term care; and the third is to shift resources from the acute care to the chronic sector, that is for the United States to organize its health care for the elderly in terms of what older people and their families want—to keep old people in the community and to enable them to have better access to home health and other supportive services. The last of these alternatives is not impossible to achieve. As Professor Peter Townsend, the British sociologist, has said:

> Society creates the framework of institutions and rules within which the general problems of the elderly emerge and, indeed, are manufactured. Decisions are taken every day in the management of the economy and the maintenance and development of social institutions which govern the position which the elderly occupy in national life, and these contribute powerfully to the public consciousness of different meanings of aging and old age.[5]

To achieve a reorganization of health care in the United States, traditional providers of medical care, physicians and hospitals, as well as policymakers, must accept the fact that health care of the elderly is not merely a medical problem, it is a social problem as well.

Comprehensive assessment of old people including evaluations of their physical and mental functioning, the environment in which they live, and their family and social support systems, help to target the special needs of individuals. Meeting those needs may require a rethinking of priorities, but it is not impossible.

Those concerned with health care and the elderly tend to focus their attention on the elderly as a problem (See 6). Life expectancy for American men and women of age 65 is now among the highest in the world, 79.5 years for men and 84 years for women. Public health measures, advances in medicine, improvements in the environment and in nutrition have achieved the "old-old," an estimated 2.6 million persons aged 85 and older in 1980. We need to take a realistic view of the elderly, whether those aged 65 and older, or that segment aged 85 and more. Are the elderly only an American problem, or should they instead be viewed as an American triumph?

REFERENCES

1. U.S. Senate Special Committee on Aging. *Long-term Care in Western Europe and Canada: Implications for the United States*. Washington, D.C.: U.S. Government Printing Office, 1984.

2. Rice, D.P. and Feldman, J.J. Tables and charts for demographic changes and health needs of the elderly. Handout from the October 20, 1982 Institute of Medicine Annual Meeting, Washington, D.C.

3. Soldo, B.J. In-home services for the dependent elderly: Determinants of current use and implications for future demand. Mimeographed (no date).

4. Shanas, E. Health care and social supports: A cross-national perspective. Paper prepared for the American Public Health Association Meeting, Montreal, Canada, November 15, 1985.

5. Townsend, P. The structured dependency of the elderly: A creation of social policy in the twentieth century. *Aging and Society*, 1:5, 1981.

6. Binstock, R.H. The aged as scapegoat. *The Gerontologist*, 23:136–43, 1982.

Medical Care for the Elderly in Other Western Countries: Lessons for the United States A Regional Policy Perspective

Charles Sprague, MD

My comments are divided into four parts. First the Texas perspective; then Region IV which is a five state area: Texas, Louisiana, Oklahoma, Arkansas, and New Mexico; a few comments directed specifically to Dr. Schroeder's paper; and last, what is going on at academic health centers in general, and specifically at The University of Texas Health Science Center at Dallas, in dealing with the problem.

THE TEXAS PERSPECTIVE

Regarding the Texas approaches to health care for the elderly, state level planners are attempting to develop a state-of-the-art needs assessment model for identifying functional and categorical health impairments as well as other social and service needs which impact demand for long term care. This model has utilized and modified nationally and internationally accepted scales of measurement of impairments. As refinement of the model moves into its second phase, continuing exchange of information with national and international scholars is critical.

In the pilot phase, which involved a study of 2,000 households with 3,500 individuals 55 years or older, several interesting patterns became apparent. More elders in Texas are living at or below the poverty level than was true in 1980. This economic change represents a substantial increase in target populations who must turn to the public sector for services. An increasing number of elders are living in single person households. If these individuals lack a support network, they may represent an increasing demand on the services sector which must substitute for family care givers. Prevalence rates for almost 40 impairments and/or chronic illnesses vary widely across Texas. The findings indicate that accurate planning for health care delivery requires local primary data bases rather than national or even state level data. By combining these individual variables into related impairment clusters, one can see where certain types of services should be clustered. For example, urban counties report a higher prevalence rate for social and emotional problems, but rural and mixed urban/rural counties report higher prevalence of chronic illness and physical disabilities. In comparisons of elders by racial/ethnic groups, there are different prevalence rates among different groups. For example, blacks have substantially more social and emotional impairments, chronic illnesses and impairments in Activities of Daily Living (ADL) than do other groups. Hispanics report more mental impairment than other groups, but this category is heavily influenced by educational barriers and, in many instances, a total lack of education reported by many elder Hispanics. This pilot study has confirmed the wide regional variations of problems within the state of Texas and supported the concept of local planning data for accurate planning of services.

REGIONAL APPROACHES

With regard to regional approaches, the absolute number and proportion of elderly persons in the Southwest is growing rapidly, including an especially rapid growth of the very old, those individuals 75 and over, a subsegment of the elderly population particularly at risk for long term care. Over the past decade, long term care has increasingly been recognized as an entire system of health and social services necessary for those individuals who as a result of chronic, physical and/or mental illness experience decreased capacity for self care. These individuals are in need of a full continuum of care which includes hospital, day care, respite care, and institutional care for individuals with chronic, physical and/or mental disorders.

Efforts in the Southwest in the past five years have focused upon expanding services and options by implementing demonstration projects in both institutional and community-based settings which most effectively respond to the unique service delivery issues experienced by the states. While these model projects have taken into consideration successful options and other nations, it has been clear in each case that such models clearly must be modified in significant ways to meet the needs of the Southwest. Adaptation must include consideration of geography and the vast territory and transportation issues, the special cultural heritage and impact on care for the Hispanic, Indian and black populations concentrated here, and the large percentage of rural counties in which limited service options are available.

A review of some of the most recent models of both community and hospital-based care in the five states includes Robert Wood Johnson Foundation hospital initiatives in long term care program. In 1984, the Robert Wood Johnson Foundation established a program to fund 25 hospitals across the U.S. to increase their involvement in long term care. One such project funded in the Southwest is at Parkland Memorial Hospital in Dallas. The project has a primary goal for the improvement of the delivery of coordinated long term services to the indigent elderly of Dallas County through the development of a geriatric assessment team. This team consists of physicians, nurses, social workers, and allied health professionals working to improve health care delivery to older persons, provide discharge planning which effectively recognizes community care alternatives to institutionalization, and improve the coordination between the health and social service system through the provision of care management centralized in the public hospital. The project has been operational since January 1985, and over the next three years, will serve approximately 300 elderly persons over the age of 70 through such expanded services. The control and experimental design, including the minimum data base for longitudinal research, will enable policy and service decisions to be made to be based on the outcomes.

The National Channeling Project

The Health Care Financing Administration and the Administration on Aging have just completed a national project on community-based long term care management of elderly persons with multiple health and social problems. One site was in western Mississippi, another was the Texas Project for Elders based in the Texas Research Institute for Mental Sciences in Houston. Through the coordination of services and the provision of case management, these community based projects were intended to assist older persons at risk of institutionalization to remain in the community in the least restricted alternative possible. The project is currently working with local health and social services agencies to identify funding and waivers which will keep its essential services viable after the project period and enable possible replication in other sites in the region.

The Arkansas Client Assessment Team

The state of Arkansas has worked over the past several years on a team model for health and social services delivery which is community based. At sites throughout the state, clients are screened for nursing home eligibility and offered the option of remaining in the community with the assistance of case management of multiple community-based services through a team of nurses, social workers and physician consultants. A recent review of the effectiveness of this model showed reduction in the overall cost of care over nursing home care for the same period of time and indicated that the single most important difference between nursing home and community based care was the availability of a family member to assist the elderly client in maintaining themselves in their homes.

The Southwest Long Term Care Gerontology Center

In 1983, the federal Department of Health and Human Services' Administration on Aging funded the last of 11 regional long term care gerontology centers; the center which serves Region IV is the Southwest Long Term Care Gerontology Center located at the University of Texas Health Science Center at Dallas. Each center is located on a health science center campus and has the mission of providing technical assistance, training, continuing education, research and development of service models in long term care for the elderly in the state in its region. The intent of these centers is to increase the number of health professionals trained in long term care geriatrics, to provide good models of long term care health and social services settings, and to implement research which would advance the state of the art in medical care policy and disease processes.

Since the inception of the Southwest Long Term Care Gerontology Center, it has worked for the five states in developing a number of services, educational and research options, which have been adapted from good models, particularly abundant in the British health care system. These projects include assistance in the development of model health promotion projects, including a drug interaction profile; an educational model in Arkansas; the evaluation of community-based care projects in several states; the development of interdisciplinary team training projects in nursing care units at several Veterans Administration hospitals; the development of a rural health and social service delivery model in northern Texas; and research focusing on epidemiological analysis of aged populations in the region using both primary and secondary data resources and a longitudinal study of the impact on community-based long term care under DRGs with national and cross-national applications for long term care for the elderly.

INTERNATIONAL MODELS

While Dr. Schroeder may be correct in his assessment of comparability between the U.S. and other western countries in the availability of physicians, it is doubtful that this holds true for the South central region of the U.S. In spite of the improvement in physician supply for the region over the last decade, there remains much ground to be covered before a reasonable degree of parity with national averages is achieved. For those who are comfortable with equating availability and accessibility, deficiencies in the number of primary and geriatric physicians will mean that the region's elderly who are less mobile and whose need exceeds other age groups will remain at a relative disadvantage.

Dr. Schroeder notes,

> Since the U.S. has both the largest utilization of expenses for health care by the elderly and the longest life expectancy for those who reach age 65, it is tempting to say that the increased U.S. life span resulted from the elderly receiving more medical care.

It is also true that the quality of life, not simply quantity of life, is an equally important consideration. Perhaps the variety of imaginative and often cost-effective alternatives of care delivery found in other industrialized countries could be introduced into our region.

For instance, countries such as Sweden, Norway, Germany and the United Kingdom reduce the need for expensive care by encouraging family care of sick elders through the provision of special allowances. The solution may appear increasingly attractive under the DRG reimbursement system. As Dr. Schroeder points out, accessibility is a major factor in utilization of health services, but this is also true for an organizational philosophy that stresses community-based rather than institutional services. When indicated, home care and ambulatory day care would be preferred to admission to a hospital, but they call for special services in the community that must be coordinated with other components of the health care system. Although public budgets are extremely tight and the supply of community services nowhere close to the quantity and variety needed, much effort is currently underway in the region to expand the long term care resource base and to coordinate the existing pool of resources.

With regard to the potential for a shift from acute to long term care, Dr. Schroeder suggests that the U.S. may have, "less flexibility in responding to the service needs of its aging population" because of our slim margin for further increasing expenditures at time of budget stringency. While this may prove to be true, expenditures on institutional long term care have been for some time the fastest growing component of the nation's health care system and most projections suggest that they will continue to escalate for some time to come. In addition, the total market for home health care is estimated to be nearly $6 billion and is expected to quadruple over the next ten years; a growth rate far in excess of institutional care.

Our region follows the national scenario fairly closely in this, but with home care alternatives a more prominent feature of other industrialized countries, it would be prudent to examine the foreign experience of integrating the home health care component into the broader system of acute and institutional long term care. One aspect of the problem of inflexibility and impediments to a shift in resources from acute to long term care noted by Dr. Schroeder, is the absence of any discussion of the differences in the age distribution of the countries he examined. Perhaps the U.S., and likewise for the regions with relatively younger age distributions, the catalyst for change will occur as a result of a dramatic increase in the frail elderly population, a shift that has already occurred in some other countries, demonstrating that need in this case may be the mother of innovation, with the European experience offering a variety of models.

ACADEMIC HEALTH CENTERS

In closing, I would like to comment briefly on something I know a little bit more about, namely what is going on at academic health centers generally, and The University of Texas Health Science Center at Dallas in particular. I think what is going on at our own institution is not dissimilar to what is going on in many institutions around the country. For example, in the last several years we have integrated geriatrics into the undergraduate medical school curriculum and it is an assigned rotation of our house staff in several specialties. Over the past two years, we have received, from private sources, endowment funds in excess of over $2 million to support the geriatric program. The gerontology program in the School of Allied Health Sciences is the fastest growing and most productive of our various programs in that school, and as I indicated, it houses the Southwest Long Term Care Gerontology Program.

Much like geriatrics has been neglected, nutrition has been as well. I am happy to say that we have a local philanthropist who has become very interested in the area of human nutrition. Recently, he brought together a group of individuals who are designated "Friends of the Center for Human Nutrition," each pledging $1,000 a year. Some 80 plus members have joined within the last month. We hope that given such support in geriatrics and nutrition, we will be able to make significant advances in both research and education. Basic biomedical research will impact increasingly upon the care of the elderly population in the years to come, and cannot be overemphasized.

Medical Care for the Elderly
in Other Western Countries:
Lessons for the United States
Panel Discussion

Dr. T. Franklin Williams: I would like to comment on the value of the geopolitical base in health care services. There are examples in this country and from abroad where such an approach works well. In the Rochester, New York area, hospital costs are about 70 percent of the national average. Blue Cross/Blue Shield charges for the same package of services are about 60 percent the national average and one-third what the same package costs in Southern California. The same applies to long term care. This community, which has long been known for local/regional planning and efforts to control and manage costs, really has been successful. If the whole country operated at the cost level of Rochester, the difference could pay for our entire Medicaid system. If one community in the country can do this, there is no reason why all can't.

We can learn similar things from abroad. What impressed me the most in terms of home support services, was the catchment area approach which I saw particularly well-organized in Australia, New Zealand, and some areas of the United Kingdom. An agency would be responsible for home care services in a catchment area of a city and the services were well organized. The costs were far lower than anything we have achieved in this country. Visiting nurse costs, for example, were about $6 per visit. In the U.S., it is $50 or $60.

There are many things we can learn from the way services are organized in other countries as well as our own, particularly at the geopolitical or local level. We could do these things if we had the will. It is a matter of public policy.

Dr. Reuel Stallones: I have a quotation from Rene Dubos that might be considered a footnote to one of Dr. Schroeder's sections and perhaps relevant to Dr. Stead's earlier commentary:

> Propounders of utopias have not even been able to agree on the value that they attach to life. Plato considered that life without health was not worth preserving, for the sake of either the individual or the community. He saw no virtue in encouraging the survival of a fellow man threatened by continuous sickness. The state physicians of his republic were to watch with care over the citizens of goodly conditions, both in mind and body. But persons who were defective, either mentally or physically, were to be suffered to die. This attitude is a far cry from the ethics of modern utopias. Life, as it is now taught, must be preserved at all cost whatever the burden of its preservation imposes on the community and on the individual concerned.

Whether this lofty ethical concept will retain acceptance if put to the acid test of social pressure, still has to be proved. Western man may rediscover the wisdom in Plato's social philosophy when the world becomes crowded with aged, invalid and defective people. He may once more rationalize himself into the belief that happiness is not possible in the absence of usefulness to the social group and that survival under these conditions is, therefore, not worth having. That might be a plea for more ice floes.

Mr. Robert Ball: I found Dr. Schroeder's three alternatives to not be exhaustive. There are really great potentials in the U.S. for providing good acute services in a cheaper way. Beyond that, we are not faced with a given pot of money as a percent of GNP for something called health services, where the trade-offs all have to be made. The trade-offs should be with everything else that society does and not just the federal budget, everything we do with our total GNP.

We are in danger of becoming victim to a current political climate that has us talking in terms of scarce resources, meaning this is a time of difficult budget constraints. This is certainly a political fact of life, but it is *only a political fact of life*. People today are contrasting the optimism of the mid-1960s, when we started things like Medicare and Medicaid, as if there were unlimited resources then, with a view that we have constrained resources now. The facts are, as compared to 1965, that after-tax per capita income in this country is about 50 percent higher now than then. We are much more wealthy, we are able to do more if we want to. The high cost of military expenditures is part of the explanation of our present difficulties. Further, this country is greatly undertaxed, and sooner or later, and not so far off I think, the population is going to say there are certain things we want and value that can be done better through public than private measures, and we are willing to spend more and pay the necessary taxes.

I return to a theme that I started with at the beginning. We have the capacity to do a lot more. If we can get to the point where we can demonstrate that what we are already doing is done efficiently, then we will find our fellow citizens willing to address this problem of long term care with additional expenditures. I don't think we are stuck with a fixed amount of public expenditures.

Dr. Eli Ginzberg: I have a lot of sympathy with the last statements of Bob Ball. It gives me an opportunity to tie them to a discussion of Gene Stead's. Dr Stead talked about the importance of trying to move slowly, experimentally, non-governmentally, towards some concept of "partial brain death," as he called. I asked him last evening, whether he knew what that was and he said no, but he still wants to move that way. That is an important comment.

One point implicit in Dr. Stead's comments is, how much do we really want to do as people get increasingly close to death? There is a legal concept called "in contemplation of death." At that point you need less support in court than you would in a normal legal case, because ostensibly a person shortly before death will not tell a lie. The problem is, what is the health care system's relationship, not to the provision of services, but to the improvement of quality of life and the extension of worthwhile life? That is really a critical issue that we have been sneaking around. Up until now, we have been a society which more or less slipped into a position in which we said "any kind of medical intervention that can prolong life is justified, especially if the family wants it, if the individual wants it, or if you are worried about some lawyers who will take you to court if you don't provide it." That is not a sustainable position. I would submit that you really should study the suicides of people on renal dialysis; the rate is disturbingly high. That means we are coming to a crisscross of curves between medical interventions and what the whole process of medical intervention should be all about, which I assume, is making a net increment to human well-being and happiness.

Dr. Stead quite correctly called attention to the fact that one cannot suddenly move the boundaries between legitimate intervention and questionable intervention. What Dr. Stead was talking about was moving toward some codification and trying to sharpen it. Physicians have always used their judgment as people get close to termination, as to whether it is worthwhile or not to take the next action. "Do not resuscitate" rules were a part of every hospital I've ever heard about. Some hospitals have established review committees, in which a physician can ask his colleagues for judgment and assistance whether he/she should continue someone on life-sustaining apparatus or take them off.

It is clear, economics has never been absent from the presence of medicine. Therefore, the poor have always been "judged a little differently from the wealthy." If you take a look at open heart procedures for blacks and whites in the country, it will blow your mind in terms of the differences. My recollection is about 10 to 1, corrected for population, white to black.

I want to get away from the medical providers and think about the patients. Patients are permitted to refuse permission so you can't do things to them, fortunately. Patients are writing living wills, which are getting reinforced by state legislatures. It was really patients who pushed for hospice care, which is one of the few modifications of the Medicare system that has occurred, because they said they did not want to be turned into guinea pigs in experimental hospitals. There are more patients getting smart enough to know that if you want to die decently, you're going to have to be at home. That is the only way to protect yourself against abuse in a hospital. A friend of mine showed me an indignant letter from a lady asking why he was doing all these things to her husband in the ICU. He wrote back, "Lady if you don't want us to do that, take him home." Now this is the Chief of Medicine in a distinguished medical school saying, "Take him home!" With this kind of event, and the suicides I have mentioned, it seems that many of the elderly don't think that this sort of medical care makes much sense.

There are other things going on in society. We have more and more professors of ethics in and around hospitals and medical schools.

We are beginning to get, out of sheer necessity, governmental rules of one sort or another, such as the Baby Doe regulations. The DRGs themselves are going to create a major modification. My own guess is that DRGs will prevent the admission of a large number of elderly complicated cases to hospitals, just like before Medicare. They are non-profitable patients. I think that is going to be one of the consequences of DRGs. What we do by not providing medical care in nursing homes, is a very unsatisfactory way of responding to those whom we have already written off, as a society, in terms of people worthwhile responding to.

How do we move from where we are to where Dr. Stead would like to go? It becomes important that all decisions about medical interventions on the elderly, especially the elder elderly, be considered, both by the elderly and the physicians, in terms of how these people perform, how much satisfaction they are getting out of their life, and what new episode brought them into contact with acute hospitalization? There's a clear difference, even with heterogeneity, between a person at 72, 82, and 92 coming in with an episode of disease "X." That much of Dr. Fries' presentation is solid. We'd better think about this problem in age-determined brackets.

My next point has to do with the family support system and the economics of the family. I know in my own situation, we turned my mother-in-law's apartment into a hospital for a year-and-a-half, because that is what her husband who died before her wanted. At $100,000 for 18 months you can do that. I thought it was ridiculous. She would have been much better off in a nursing home. It is not a suicide problem if you have that kind of money and you want to blow it that way.

The next issue that Dr. Stead spoke about was that patients vary as to how they want to be treated, and whether they want to live or die dependently. One of my earliest recollections is visiting a Brooklyn state hospital about 1948 just after the antibiotics came in, and seeing almost a thousand psychotic patients who used to die of pneumonia strapped to their beds, being kept alive. It was one of the most gruesome sights I have ever seen. Total insanity. Psychotic patients, who under no terms would have come out of that hospital alive, strapped to their beds and given antibiotics in order to keep them alive. I would say that the patient's preferences, with respect to whether they are willing to be dependent or not is a very important part of this.

Finally, it is not unreasonable to say to elderly people who have some money, "Hey grandma, do you want to live another month, or do you want your two grandchildren to go comfortably to college?" That is the trade-off at some point in time. Going into the hospital, for the extra 60 days, which is where half of all the dollars that are spent during the last year, is that worth anything to you? That would make more sense. Gene Stead put on the table very important questions, which if we don't solve, will assure that we won't get public support to handle the problems of the elderly. The money is there, but as long as these issues remain unresolved, we may not be able to get the public to think sensibly about this problem.

Dr. Carroll Estes: Don Young spoke about the propensity toward deinstitutionalization that is encouraged by the prospective payment and the growing cost problems. In this context, it is important to examine the extent to which trade-offs are occurring between the medical and social services and their availability in the community care system.

About seven years ago, Steve Brody estimated the ratio of medical dollars to social services dollars at about $30 to $1—that is, for every one dollar of social services funding, thirty dollars are available for medical services. We have estimated currently that the imbalance between social and medical services has grown to about $40 to $1. Given the trend toward deinstitutionalization promoted by cost containment, there is a growing population in need of the social aspects of care and support at the community level.

Dr. T. Franklin Williams: I cannot let Dr. Ginzberg's or Dr. Stead's remarks go unchallenged. The view that we are spending inordinate amounts of money for the terminal care of hopeless people is based on no careful studies that I know of. Dr. Stead and I have talked about this and he states you simply have to walk around some facilities and see people being maintained this way when nobody thinks they should be. I grant that right away. I am entirely in agreement with Dr. Stead and Dr. Ginzberg about the importance of making prudent decisions, participated in by everybody, first of all the patient, and secondly the family and professionals, about what to do or not do about sustaining measures.

I know of only one study on this issue, and that is where a medical student and I examined 20 patients in a long term care facility and 20 on the medical services of an acute hospital who were judged to be terminally or extremely ill. We identified these patients, got all the medical, nursing, social and family information together, and got an independent panel of judges to review this information from a number of points of view. One of them was the question of whether inappropriate curative efforts were being continued or not. In 38 of the 40 instances, the judgment was that they were not being continued. That is, the shift to care rather than cure had been made. The other two cases involved instances where the families insisted on continuing heroic measures. It is an error to start with the assumption that a large proportion of high costs are because of inappropriate care in the last stages of life.

Dr. Robert Kane: Two pieces of data bear on the question of the euthanasia approach to handling medical costs. In a study by Bernard Linn and his colleagues in Miami about twelve years ago on burn victims, the patients were given information about the probability of their survival and asked to make decisions about whether they wanted to have heroic measures taken. The implication was given to them that if they didn't spend the money, it would be available to their heirs. About two thirds of them elected not to undergo heroic treatment. If you compare the survival rate of that study which was done in about 1972, to the current survival rate of burn therapy, you will find that a lot of those people could have survived today. Technology has changed rather dramatically, even in a decade, in terms of the management of burn cases.

Steve Schroeder presented some data earlier in his presentation about end-stage renal disease. It is very interesting to remember that the only group that was covered for end-stage renal disease prior to 1972 was the elderly. The increases in utilization of end-stage renal disease therapies, primarily dialysis, changed dramatically for the elderly once everybody else was entitled to get that therapy, and there was an excess of supply. Prior to the universalization of payment for end-stage renal disease, we rationed care for the elderly very differently than we ration it now. We did it because there was a constraint of supply, because of the constraint on funding.

My concern is that if we are going to make these kinds of decisions about people, we need good criteria on which to make them. We are dealing with stereotypical thinking about nursing home patients. We say nursing home patients behave atypically, when, in fact, they behave like people. There was a conference in March, 1985, that Frank Williams' wife and my wife were at, organized by advocates of nursing homes patients. These patients flew in to Tampa and participated in the national conference about how nursing home patients should be treated. They behaved just like ordinary people. In our research, we have discovered that a great many people who are written off as demented and uncommunicative in nursing homes, profit by discontinuing most of their drugs. When you talk to them, they are able to articulate what it is they want out of life. People should have more of a say about their life and death.

We have talked about trying to develop scenarios for making these value judgments. What it comes down to in the end, is the issue of residual responsibility. If we were omniscient enough to decide if somebody had a certain percentage chance of survival at a reasonable quality of life for X number of years, and we could calculate out what the cost to society was, we would say to that individual, "Okay, you are going to cost us $10,000 before you die, how about if we give you a $9,500 cash settlement straight across the board? You go off and have a good time for yourself, then go out with a bang." We would never enter into those kinds of arrangements with people. The basic reason is, what if the patient spent the money and then didn't follow through. We don't have the social sanctions to honor the other side of the deal. That has held us back from doing a large number of these kinds of things.

Dr. Eugene Stead: I know many people, and think the rest of you do too, who, when they see what is happening to people who don't know where they are or what they are doing, can't recognize any of their friends, and have no motivation to make any kind of move, the thing that they say is

> Gene, can you fix it so that won't happen to me? If I am at home and I am like that, just put some food and water around and don't do anything else. If I happen to get into an institution, can you build up a system in which the people who are there could let me die? I don't want to have influenza vaccine, I don't want to have a lot of drugs. If I get pneumonia, be thankful, don't get out any antibiotics.

I am looking first at not making any dramatic changes in the system, I am trying to find a little niche in which we can begin to think a little bit. I got caught by my friend who said "I think maybe you are using a word like 'partial brain death' without yet having defined it." I don't really have that definition. I am not interested in compulsory systems. It would be nice if those who wanted to keep people alive in those circumstances paid for it. I would be a great proponent of the anti-abortion movement, if those people who are against abortion put the money on the table to take care of those kids. It would be nice if we could put some personal responsibility back in the kinds of decisions where somebody says "Let the state pay for it," and then disappears and does not come back for three years. I don't know how to do that.

When I take care of any elderly person, I always take care of him like he has a chronic illness. I don't care what the diagnoses are or how healthy somebody else says he is, to me he has a chronic problem and the most likely thing about him is that he will go broke. So, from the very beginning, I start to look at the resources that are there, what he wants to do, what the family wants to do. I am very aware of the fact that I would much rather have my grandchildren have a certain amount of worldly goods than to spend them on care for me if I did not know where I was. That is as far as I think we can go at the present time, and even going this far will raise a considerably outcry. I think the time has come where I am going to produce that definition of "partial brain damage."

Rebuttal

Steven A. Schroeder, MD

The discussion included a very wide-ranging set of comments. I don't want to offer a rebuttal because I really don't quarrel with much of anything. I want to make a couple of comments, however. In our discussion of long term care, we romanticize the European models. I am most familiar with the English one. To the extent that it works, it does so because of the mandatory assignment of all patients to a defined general practitioner, and because the district makes available money for a wide set of social services. Those are structural issues unique to the British health care system. It is going to be very hard for us to get from here to there. Additionally, the social and health care systems in Britain are integrated much better than ours. However, I should point out that the United Kingdom has essentially no public support for nursing homes. They are beginning now to expand in a private market and to begin considering experimentation with public support. But, as in the U.S., nursing homes are mainly private.

Why do we live longer in the U.S.? I don't know the answer to that, but I know that 10 or 12 years ago, public health experts were saying what a bad medical care system we had because it was so expensive and we didn't live as long as people in other countries. And now that we are living longer, I still read comments from public health leaders who say that our system doesn't work because we don't do as well as other nations. I think they're behind. I think we ought to catch up in our rhetoric. I would suspect that some of the credit for longer life expectancy goes to the health system, but I don't know how much. It would be nice to know, for example, why heart disease rates are falling. It is difficult to partition out how much is attributable to lifestyle and how much to medical care.

I agree totally with the need for local coordination of social services, that was mentioned by several speakers. That is a major problem in our country. It was a major problem in the U.K.,

Australia, and Canada; nobody thinks they are coordinating local services very well, but we are probably doing it worse than most.

Dr. Shanas is absolutely right that the family is the major source of long term care in most communities in this country. The U.S. is a little different from most western countries in that we probably have greater mobility. Many people I know in San Francisco have parents living on the east coast. That is different from England, Denmark or the Netherlands, where people live very close together. The fact that more of our women work means there is a double hazard for the family not being as able to take care of the elderly parents.

Dr. Ethel Shanas: The facts are that people who live at great distances very often have one child that lives close by. Middle class adult children are more likely to live at a great distance from elderly parents than blue collar workers. The facts are, that now-a-days with the airplane, nobody is really at a great distance in case of need.

Dr. Steven Schroeder: In case of need, yes, but in terms of ongoing care, it is harder. There is another factor that nobody has mentioned: 50 percent of all marriages end in divorces. Who is responsible for the former in-law?

I worry that we are moving to a two-class, or rather, that we are intensifying the two-tiered system of hospital medical care. We are going to go to a system where the middle class can buy those services and again, the problem of long term care is going to be increasingly a problem for the elderly poor. We may be moving to a system where those elderly who can pay $100,000 a year will stay where they want, and those who can't will wind up getting warehoused. This should be a concern for us.

Dr. Williams mentioned the need for regional coordination and hinted at the fact that, just as there are cross-national differences in utilization, so are there differences across counties and states, and the potential to save money is tremendous. Let's not forget that if we prevent one coronary artery bypass surgery, we can buy two home health aides, full time.

Mr. Ball, I really respect your wisdom, and I wish I had your optimism about the political situation. It would be nice if we could tax more and if there was more equity and solidarity. There needs to be a political background for that. I don't think we have done too well in the last years on that. You clearly posed a political challenge to all of us. I don't feel very optimistic about that in the short run, as I watch the growth of "yuppiedom." I hope you are right. I wish I could be as sure about it as you are.

Just a few concluding comments on the issue of "partial brain damage" or whatever you want to call it. We start with the sense that we do a lot more care of the kind that Dr. Stead thinks is too much than any other country. If we do want to cut back, we have some room. Right now we are in an interesting situation of counteracting trends. We have, on the one hand, prospective payment, which is creating some financial disincentives to putting everybody into the intensive care unit. We have the right to die movement, the hospice movement. On the other hand, we have the technologic imperative and the tremendous investment in specialist and acute care hospital capabilities. I still think that, in an arm wrestling match, they are stronger, but it is a little more of a contest now. I am surprised, in my role as a personal physician, how many patients I think would not want to go on, do want to go on when I ask them. Sometimes it is for them, sometimes it is for hope, sometime it is for their family. The legacy of guilt that we leave a family with when we say "don't they think we had better turn off the machine?", particularly if unresolved intergenerational or spousal problems have not been resolved, is tremendous. And that may lead people to want to go on.

I feel that there is enough room to economize on the rest of our economy, without having to, as Eli Ginzberg suggested, pit grandparent against grandchildren going to college. As wealthy as this country is, and as much as we spend on all the things that we do, I hope we are a far distance away from that type of choice.

Summary

Stanley Joel Reiser, MD, PhD

There is a children's tale about a young boy who wakes up one morning and finds seated next to his bed a small dragon. They wink at each other. The dragon jumps upon the bed and the boy is struck with the feeling of reality about his new friend. Enthusiastically, he runs down stairs to tell his mother the news. His mother responds, "There are no such thing as dragons." When the dragon comes down to breakfast, Mother doesn't say anything. Gradually, the dragon begins to grow and grow, enlarging to the size of the dining room, then to the entire house and soon the house is a small bump on the dragon's back, and is being carried down the block. Finally, the mother says, "Maybe there is such a thing as a dragon." At this point, the dragon begins to diminish in size, becoming smaller than the house, and finally, reduced to the size it had been in the beginning of the story. Reflecting on the matter, the mother asked, "Why did dragon grow so much?" The young boy ends the story by saying "Perhaps he wanted to be noticed."

In many ways, the story of the elderly is the story of the dragon wanting to be noticed. It is extraordinary, as we look back, to think that in the 1950s we did not notice elderly people. They were all about us, but we did not notice them. Part of the Civil Rights movement has been an attempt to recognize them. I still don't think we notice them to the extent we should, although certainly more than we did 20 years ago. An extraordinary number of things have occurred around this issue of non-recognition. For example, if you wanted to look foolish as a medical scientist in the early 1950s, you could say you were doing research on the process of aging. This activity was thought to be ludicrous, because affecting that process was believed to be impossible. As I reflect on that history, it seems we did the same thing in respect to aging that we did in the 19th century, when we said to those who were experimenting with ether and other anesthetic gasses, "There is no way for a surgical knife and pain not to be linked." We are still exploring the idea of what is possible and trying to recognize the elderly as the vital segment of our society that they are.

The papers and discussion have been interesting because they spread into all channels of scholarship bearing on the issue of health policy for the elderly. I am very much struck, in discussing the issues of education, that often the failures of education result in challenges to policy. When we fail in education, we simply push the problem to the policy-making organs of our society. Thus, the educational issue of how to teach students about all dimensions of health care of the elderly is critical.

As we had the discussion about the history of the teaching nursing home, it recalled to me the history of the mental hospital. We made a self-conscious decision in the 19th century to segregate the chronically mentally ill into hospitals separate from those devoted to physical medicine. Looking back upon that, it was a bad decision, for a number of reasons. It became clear during the 20th century that many medical students and nursing students understood the problems of mental health only in terms of seeing a cohort of patients in mental hospitals—the types of patients who did not get better. I fear that if we look upon the nursing home as the main locus of education, we will again be making the same error. This does not mean we should discard the concept of a teaching nursing home, but rather reflect upon the experience we had with segregating one portion of the patient population, the mentally ill, and determining whether we want to replicate that education experience with the elderly. I don't think we should.

Dr. Fries' thesis on the compression of morbidity is one of the most interesting to come along in this decade. It was clear, however, that many people around the table were skeptical about the evidence for the existence of this compression of morbidity. There also was much discussion that centered on the issue that if the theory indeed were true, so what, where does it get us? What does it tell us about formulating health policy for the elderly?

If morbidity is compressed, and our hospitals become crowded with very ill patients whose organ reserve is at an end, two things must happen. First, there is a need to develop adequate prognostic indices, so we understand just what level of organ failure these patients are experiencing. Second, as Dr. Ginzberg and others noted, we have to deal more often with the ethics of trade-offs. I believe we have the intellectual tools to make those decisions now. I see them in practice on wards of the U.T. Medical School when we have ethics rounds. I believe we can teach and use these intellectual tools.

In order for health professionals to make effective and humane ethical decisions, the court system must be reformed. In the early 1970s, with good reason, the courts began increasingly making decisions about medical care. When one looks at those court decisions, one repeatedly finds the statement that the courts are the only place in society where dispassionate, objective formulations of what is right and wrong can be made; the doctors and the parents and the patients are too involved. That is an erroneous belief and misinterpretation and fear of the law has created confusion among practitioners and families and led to bad decisions. We must settle this issue with the courts. The government has a legitimate role in health care, but its role now in respect to end-of-life situations is much more confusing than it is settling.

Robert Ball presented a fascinating account of the development of national health insurance and Medicare. I have always been fascinated by one element of that. Was Medicare a true policy breakthrough or was it a traditional response to health care problems? I am really more persuaded it was the latter. If one looks at the history of medical care in this country, one finds that government has traditionally focused on individuals who are in special need of care, rather than across-the-board help to all members of society. This is in consonance with the values of our society. The reason we funded mental health institutions and tuberculosis hospitals in the 19th century was because of the chronicity of the disease, the expense of dealing with it, and the inability of families to handle it. In a certain way, the elderly represent the same delimited population with special needs that society can coalesce a policy about. Thus, in order to expand Medicare, fundamental value changes in this society will be necessary. The issue of developing the minimum floor, by which all of us are supported, will be very hard to accomplish.

The discussion about home care versus hospital care was a particularly fascinating one, because, in my view, the era in which the hospital stood alone and pre-eminent is at an end. We must remember that the hospital is really a very modern institution. Although it was created in the early Christian era as a fundamental institution of health care, it has only been the central institution for about 80 years. It was in about 1900 that hospitals began to be built in great number in the United States, very dramatically and very quickly. Therefore, we are not talking about something that has an extended history, nor do I think we are talking about something that will exist forever into the future. Technological possibilities, economic changes, and social issues will create a tendency to decentralize and move patient care outside of the hospital to other loci. What the hospital becomes will be fascinating to watch, it certainly will not be what it was. I think this transformation will happen rather quickly.

The issue of health promotion and taking responsibility for one's health seems to be a very difficult one for the elderly, because of the dilemmas associated with being old and trying to support oneself easily outside of the hospital. The question of whether the health promotion activities are equally applicable to the elderly and the younger seems still to be a matter in need of much research.

There still seems to be inadequate knowledge as to whether or not DRGs and PPS are going to result in a net gain or net loss for the elderly population. Interestingly, when one looks at how England allocates resources, it seems that they use a relatively similar level of care for those techniques that are proven quite effective. The great dividing line is not so much between their use of these effective techniques, but rather their failure, or wisdom, in not using the techniques that are more marginal, for which good technology assessment has not yet been done. One wonders, therefore, whether or not in this country in order to deal with these marginal technologies, we will have to engage in a much more sophisticated exploration of assessment, if we are to have any hope of reducing health care costs.

Finally, in the end, perhaps the greatest influence of this focus on the elderly will be to improve health care for us all. It is impossible to contemplate the needs of the elderly without taking into much greater account than we did before, the sociological variables that are part of all illness. The elderly will cause us to refocus the attention of medicine on the larger social and economic questions of health care and thus, generate benefits for every one of us.

Index